I0060876

Epidemiology II

Theory, Research and Practice

Epidemiology II – Theory, Research and Practice

Publisher: iConcept Press Ltd.

ISBN: 978-1-922227-76-8

This work is subjected to copyright. All rights are reserved, whether the whole or part of the materials is concerned, specifically the rights of translation, reprinting, re-use of illustrations, recitation, broadcasting, reproduction on microfilms or in other ways, and storage in data banks. Duplication of this publication or parts thereof is only permitted under the provisions of the authors, editors and/or iConcept Press Ltd.

Printed in the United States of America

Copyright © iConcept Press 2015

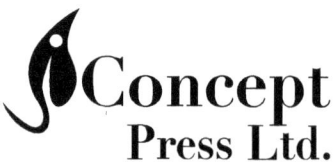

Concept Press Ltd.

www.iconceptpress.com

Contents

Preface

Epidemiology is the study (or the science of the study) of the patterns, causes, and effects of health and disease conditions in defined populations. Epidemiology has developed into a vibrant scientific discipline that brings together the social and biological sciences, incorporating everything from statistics to the philosophy of science in its aim to study and track the distribution and determinants of health events. *Epidemiology II – Theory, Research and Practice* presents the latest epidemiological principles, concepts and research outcomes as well as the practical uses of epidemiology in public health and in clinical practice.

There are totally 11 chapters in this book. Chapter 1 introduces a P3 laboratory. A P3 laboratory allows handling of microorganisms that can be spread through inhalation. The laboratory's structure is constructed using material that is resistant to any form of corrosion. Chapter 2 illustrates the importance of assessing mixtures in drinking water as risk factors for disease, especially when exposure to the mixture can result in a reaction product that is more toxic than the contaminants alone. It reviews nitrosamine metabolism and carcinogenesis as well as provides an assessment of nitrate and atrazine in Nebraska groundwater. In Chapter 3, a linked Surveillance, Epidemiology, and End Results (SEER)-Medicare database analysis was conducted to evaluate treatment patterns, survival, and frequency of complications among elderly patients undergoing treatment for metastatic colorectal cancer (mCRC). The results provide real-world confirmation of clinical trial data in younger patients and imply that age should not discourage the use of guideline-recommended therapies for mCRC. Chapter 4 describes an observational retrospective study concerning the implementation of laparoscopic surgery for rectal cancer within a fast track recovery setting. The clinical and oncological outcomes are analyzed.

Chapter 5 explores the use of social quality theory for researching and understanding the social determinants of health. In this chapter, the authors use national data from Australia to analyse the social determinants of health using social quality theory. Chapter 6 discusses the applicability of stopped-flow light scattering analysis as a new methodology for determining stability of the enveloped viruses. It demonstrates how the technique can be used to qualitative and quantitative evaluate the stability of the influenza virus. In Chapter 7, it discusses recent studies revealing that the exchange of genetic information between hosts and pathogens is more frequent and has a larger impact in their genomes than formerly thought, even in previously unsuspected species. This horizontal gene transfer has important implications in the evolution of hosts, pathogens and the relationships between them. Chapter 8 discusses Avian influenza virus (AIV). It can cause a variety of diseases in domesticated poultry ranging from asymptomatic to severe systemic infections with 100This chapter reviewed in details the chemotherapeutics, natural antivirals and probiotics on AIV. Approaches for the control of the disease in poultry using advanced molecular techniques and development of transgenic chickens were also addressed.

Chapter 9 shows that ecology of *Babesia microti* group, a tick-bone erythrocytic protozoan, can be elucidated by well-designed epidemiological survey and molecular analysis, by demonstrating phylogenetic relationship of the parasites within the group and specific associations of Hobetsu and U.S. lineages with sympatric ticks, *Ixodes ovatus* and *I. persulcatus*, respectively, in Japan. Chapter 10 focuses the community-based intervention employing the cluster randomized balanced design and discusses the interconnected links between epidemiological surveillance of dengue vector breeding, extensive evidence-based research findings and concerted community efforts for integrated vector management within the context of multiple stakeholder environment. Chapter 11 discusses molecular and cell culture methods for evaluating viral contamination in environmental samples. It proposes to indicate the human adenovirus as a model of enteric virus to assess the efficiency of disinfection processes and as a biomarker in sanitary quality studies.

Editing and publishing a book is never an easy task. Each chapter in this book has gone through a peer review, a selection and an editing process so as to guarantee its quality. Without the supports and contributions of the authors and reviewers, this book can never be able to complete. We would like to thank all of the authors in this book and all of the reviewers who participated in the reviewing process: Francisco J Alarcon-Chaidez, Mohammad Ali, Muhammad Yunus Amran, Raghupathy Anchala, Teresa Kisi Beyen, S Bhattacharyya, Silvia Bofill-Mas, Vincent Bourret, Gioia Capelli, Yin-Hsiu Chien, Claudia Consales, Kennedy Daniel Mwambete, David N. Frick, F Geurs, S. Gill, Hongxiong Guo, Ubydul Haque, Sharifah S Hassan, Akihiko Hata, Andres F. Henao-Martinez, Marta Hernández, Madiha Salah Ibrahim, Simon Kaja, Sang Sun Kang, Anu Kasmel, Marwa Khairy, Maciej Kurpisz, Byungsuk Kwon, Audrey OT Lau, Susan Madison-Antenucci, Savi Maharaj, Maurie Markman, Luiz Carlos Porcello Marrone, Abdul-Wahed N. Meshikhes, M J Molina-Garrido, Franco M. Neri, Timothy P. Newsome, Moses N Ngemenya, Hermenegilde Nkurunziza, Nicolas Padilla-Raygoza, Johanne Poudrier, Ambepitiyawaduge Pubudu De Silva, Jialan Que, Muthukumaran Rangarajan, J.A. Reis Neto, Sharon Rainy Rongpharpi, Anna Ruggieri, Lara Saraiva, E A Sherer, Sonica Singhal, Francisco Sobrino, Jae-Min Song, Cameron R. Stewart, Ching-Ho Wang, Orlando P Zacarias and Yun Zhang. We hope that you, the reader, will find this book interesting and useful. Any advices please feel free and are always welcome to tell us.

iConcept Press Ltd.
June 2015

Operations at Biosafety Level III: The P3 Laboratory

Yoshio Ichinose, Shingo Inoue, Masaaki Shimada, Gabriel Miring'u, Betty Muriithi, Angela Makumi, Ernest Wandera, Martin Bundi, Chika Narita, Salame Ashur, Allan Kwalla, Amina Galata, Erick Odoyo, Sora Huqa, Mohammed Shah, Mohammed Karama, Masahiro Horio

1 Introduction

Biomedical research on pathogenic agents has steadily grown within the past decade, with increasing disease burden necessitating intensive research on highly infectious agents as well as organisms of unknown pathogenicity. Coupled with the need to ensure public health, protection of laboratory staff and the environment at large are of utmost importance, hence formulation of biosafety guidelines and subsequent development of containment laboratories.

Institution of biosafety strategies can be traced back to the mid-20th Century, when the first instances of laboratory–acquired infections occurred due to unsecured laboratory operations (Pike, 1979; Vesley & Hartman, 1988; Pedrosa & Cardoso, 2011). These stimulated the World Health Organization (WHO) to design biosafety guidelines that would guide development of codes of practice for safe handling of pathogenic microorganisms (WHO, 2004). Given varying pathogenicity of different microorganisms, differentiation of laboratory facilities into cumulative containment levels and Risk Group (RG) classification of microorganisms were developed. There are therefore four Biosafety Levels (BSL), or Protection levels; BSL-1, BSL-2, BSL-3 and BSL-4, each having specific design features, containment facilities, practices and operational procedures.

A BSL3 laboratory (or P3) laboratory is a medium containment facility that enables isolation and manipulation of pathogens that can be transmitted through aerosol (WHO, 2004). P3 laboratories apply BSL-3 principles and utilize various biocontainment strategies to provide total physical separation between a laboratory worker and a possible source of contamination. They have unique design and engineering features that facilitate containment in addition to biosafety equipments, all strategies aimed at ensuring maximum containment of infectious materials.

P3 laboratories can be found in hospitals, research institutions and food industries, and their importance ranges from securing laboratory procedures to protecting the public and the environment. Generally, disease burden is steadily rising, necessitating accurate diagnosis especially for diseases related to level three organisms, or even specimens suspected to be having microorganisms of unknown pathogenicity. There is also need to carry out intensive research on level three microorganisms alongside emerging and re-emerging infectious diseases, procedures which need comprehensive analytical processes and user protection strategies that can only be found in P3 laboratories. Moreover, occupational and environmental safety has to be observed when dealing with extremely dangerous microorganisms. These are coupled with the fact that health sectors have now boldly embraced evidence-based practices, broadly informed by research. A P3 laboratory is therefore of outmost importance since it guarantees user and environmental safety, as well as safety of research procedures. In addition to these, a P3 facility generally creates a good working atmosphere by assuring safety of laboratory workers. Since the core purpose of a P3 laboratory is to contain contaminants, people working within it are guaranteed of optimum safety, even in case of an operational error. Further, P3 laboratories enhances adherence to biosafety rules and guidelines while strengthening vigilance against laboratory acquired infections.

A P3 laboratory is mainly used for manipulation of RG3 microorganisms such as *Rickettsia typhi, Bacillus anthracis, Brucella abortus,* Yellow Fever Viruses and other arboviruses, and MDR-TB strains, among others. Generally, microorganisms are categorized into four risk groups (RG 1, RG 2, RG 3 and RG 4) based on their relative hazard (WHO, 2004). RG 1 comprises of microorganisms that are unlikely to cause any human or animal disease (WHO, 2004). RG 2 includes low risk microorganisms that can cause diseases in humans through percutaneous injury, ingestion or mucous membrane exposure, but which pose minimal risk to laboratory staff or the environment. (Schaechter, 2009; CDC, 2009). Laboratory exposure to RG 2 biological agents does not cause serious disease, risk of spread is minimal and therapeutic treatment is available (CDC, 2009). These organisms are normally manipulated on open benches though biosafety cabinets can be used for the more contagious ones. RG 3 microorganisms are agents that can be spread through aerosol. They cause serious but treatable human diseases and present a high individual risk but low community risk (Schaechter, 2009). Biosafety cabinets and other primary protective devices are required for safe manipulation of RG 3 microorganisms. Lastly, RG 4 organisms pose high individual and community risk, with directly and indirectly transmissible diseases, which have no effective treatment or preventive measures (WHO, 2004; Schaechter, 2009). They are best manipulated in Class III biosafety cabinets or in Class II biosafety cabinets combined with positive pressure suits.

In addition to RG3 microorganisms, WHO (2004) also recommends that large quantities or high concentrations of RG-2 organisms should be manipulated at BSL-3 due to increased risk of aerosol spread. Further, unknown specimens for either research or diagnostic purposes should be processed in a P3 laboratory.

2   Establishment of a P3 Laboratory

The process of establishing a P3 laboratory can be quite lengthy, due to high costs and biosecurity concerns that surround such facilities. Any institution setting up a containment facility is therefore required to adhere to recommended construction and operation guidelines, since the laboratory can pose a biosecurity threat in case of a technical or operational error. A P3 facility is purchased from certified medical and chemical equipments suppliers, certified by local and international bodies upon meeting set safety and quality standards. Initial staff training and regular technical maintenance are carried out by the supplier.

P3 laboratories are purchased as a pre-finished casework ready for installation. The case is made and finished using a non-corrosive water tight material, complete with a ceiling, a floor and provisions for creating necessary openings, using measurements of the actual room into which it will be installed. Interior surfaces of walls, floor and ceiling are therefore easy to clean and resistant to corrosion by laboratory reagents and cleaning detergents. Upon installation, power and air conditioning lines and systems are drilled into the walls or ceiling and any cracks or gaps sealed airtight.

As shown in Figure 1, biosafety cabinets are the most dominant features of a P3 laboratory due to their role in containing infectious material during sample processing. They are best installed in areas with limited movement and away from the door in order to enhance directional flow of air necessary for the cabinet to function optimally (WHO, 2004). At the middle is a work surface located in close proximity to other equipments, especially the biosafety cabinets to ease movement and reduce the risk of breach of containment. An autoclave is also an important component in the P3 laboratory, as a tool of managing contaminations. It is best located at the furthest edge of the laboratory, away from work benches to reduce chances of contamination. Beside the autoclave is a pass box used to move samples and small equipments into and out of the laboratory. Other equipments should be arranged in a manner that will assure sufficient working space and ease of access.

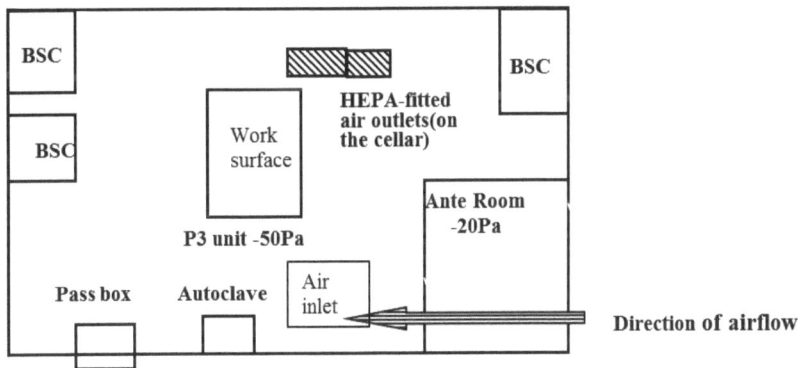

Figure 1: Basic layout of a P3 laboratory.

Basically, a P3 facility should be installed in a segregated location to allow for physical separation from areas of unrestricted traffic. Upon installation, necessary utilities and equipments are fitted, including analytical and biosafety equipment to allow the laboratory to function as an independent unit, and maintain containment by minimizing movement of specimens and equipments into and out of the laboratory. Major functional areas of the laboratory can be computerized in order to make it more efficient and easy to maintain.

3   Features of the P3 Laboratory

3.1   Physical Features

3.1.1   Door Interlock

The door interlock is a double door structure that functions in maintaining negative pressure and optimum temperatures. It also locks in potentially contaminated air, preventing it from spreading to the environment. The interlock system includes the outer door that opens into the ante-room and P3 room door. The doors are controlled by an interlocking sensor, are self-closing, and cannot be opened at the same time. The P3 room door has to be well closed for the ante-room door to open.

3.1.2   Air Conditioning System

P3 laboratories operate at a particular temperature range since extreme temperatures can yield discomfort for users, interfere with normal operation of equipments, or impede analytical processes. The air conditioning system therefore functions to maintain optimum temperatures.

3.1.3   Ventilation System

This is an aeration system that maintains a steady supply of fresh air into the facility alongside removing circulated, potentially contaminated air. Generally, air is drawn from the environment into the water-air purification system, where particulate matter is removed before being channeled into the pre-filters, and finally through intermediate filters; the last stage of air purification. Purified air is then passed through the air conditioner where its temperature is adjusted to room temperature then channeled into the prep room and the P3 room through cellar fans. Recirculated air on the other hand is drawn out through cellar and Class IIB2 exhaust routes. The cellar exhaust route draws out air from within the laboratory at about $720m^3$/hour. Biosafety cabinet, class IIB2 exhaust route also utilizes a negative pressure system, drawing out air at about $1380 m^3$/hour. Both routes are supported by dampers that regulate rate of flow of air. The two also have a sterilization bulb that decontaminates air before it can be removed into the atmosphere and are fitted with High Efficiency Particulate Absorption filters (HEPA filters). For increased efficiency, the exhaust ventilation system can be fitted with an automated double damper system capable of automatically switching to a reserve damper in case of failure of the default one.

   The role of the ventilation system is to maintain steady supply of clean air, hence preventing contamination of laboratory procedures by contaminants of environmental origin as well as enhancing biocontainment by maintaining directional flow of air and negative pressure.

3.1.4   Glass Windows

These are large screens, located on separate locations around the laboratory. They allow people outside the P3 laboratory to view the inside, communicate or observe its general condition without necessarily having to get in. The screens also serve as an emergency exit as they are provided with a hammer from within the laboratory that can be used to break the window, creating an exit route in the event of an emergency.

3.1.5   Interphones

These are communication gadgets located in the P3 and ante-rooms that are also connected to the rest of the telephone network within the institution. Interphones allow communication between the laboratory rooms, and to or from other offices and laboratories within an institution. Further, they can serve as a security measure since they can be used to alert staff in case of an accident.

3.1.6 Pass-box

A pass-box is a big window-like structure that opens to adjacent laboratory units such as the cell culture room. It acts as a link between the P3 room and an adjacent laboratory, providing an entry and exit route for samples, small equipments, and waste materials. By providing a passage route, it eliminates the need to constantly open the main door which would otherwise interfere with directional airflow and negative pressure hence compromising containment. The pass-box also has interlocking glass doors.

3.1.7 Generator

A generator provides power back-up for a P3laboratory, ensuring uninterrupted functioning of the laboratory while upholding containment. The generator should have sufficient capacity to cover essential components; mainly the air conditioning system, freezers, incubators, ventilation system and the negative pressure system. Like all power supply systems, it should be connected to a current stabilizer in order to protect equipments from damage by fluctuating electric currents.

3.1.8 Water-air Filtration System

Normally, air for a P3 facility is drawn from the environment then passed through the normal air filtration system. However, in some instances, the environment could be heavily laden with dust particles and particulate matter that rapidly clog the air inlets, necessitating regular changing of the intermediate filter, which significantly increases maintenance costs. A water-air filtration system (NIHON IKA Chemical Company), an improvisation which capitalizes on the ability of water to trap fine pollutants and particles can however be installed on the air inlet to filter off excess particulate matter before it enters into the main filtration channel. This improves efficiency of the air filtration system while reducing frequency of intermediate filter change-over.

As shown in Figure 2(b), water runs down a filter, made of special fibrous material, wetting its filaments while providing a medium for initial cleansing of air before it is drawn into the main air filtration system. The structure consists of a water storage tank, arranged in a manner that enables recycling of water. Air drawn through this system has a lower amount of particulate matter, therefore the rate at which the intermediate filters get clogged is lower hence they can be used for a longer duration.

Figure 3 shows intermediate filter consumption of a system before and after installation of a water-air filtration system. In the absence of the filtration system, the intermediate filter is consumed within 6-9 weeks. After installation of the system, it can take more than 12 weeks for the manometer to reach the 150Pa mark, hence less frequent intermediate-filter change over, translating to reduced maintenance costs. Though quantity of particulate matter in the environment is the main determinant of the rate of consumption of the intermediate filters, use of water-air filter significantly lengthens duration of usage of intermediate filters.

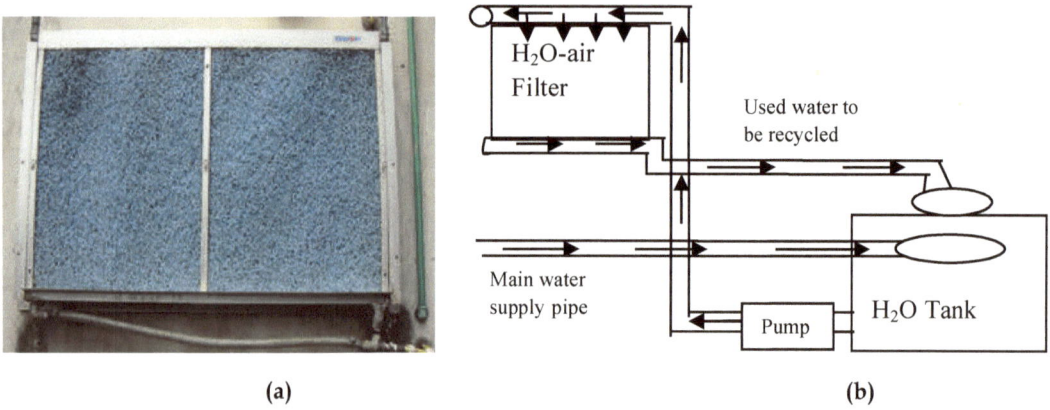

(a)   (b)

Figure 2: (a) The water-air filtration system, and **(b)** its water supply schema.

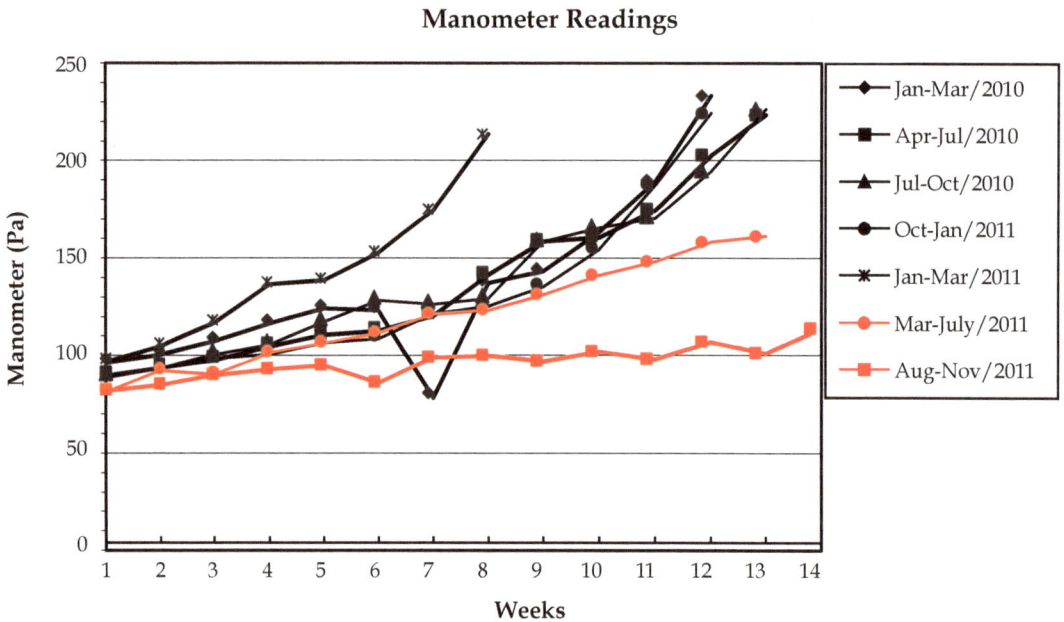

Figure 3: A graph showing manometer readings before and after installation of water-air filtration system.

3.2   Operation features- General features

3.2.1   Run mode

Run mode is the normal operation mode activated during the day, when the facility is in use or when it is being prepared for use. It is activated using a manual switch button on the display of the control panel. At run mode, the laboratory operates optimally with maximum power consumption.

Eco mode, an alternative operation mode can also be installed to achieve energy efficiency. It is a modified operation feature that subjects the entire facility into a power saving mode, and is turned on manually when the laboratory is not in use. Eco mode maintains normal power supply to vital equipments and minimal supply to those that require power to function but can operate on minimal power supply when not in active use. It also stops supply of clean air into the ante-room and maintains temperature in the P3 room at 30° Celsius, hence eliminating the need for air conditioning, which saves power consumption in the facility by at least 30%.

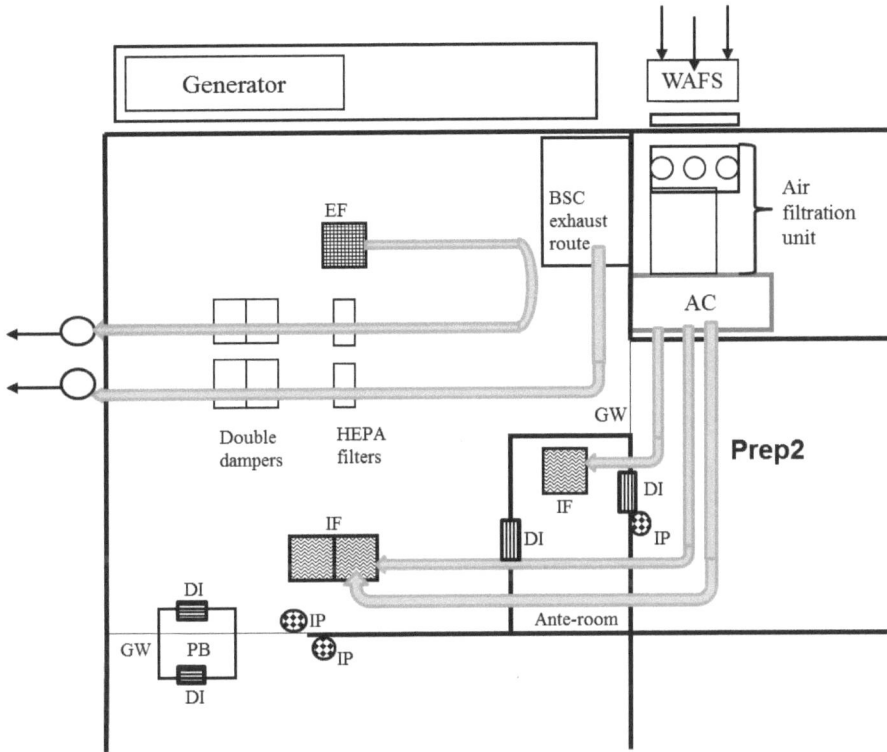

Figure 4: Physical features of a P3 laboratory; DI-door interlock, AC-air conditioner, IF-inlet fan, EF-exhaust fan, HEPA filters-high efficiency particulate air filters, GW-glass window, IP-interphones, PB-pass-box, WAFS-water-air filtration system.

3.2.2   Directional Air Flow

This refers to directed flow of air in and out of the P3 facility. Purified air flows in through the inlet system into the ante-room and the P3 room through ceiling ducts. Circulated air on the other hand is exhausted through an exhaust ceiling duct and the BSC Class II B2 exhaust route, all fitted with HEPA-filters. Directed flow is further enhanced by the air-tight nature of the facility that limits flow of air to designated routes.

P3 facilities operate under negative pressure, achieved by maintaining a rate difference between exhaust and inlet air flow, which generates a higher exhaust speed relative to inlet speed. Both directional air flow and negative pressure facilitate biocontainment. Efficiency of such a pressure system can be increased through computerizing operation of inverters, by connecting these to control gadgets, which automatically run inverters at the air inlets. The gadgets have a display screen and control buttons that allow resetting and calibration of the system without having to modify the actual inverters.

These and other automated features of a P3 laboratory are controlled from the control panel whose display panel is shown in Figure 5. The operation mode system is inbuilt within the panel from where it can be operated through a switch on the panel's display. Temperature and pressure control functions are also controlled from the control panel. The control panel therefore runs operation components of a P3 laboratory, with its display panel facilitating easy monitoring of functioning of the facility by displaying all vital readings.

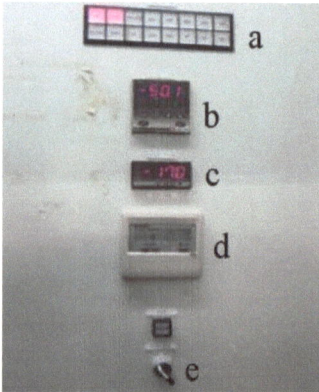

Figure 5: Control panel; a) Operation mode display, b) P3 room pressure, c) Ante-room pressure, d) Temperature display, e) Eco/run mode switch.

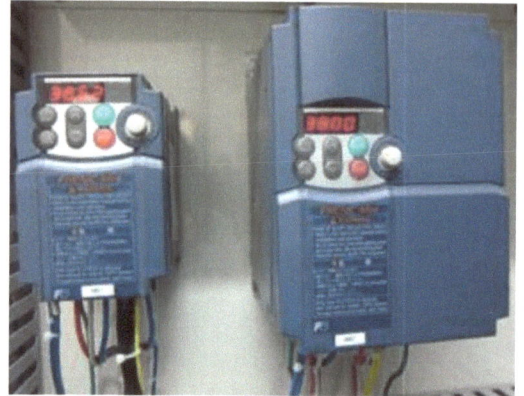

Figure 6: Inverter control gadgets.

4   Equipments

A P3 laboratory can be equipped with a range of equipments depending on intended usage, with biosafety equipments being the main basic necessities. Among these, biosafety cabinets and autoclaves are the most important. General laboratory equipments such as incubators, ELISA machines, PCR machines among others can be installed based on the laboratory's operation protocol. A freezer is also considered a basic equipment since some specimens must be maintained under BSL-3 conditions. P3 equipments maintain physical containment or minimize chances of transmission of contaminants.

4.1   Biosafety Equipments

Safety equipments form the core of biosafety, and biosecurity and containment cannot be achieved without a full set of these. They provide a physical primary barrier between the user and the source of contaminants, since aerosols are bound to be produced even after biosafety procedures have been followed. Major safety equipments include biosafety cabinets, autoclaves and protective clothing, though other safety enhancing equipments can be provided based on a laboratory's function or research protocols.

Biological safety cabinets are a major component of a P3 laboratory due to their ability to contain aerosols, conferring protection to both the user and specimens being processed. There are three classes of biosafety cabinets; class I, II and III. Class I cabinets are open-front safety cabinets, fitted with exhaust HEPA filters only, and exhausts all air to the outside or into the laboratory room (CDC, 2009). These cabinets protect the environment but offer minimal protection to specimens within the hood. Class II cabinets have considerable negative pressure, have HEPA filters at the exhaust route only and provide protection for both the environment and the specimens being manipulated (Maier, Pepper, & Gerba, 2009). Class II A1 recirculates 70% into the cabinet and exhausts 30% into the room or outside while class II B1 recirculates 30% and exhausts 70%. Class II B2 exhausts all air to the outside while Class II A2 are similar to A1, but with a higher face velocity (100 lfm) (CDC, 2009). Moderately risky pathogens such as *Clostridium spp., Shigella spp., Microsporum spp., Entamoeba spp.,* adenoviruses and influenza viruses among others can be manipulated in Class II cabinets (Maier, Pepper, & Gerba, 2009). Class III cabinets are total containment cabinets that enable safe manipulation of high risk pathogens. They are fitted with one inlet filter and two outlet filters and have attached rubber gloves through which all work within the cabinet is performed (Maier, Pepper, & Gerba, 2009). Microorganisms such as *Brucella spp., Rickettsia spp., Mycobacterium tuberculosis, Coccidioides immitis* and Dengue virus among other high risk pathogens can be safely manipulated in class III cabinets. Class IIA1, A2 and B1, B2 and class III safety cabinets are the most recommended for a P3 laboratory, though class IIB2 cabinets are more popularly used in place of class III.

Autoclaves on the other hand function in sterilization of infectious or contaminated materials for disposal or reuse. Preferably, an autoclave should have different inbuilt operating programs to allow for decontamination of a range of materials with varying levels and types of contaminants. Further, the laboratory should be sufficiently supplied with all the necessary Personal Protective Equipments (PPE) (Figure 7). PPE is normally stored in the anteroom, from where it can be worn before entering the P3 room and removed upon exit. Other safety equipments may include centrifuge cups, pipette aids and leak proof collection containers among others, which serve in containing hazardous materials (WHO, 2004).

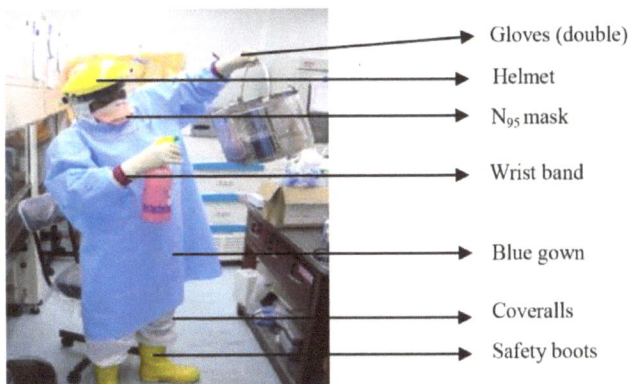

Figure 7: Personal protective equipment.

4.2   Emergency Response Equipment

These are gadgets that enable laboratory workers to manage accidents or incidents, mainly fires, power failures and leakage of laboratory gases. Fire detectors, fire extinguishers, gas detectors and emergency lighting are the most essential emergency response equipment.

Fire extinguishers are preferably carbon dioxide type or powder type, located within the P3 room and in the ante-room. These should be conditioned regularly, strategically stationed and have a user instruction manual attached. The gas detector is normally fixed on top of a biosafety cabinet and has an alert component that goes off in case of any gas leakage. The fire alarm can be inbuilt within the laboratory from where it activates fire alerts at the onset of a fire. A hammer is provided on each glass window to be used to break the glass and provide a safe exit route, in addition to conventional emergency exits.

Lack of lighting during power outages can be quite disastrous and a generator back-up power can fail. It is therefore necessary to provide emergency lighting by installing a fluorescent lamp supported by a rechargeable battery. The bulb automatically switches on for one hour, following a total power failure to allow users to finish-up their experiments or undo set-ups and evacuate.

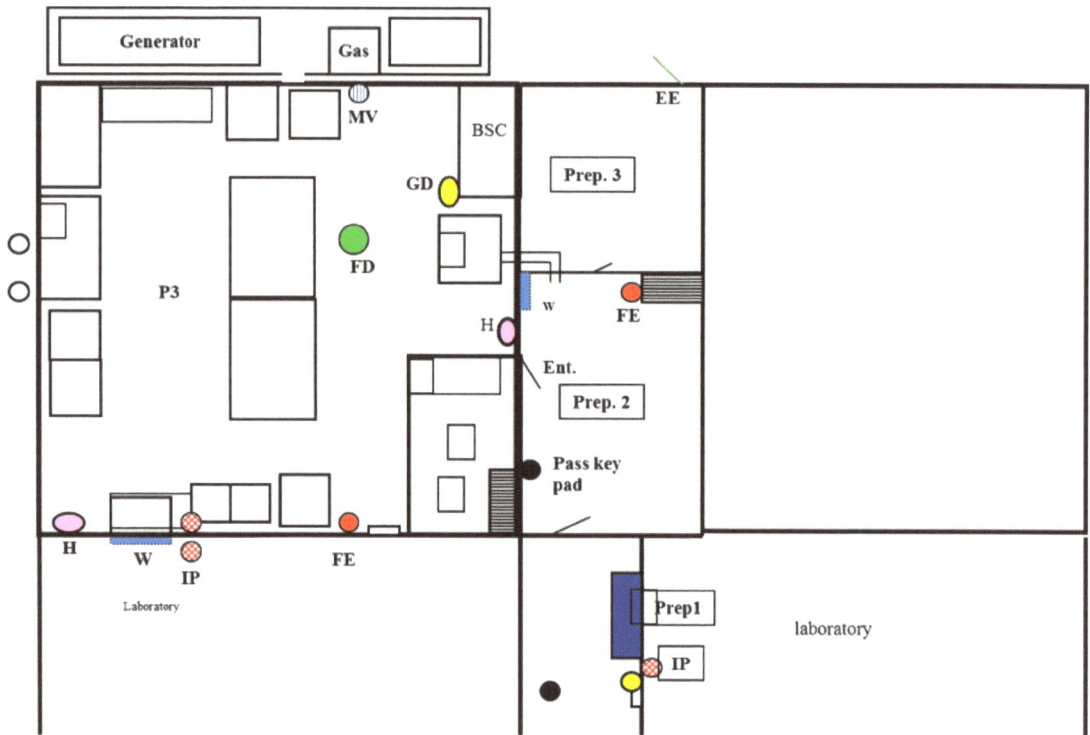

Figure 8: Aerial view of location of emergency response equipments within a P3 laboratory; GD-Gas detector, FD-fire detector, EE-Emergency exit, H-Hammer, IP-Interphone, FE-Fire extinguisher.

5   Maintenance

Maintenance of P3 facilities is a key aspect of biosafety management systems because use of faulty and unconditioned equipments can cause contamination. A P3 laboratory can increase the risk of transmission of biohazards due to the nature of pathogens handled in it hence regular maintenance is of utmost importance. For easy maintenance and optimum functioning of the laboratory, daily, weekly, monthly and yearly maintenance routines are carried out, overlapping maintenance with daily usage rather than having to repair systems only when they breakdown.

5.1   Daily Maintenance

Daily maintenance mainly involves floor cleaning, disinfection of handles, waste removal, and monitoring of vital parameters at the control panel display as well as documentation of observed off-readings. Additionally, biosafety cabinets are decontaminated after each use by Ultraviolet (UV) light. The entire P3 room must also be decontaminated daily after work for at least an hour using UV light.

5.2   Weekly Maintenance

Changing of pre-filters is carried out weekly. Being part of the initial air filtration stages, the fibrous pre-filters trap large quantities of dust and fine particles. It is therefore necessary to change them every week in order to minimize chances contaminating or damaging the entire system. The pre-filters are washable hence their maintenance basically involves removal of dirty filters from the panels as shown in figure 9 (a) and replacement with a clean filter. The generator is also maintained weekly. Its control panel is programmed to turn on the generator once every week for ten minutes or so, to allow for routine maintenance, mainly checking and recording of vital operating parameters and battery recharge.

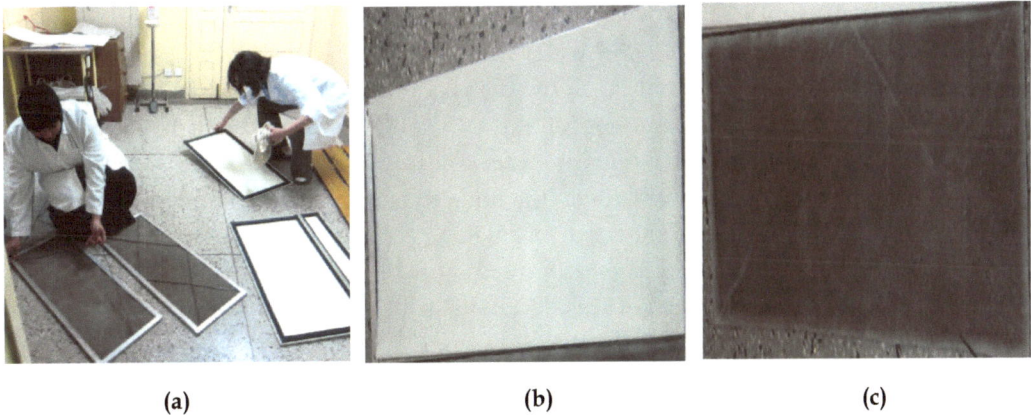

| (a) | (b) | (c) |

Figure 9: (a) Changing of pre-filters, **(b)** A clean pre-filter, **(c)** A soiled pre-filter

5.3   Monthly Maintenance

Monthly maintenance is applied on the air filtration system, depending on manometer readings. It involves replacement of intermediate filters since they get clogged with dust particles in the course of usage. The manometer in Figure 10 (a) monitors the condition of these filters and indicates when they are due for replacement. The black arm of the manometer shows meter readings, indicating how much of the intermediate filter has been consumed while the red arm shows maximum consumption, at which the intermediate filter should be changed.

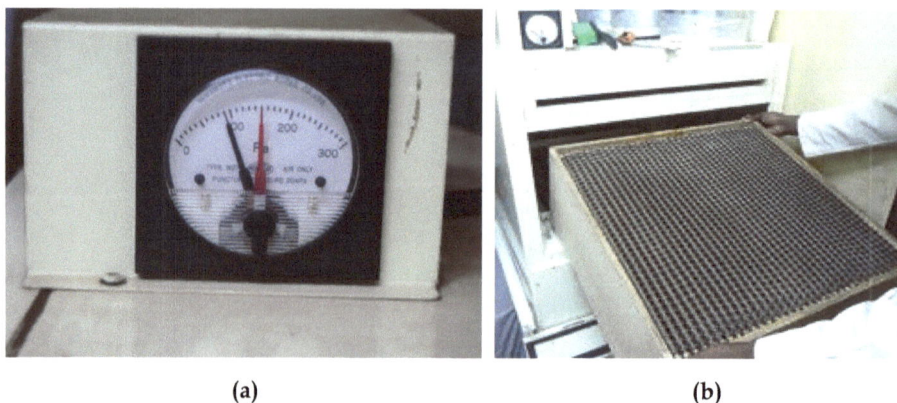

(a)   (b)

Figure 10: a) The manometer, b) A used-up intermediate filter being removed from the filter chamber for changing

5.4   Yearly Maintenance

Every year, core P3 facilities are serviced, preferably by trained experts or by suppliers. Yearly maintenance mainly focuses on fumigation of biosafety cabinets and changing of HEPA filters. Fumigation uses a bactericidal principle to get rid of aerosol contaminants that accumulate within the inner spaces of a biosafety cabinet in the course of its usage. It is carried out using paraformaldehyde and water, followed by neutralization using ammonium hydrogen carbonate. Hotplates holding the fumigants are placed within the hood as shown in Figure 11 (a). The front panel of the cabinet is then removed and the cabinet sealed using a thick film. Humidification with the fumigants is initiated within the sealed cabinet by switching on the hotplate containing paraformaldehyde and water for a while, while switching the biosafety cabinet on and off for at least one minute to allow the gas to circulate within the plenum. Following humidification, fumigation continues for at least twelve hours after which neutralization is carried out for about one hour using ammonium hydrogen carbonate. HEPA filters are then changed as shown in Figure 12 and their functionality confirmed using air velocity and air particle count tests. Figure 13 (a) shows the air velocity test that examines the rate of flow of air into and within the cabinet. Final velocity reading is the average of several readings taken at different points within the cabinet. Inside air velocity should be between 0.3 to 0.4 m/s while that at the entrance ranges between 0.7 to 0.8m/s. Air particle count shown in Figure 13 (b) confirms efficiency of fitted HEPA filters, by measuring penetration of the filter. Caution should be observed when changing HEPA filters because these could still be bearing contaminants, hence personal protective equipments should be used.

    Yearly routines also cover major technical functions of the laboratory. Pressure, ventilation and air conditioning systems are checked alongside electrical systems, and repairs and maintenance undertaken where necessary. Breaks are also checked for within the P3 structure to ensure that there are no air spaces that could compromise its air tight function.

6   Safety and Security Features

Operations in a P3 laboratory call for adherence to strict safety and security measures. While physical features of the laboratory provide necessary secondary barrier in addition to primary

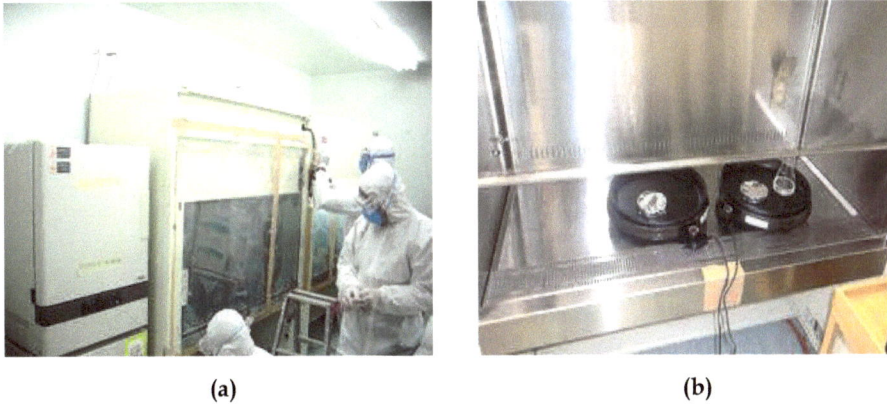

(a)   (b)

Figure 11: Positioning hotplates **(a)** and sealing biosafety cabinets **(b)** in preparation for fumigation.

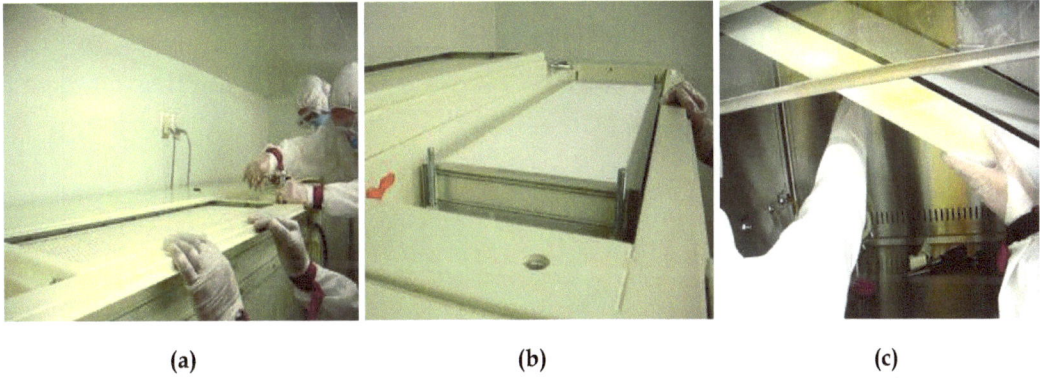

(a)   (b)   (c)

Figure 12: (a) Removal of exhaust covers during replacement of HEPA filters, **(b)** Aerial view of old exhaust filter, **(c)** Fitting of new inlet filter.

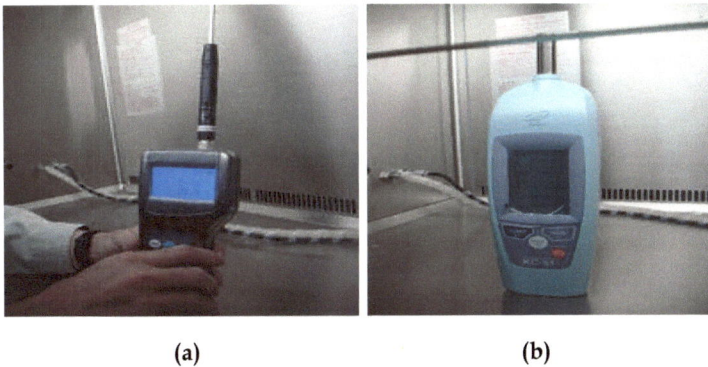

(a)   (b)

Figure 13: Confirmation of efficiency of fitted HEPA filters using **(a)** air velocity testing, and **(b)** air particle counting.

safety provided by safety equipments, additional safety and security features can be incorporated to enhance biosafety. For physical separation, the laboratory should be located in an area with minimal movements. Further, only authorized persons can access the laboratory, a measure that can be reinforced by use of an automatic locking pad operated using a password that can be changed regularly. Only trained laboratory staff can use the P3. In case untrained persons need to use the facility, they should be accompanied by trained personnel. A register is provided and maintained to track activities in the P3 laboratory. Such a register can also be used for follow-up in case of any irregularity.

Other safety features include safety signs and labels that aid in identification of hazardous areas or materials or remind users of recommended safety procedures. A biohazard label is the most dominant safety signage in P3 laboratories. It bears a biohazard symbol and is affixed on the P3 room door, waste containers, refrigerators and freezers containing hazardous materials and on any equipment that may be contaminated. An exit sign is yet another safety label that directs users to a safe emergency exit route in case of any accident. Activated pathogen tags on a pre-printed chart can also be affixed on the door to inform users on particular pathogens being handled in the laboratory at any given time. Some P3 laboratories also have custom made biosafety symbols to fit its safety policies. For example, a limited entry symbol can be used to limit entry of unauthorized users into the P3 area, alongside other more specific symbols on P3 laboratory etiquette or even PPE usage.

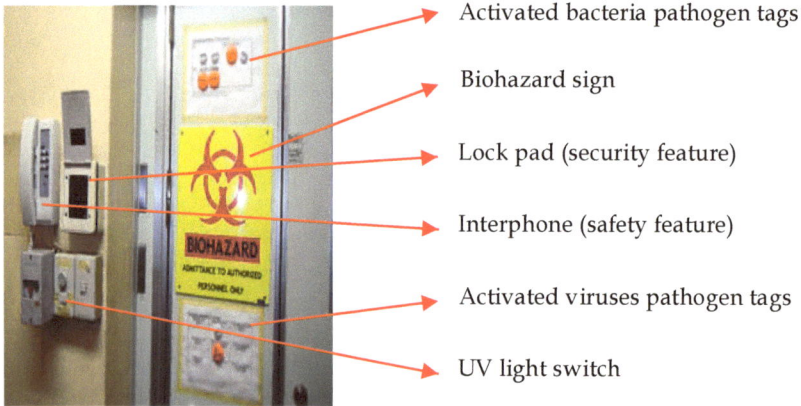

Figure 14: Safety and security features.

Given the level of hazard associated with P3 laboratories, decontamination by ultraviolet light after each work session is necessary. The UV light switch bulb enables easy decontamination of the laboratory since it is preset to run for a pre-determined duration, sufficient to fully sterilize the laboratory. Interphones are also provided to enhance safety by easing communication in the event of an accident.

Labels and signs are openly affixed on any hazardous or potentially hazardous area within the laboratory, or where extra caution needs to be observed. Most importantly, areas of multiple hazards are clearly indicated using multiple signs as on Figure 14, each signaling individual hazard that users are likely to encounter. All signage features follow universal specifications in terms of color scheme and images, for easy recognition.

7 Documentation

Documentation is a critical feature of safety management procedures. Biosafety management systems recommend design and utilization of records that capture information on users and activities intended to be carried out in the laboratory in a particular session. Generally, these records track activities in the P3 laboratory, movement in and out of the laboratory and usage of laboratory equipments. Such records include:

7.1 P3 In/Out Record

This is a general record on utilization of P3 laboratories. It records information on daily activities in P3, the number of people using it and usage of P3 facilities. It captures the name of laboratory staff, time in and out; number of biosafety cabinets used per session, purpose of using the laboratory and pathogens intended to be manipulated.

7.2 Biosafety Cabinet Usage Record

This is a record specific for usage of biosafety cabinets. It captures information on duration of usage, pathogens being handled in the facility and specific biosafety cabinets intended to be used. The record can be used to schedule maintenance activities, especially in cases where the biosafety cabinets are frequently being used.

7.3 Daily Check-point for Ante-room

This is the ante-room record in which daily observations made on the overall working condition of the P3 laboratory as shown on the control panel are entered. It documents pressure reading on inverters I and II, P3 pressure, ante-room pressure and temperature readings.

Item \\ Date							
Inverter I							
Inverter II							
P3 Pressure							
Ante Pressure							
Room Temperature							
Remarks							

Table 1: An ante-room checklist.

8 Biosafety Rules and Standard Operating Procedures (SOPs)

Failure to adhere to good laboratory practices, laboratory worker error and misuse of equipments accounts for majority of laboratory injuries and laboratory-acquired infections. Consequently, good laboratory practices and SOPs must be in place to prevent laboratory-acquired infections, minimize laboratory accidents and maintain biosafety and biocontainment. A biosafety manual provides a code of conduct in compliance with good laboratory practices, whose proper implementation reduces occurrence of hazardous incidences. WHO (2004) provides a basic code of practice that can be adopted and fine-tuned to fit institutional needs. A good manual should define access requirements; restricting entry to only authorized persons, biosafety practices in daily utilization of laboratory facilities, personal protection and laboratory etiquette (WHO, 2004). For example, one should not eat or store food in the laboratory, personal protection equipments should be worn and used appropriately, biosafety protocols must be followed, and biosafety symbols must be used as necessary and should follow universal specification.

SOPs on the other hand should document analytical and maintenance procedures as well as safety procedures that can be applied in case of an accident or in order to avert a would-be incident. Biosafety management SOPs include accident and incident reporting procedure, disinfection and decontamination of work surfaces, entry and exit procedures and waste disposal among others (Zaki, 2010). Further, each equipment in P3 should have an SOP, for use within the laboratory and for facilitating training of new staff. SOPs provide a brief description of the equipment, how to operate it and guidelines on its maintenance and calibration routines where applicable. Each research project utilizing a P3 laboratory should also have an SOP.

9   Waste Management

P3 laboratories generate a variety of infectious wastes necessitating development of proper waste disposal system in order to minimize potential for exposure of laboratory workers who must handle the material. In most cases, institutions usually develop their own waste disposal protocol that fit their needs. A protocol defines wastes into various categories, provides a unique color of waste container and liner, and provides a set of handling and disposal policies for each category. A set of policies are also provided for each category, instructing laboratory workers on how to handle and dispose various types of wastes.

To ease waste disposal, P3 laboratory users initiate the disposal process, by autoclaving wastes where necessary and segregating wastes into respective waste containers. Following initial treatment, wastes are disposed as per the institution's waste disposal protocol by designated staff.

10   Training

Usefulness, efficiency and safety of a P3 facility depends on the level of awareness and expertise among researchers, hence the need for training. The training component of a P3 laboratory is of utmost importance not only because of the need to develop manpower but also because of the relevance of P3 facilities in securing laboratory procedures.

An ideal P3 training curriculum covers biosafety and personal safety, and is delivered through lectures and practical demonstrations. Participants are first introduced to the concept of biosafety and the P3 laboratory in general before being instructed on operations at biosafety level three. Most specifically, training focuses on informing participants on the hazards associated with the facility and possible ways of eliminating personal harm while minimizing the risk of exposing other people to danger. Maintenance and management of a P3 laboratory is also covered. Effectiveness of the training session is evaluated through an assessment test whose outcome can inform the institution on gaps of knowledge and areas of weakness, for which refresher courses can be scheduled.

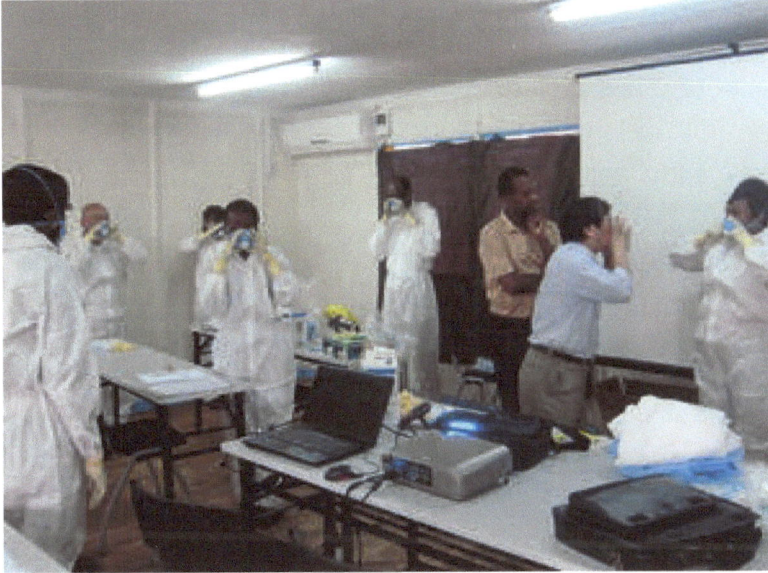

Figure 15: A training workshop's practical session.

11   Biosafety Committees and Biosafety Meetings

For a P3 laboratory, need to develop, implement and adhere to biosafety policies cannot be overemphasized, functions that are executed through biosafety committees and meetings. A biosafety committee can be a group of laboratory staff who have undergone intensive training on biosafety and biosecurity systems to acquire sufficient capacity to manage P3 laboratory security systems. It is in charge of ensuring that biosafety guidelines are adhered to, carrying out risk assessments on new projects utilizing P3 facilities, supervising laboratory maintenance routines, responding to alarms and emergencies, chairing biosafety meetings and training new users (Zaki, 2010). Led by a biosecurity officer, it is also the responsibility of the biosecurity committee to manage P3 facilitates and to ensure sufficient supply of laboratory consumables. Apart from training laboratory users, the committee creates awareness on matters of biosecurity within the institution to assure occupational safety of other workers.

Biosafety meetings are an output of biosafety committees. These are usually monthly meetings that bring together researchers who have used the P3 laboratory within a particular month and other trained users. The meetings provide a forum for attendees to share their experiences with regards to using the P3 laboratory, identify and discuss areas of difficulty, update each other on recent occurrences or new installations and get informed on ongoing activities. Occurrences, especially alarms or system breakdowns can be communicated and discussed to identify their causes and generate preventive measures against these and other would-be occurrences.

Attendees are also reminded of basic safety rules and practices, emphasizing on the need to observe personal safety and safety of other people around the institution. It should be mandatory for all users and trained staff to attend and participate in the meeting.

12   Accreditation

Given the complexity of operations in a P3 laboratory coupled with increasing public health threats, a P3 laboratory has to always be in optimum working condition and in a position to manage emerging challenges. Laboratory accreditation is therefore necessary since it assures that all recommended physical and operational features of a P3 laboratory are in place and well maintained and that biosafety guidelines are being adhered to. Moreover, an accredited laboratory instills confidence in users and assures them of personal safety and safety of their research procedures, as well as quality of their research outcomes. A P3 laboratory is first accredited by default by the supplier, since a containment facility manufacturer has to be certified before it can be allowed to supply. However, the laboratory must obtain more authentic accreditation by in-country and international bodies, though this can be quite a lengthy process especially in countries lacking proper accreditation systems.

13   Conclusion

Several uncertainties surround laboratory acquired infections. It is not only difficult to determine the actual risk for infection after exposure but it is also difficult to determine the actual source or mode of infection (CDC, 2012). Further, laboratory workers are at a greater risk of exposure to pathogens than the general public. Biosafety facilities therefore aim at minimizing the risk of exposure to infectious agents, in order to enable proper disease diagnosis or specimen processing the in case of research laboratories. Proper construction, utilization and maintenance of a P3 laboratory provides users with optimum safety necessary when handling risk group three organisms. However, equipments only cannot guarantee biosafety. Capacity to utilize the facility has to be developed continuously, while entrenching good laboratory practices among laboratory workers, to responsibly undertake biosafety observance.

Acknowledgements

Establishment of our P3 facility would not have been possible without the support of many partners. We wish to acknowledge the Director of Kenya Medical Research Institute (KEMRI) for the continued support and in particular, the Center for Microbiology Research who are hosting our laboratories. Special thanks to Nagasaki University (Japan) for supporting our research activities technically and financially. Finally, we thank Nippon Medical &Chemical Instruments Company (Japan), the suppliers of our P3 facility for providing labor for continuous maintenance of the laboratory.

Authors

Yoshio Ichinose, Shingo Inoue, Masaaki Shimada, Gabriel Miring'u, Betty Muriithi, Angela Makumi, Ernest Wandera, Martin Bundi, Chika Narita, Salame Ashur, Allan Kwalla, Amina Galata, Erick Odoyo, Sora Huqa, Mohammed Shah, Mohammed Karama, Masahiro Horio
Institute of Tropical Medicine, Nagasaki University, Nairobi, Kenya, Japan

References

Centers for Disease Control and Prevention (2012). *Guidelines for safe work practices in human and animal medical diagnostic laboratories. Morbidity and Mortality Weekly Report, Supplement/Vol.61, 1- 103.*

Centers for Disease Control. (2009). **Biosafety in microbiological and biomedical laboratories, 5ᵗʰ edition. Centers for Disease Control.**

Maier, R. M., Pepper, I. L. & Gerba. P. (2009). *Environmental Microbiology, 2ⁿᵈ edition. Elservier Inc., United Sates of America.*

Pedrosa, P. B. & Cardoso, T, A. (2011). *Viral infections in workers in hospital and research laboratory settings: a comparative review of infection modes and respective biosafety aspects. Int Journal of Infect Dis., 15(6), 366-76.*

Pike, R. M. (1979). *Laboratory-associated infections: incidence, fatalities, causes, and prevention. Annu Rev Microbiol., 33, 41-66.*

Schaechter, M. ed. (2009) *Encyclopedia of microbiology. United States of America: Elservier Inc.*

Vesley, D., & Hartmann, H, M. (1988).*Laboratory-acquired infections and injuries in clinical laboratories: a 1986 survey. Am J Public Health, 78, 1213-5.*

WHO. (2004). *Laboratory Biosafety Manual, 3ʳᵈ ed. Malta: World Health Organization.*

Zaki, N. Adel. (2010). *Biosafety and biosecurity measures: management of biosafety level 3 facilities. International Journal of Antimicrobial Agents, 36S, 570-574.*

Evaluating Mixtures in Drinking Water Supplies as Risk Factors for Cancer: A Case Study of Nitrate and Atrazine

Martha G. Rhoades, Jane L. Meza, Cheryl L. Beseler, Patrick J. Shea,
Andy Kahle, Julie M. Vose, Mary E. Exner, Roy F. Spalding

1 Introduction

Non-Hodgkin lymphoma (NHL), a cancer first recognized in the 1800s, is currently the fifth most common type of cancer in the United States. NHL incidence in the Midwestern United States is among the highest in the country. Several studies have reported increased risk of NHL to be associated with some phenomenon related to agriculture, and at the forefront in epidemiological research, has been exposure to nitrate in drinking water and exposure to pesticides. Groundwater supplies about 50% of the drinking water in the U.S. and over 85% in Nebraska. Nebraska is an agricultural state with more groundwater than any other state, largely due to the High Plains Aquifer. Groundwater used for irrigation is four times that of surface water irrigation, livestock, industrial, public and domestic water supplies combined. Vulnerability to leaching and agricultural practices over the last 50-60 years has led to increased nitrate and pesticide contamination of drinking water supplies. Atrazine (6-chloro-N-ethyl-N'-(1-methylethyl)-1,3,5-triazine-2,4-diamine), a herbicide commonly used since the early 1960s, is the most prevalent pesticide detected.

The Environmental Protection Agency recently began reevaluating the maximum contaminant level of atrazine (3μg/L) due to research findings suggesting it may be responsible for some cancers, and reproductive and developmental disorders. Studies have also reported that adverse health effects due to nitrate in drinking water may be a result of the formation of N-nitroso compounds *in vivo*. Nitrite (produced from the reduction of nitrate) reacts with nitrosatable compounds in acidic environments. Atrazine is such a nitrosatable compound. It is a secondary amine that readily nitrosates in an acidic environment with excess nitrite to form a nitrosamine, N-nitrosoatrazine (NNAT). NNAT forms easily at pH 3 to 3.5, is fairly stable, and has been shown to cause chromosomal abnormalities in lymphocytes *in vitro*. Atrazine has two nitrosatable secondary amine moieties and its degradation products, deethylatrazine (DEA) and deisopropylatrazine (DIA) (also found in groundwater), are nitrosatable. Where atrazine is found, the concentration of DEA and DIA is typically at least equal to that of atrazine and the toxicity of their nitrosated products may be similar or greater than nitrosated atrazine.

This chapter describes the scientific basis for, and the methodology used, to test the hypothesis that individuals who drink water contaminated with nitrate and atrazine are at increased risk of developing NHL when compared to individuals not having the co-exposure. A summary of NHL and its risk factors is provided as well as the biological plausibility of how co-exposure to nitrate- and atrazine-contaminated drinking water can lead to developing NHL. Monitoring and regulation of these two drinking water contaminants are summarized and the atrazine and nitrate groundwater situation in Nebraska illustrated. The details of an ecological study using Bayesian analysis and a case-control study to confirm/refute the findings of the Bayesian study are provided. We discuss the results, strengths and limitations of our studies and conclude the chapter with suggestions for future research.

2   Non-Hodgkin Lymphoma

Several types of lymphatic system tumors are classified as NHL, a lymphatic malignancy resulting from genetic events occurring in the peripheral organs (Weisenburger, 1992). On presentation, NHL patients generally have complaints of enlarged lymph nodes, fever and weight loss (NCI, 2010). NHL is characterized by genetic alterations including translocations, deletions and other nonrandom aberrations, the most common being t(14;18)(q32;q21) which results in inhibition of apoptosis (Meijerink, 1997, Chiu *et al.*, 2006). In this translocation the immunoglobulin-heavy chain promoter on chromosome 14q32 is coupled with the *bcl-2* oncogene on chromosome 18q21, resulting in overexpression of the anti-apoptotic *bcl-2* protein, important early in NHL development (Meijerink, 1997, Chiu *et al.*, 2008). The t(14;18) aberration is found in nearly 90% of follicular lymphomas (Meijerink, 1997).

Lymphoma classification began in the 1930s and several protocols to classify NHL have been written over the ensuing 60 years. In 1991, the International Lymphoma Study Group formed and proposed the Revised European-American Classification of Lymphoid Neoplasms (REAL). In 1997, the new official classification of the World Health Organization (WHO) was published and is currently used by researchers and clinicians.

In the U.S., and specifically the Midwest, diffuse large B-cell lymphoma (DLBCL) and follicular lymphoma are the most frequently diagnosed subtypes (Anderson *et al.*, 1998; Abelhoff *et al.*, 2004); but little is known about the risk factors associated with these two types of NHL. One-fourth to one-half of all lymphomas present as extranodal disease. Etiology of extranodal NHL is multifactorial and includes congenital, acquired and iatrogenic immune suppression, autoimmune disease, infections (both viral and bacterial), and exposure to pesticides and other environmental agents.

NHL subtypes can be categorized as aggressive B-cell, indolent B-cell or T-cell lymphoma (Vose *et al.*, 2002). Aggressive B-cell lymphoma includes DLBCL, mantle cell lymphoma, and Burkitt lymphoma. The increasing incidence of NHL is due in part to an increase in DLBCL, the most common NHL in the world. Follicular lymphoma, an indolent lymphoma of follicle center B-cells (centrocytes and centroblasts), is the second most common lymphoma in the U.S. Cutaneous B-cell lymphoma, mucosa associated lymphoid tissue (MALT) lymphoma, marginal zone and chronic lymphocytic leukemia/small lymphocytic lymphoma are also classified as indolent B-cell tumors. The most common B-cell primary tumor of the skin is follicular lymphoma, followed by marginal zone cutaneous lymphoma. Extranodal marginal zone B-cell lymphoma of MALT is the third most common NHL and is predominantly found in the stomach. Nearly 50% of lymphomas found in the stomach are of the MALT type. MALT lymphoma is likely related to *Helicobacter pylori* with more than 90% of MALT cases having *H. py-*

lori infection (Mauch *et al.*, 2004). The association between MALT lymphoma and *H. pylori* could be related to nitrosatable medications typically taken for this condition (Brambilla *et al.*, 1985) or the *H. pylori* bacteria reducing nitrate to nitrite, increasing the concentration of nitrite in the stomach.

T-cell lymphomas are rare in Nebraska and there is scant information linking T-cell lymphoma etiology to environmental exposure. Mycosis fungoides, the most common cutaneous T-cell lymphoma, is rare and the etiology is not known. Cutaneous anaplastic large cell lymphoma arises in the skin, is difficult to diagnose and also occurs rarely. It is strongly associated with mycosis fungoides and Hodgkin disease. The etiology for T-cell large granular lymphocyte leukemia is not known but this cancer is more common in patients with autoimmune disease and is found in 25% of rheumatoid arthritis patients. Peripheral T-cell lymphomas represent about 7% of all NHL tumors, display T-cell or natural killer cell immunophenotypes and occur more often in patients with ataxia telangiectasia (Mauch *et al.*, 2004).

2.1 Risk Factors

Occupational. Several occupations have been associated with NHL, likely due to environmental exposure in the workplace. Hardell *et al.* (1981) reported an association between organic solvents, chlorophenols and phenoxy acids and risk for malignant lymphoma, contradicting Kato *et al.* (2005), who reported an increased risk of NHL only for participants whose first exposure occurred before 1970. Exposure to benzene, xylene and toluene are reported risk factors for NHL (Smith *et al.*, 2007; Vineis *et al.*, 2007), as is trichloroethylene (TCE) exposure (Mandel *et al.*, 2006). Toolmakers, machine tool operators and workers in leather and leather products had increased risk of NHL (Schenk *et al.*, 2009), possibly related to the use of TCE in leather tanning and as a degreaser in machining. TCE is a common point source contaminant of drinking water due to the improper disposal of used TCE around manufacturing plants. In Australia, workers exposed to 50/60 Hz magnetic fields were at slightly increased risk of NHL (Karipidis *et al.*, 2007). Printers, wood workers, farmers (especially farmers involved in animal husbandry) and teachers are at increased risk for developing NHL (Boffetta & de Vocht 2007). Exposure to some congeners of polychlorinated biphenyls increase the risk for NHL risk (De Roos *et al.*, 2005; Engel *et al.*, 2007a,b; Freeman and Kohles, 2012).

Genetic translocation and risk factors. Family history is an accepted risk factor for most cancers. Lymphoma risk is increased when first degree relatives have a hemolymphopoietic cancer (Negri *et al.*, 2006; Wang *et al.*, 2007a; Mensah *et al.*, 2007). Men with a family history of nonhematopoietic cancer and hematopoietic cancer in first degree relatives are at increased risk for NHL, especially small lymphocytic NHL (Chiu *et al.*, 2004).

Studies investigating genetic factors have reported that smoking is not associated with risk of t(14;18)-positive or negative NHL in men but family history of hematopoietic cancer increased risk of both t(14;18) defined NHL subtypes in men and women. Women who had ever smoked cigarettes were at increased risk for t(14;18)-negative NHL and risk increased with longer duration and early initiation. There was no association with ever smoking and t(14;18)-positive NHL (Chiu *et al.*, 2007a). Risk of t(14;18)-positive NHL was higher in farmers who used insecticides during animal production or applied insecticides, herbicides and/or fumigants to row crops and increased with duration of use. None of these pesticides were associated with t(14;18)-negative NHL (Chiu *et al.*, 2006). Organochlorine exposure and immune gene variation have been associated with NHL risk (Colt *et al.*, 2009). A study to evaluate sun exposure and the vitamin D receptor gene (Purdue *et al.*, 2007a) found an inverse association between UV exposure and NHL risk. B-cell NHL patients and patients with autoimmune disease have been found to have elevated B-cell activating factor serum levels (Novak *et al.*, 2009). NHL risk was increased among subjects with an autoimmune condition and tumor necrosis factor (TNF) genotype when compared with those subjects not having an autoimmune condition (Wang *et al.*, 2007b). Results were similar for DLBCL and follicular lymphoma. Risk of NHL has been associated with folate metabolizing genes (Lightfoot *et al.*, 2005). Caspase gene variants were protective against developing NHL (Lan *et al.*, 2007). Genes responsible for DNA double strand base repair may influence susceptibility (Novik *et al.*, 2007) as might variation in the IL10 and TNF loci (Purdue *et al.*, 2007b). Genetic variations that result in the generation of reactive oxygen species were reported to increase risk of NHL and its major subtypes, particularly DLBCL (Wang *et al.*, 2006).

Demographic and lifestyle factors. Lifestyle habits have been associated with NHL risk. Physical activity decreased risk but obesity and caloric intake increased risk in both men and women (Pan *et al.*, 2005). A higher adult body mass index (BMI) was associated with NHL risk (Chiu *et al.*, 2007b). Women having a history of sun tanning are at greater risk for developing NHL and risk increases with time spent in strong summer sunlight (Zhang *et al.*, 2007). NHL risk was lower among those drinking alcohol than for nondrinkers and for former or current smokers than nonsmokers but severe obesity (BMI ≥35) and taller height were moderately associated with NHL (Lim *et al.*, 2007b). The use of dark, permanent dyes before 1980 was associated with NHL risk (Morton *et al.*, 2001; Zhang *et al.*, 2004, 2008; Sanjose *et al.*, 2006). As birth order increased, DLBCL risk increased but follicular lymphoma risk was not increased (Cozen *et al.*, 2007). Participants living in less crowded, cleaner areas had fewer childhood infections but had greater risk for NHL later in life (Bracci *et al.*, 2006). Compared to subjects having no siblings, having four or more siblings was associated with moderately increased NHL risk (Smedby *et al.*, 2007). Pet owners have decreased risk for NHL and DLBCL than participants who had never owned a pet (Tranah *et al.*, 2008) but exposure to cattle for greater than or equal to five years or exposure to pigs was associated with increased NHL risk. Residents whose homes were treated for termites before the chlordane ban in 1988 had elevated NHL risk (Colt *et al.*, 2006).

Other risk factors. Medications such as aspirin, nonsteroidal anti-inflammatory medications, and antibiotics produced inconsistent results relative to NHL risk (Cerhan *et al.*, 2003; Chang *et al.*, 2005; Flick *et al.*, 2006; Hoeft *et al.*, 2008). Antipsychotics and antidepressants have been associated with chromosomal aberrations in lymphocytes and many of these pharmaceuticals are nitrosatable (Brambilla & Martelli 2007; Brambilla *et al.*, 2009). Reproductive hormones were protective against DLBCL in women (Lee *et al.*, 2008) and no evidence was found linking increased risk of NHL to women using postmenopausal hormone replacement therapy (Norgaard *et al.*, 2006). Gaikwad *et al.* (2009) reported men with NHL had higher concentrations of estrogen-DNA adducts in their urine compared to healthy controls and suggest that catechol estrogen quinones reacting with DNA may be inducing NHL tumors. Dietary factors, including animal protein, B and C vitamin and carotene intake, consumption of vegetables, alcohol intake, milk products and trans unsaturated fat have been studied as possible risk factors for NHL (Ward *et al.*, 1994; Zhang *et al.*, 1999; Lim *et al.*, 2005; Chang *et al.*, 2006; Cross *et al.*, 2006; Lim *et al.*, 2006; Chiu *et al.*, 2008; Koutros *et al.*, 2008) suggesting the role of dietary factors in developing NHL.

Risk of NHL was not associated with sexually transmitted infections, sexual behavior, blood transfusions, influenza, acne and either occupational or domestic exposure to zoonotic infections (Vajdic *et al.*, 2006). However, some viruses, HIV and some infections were found to increase NHL risk (Engels, 2007). An inverse association between HDL cholesterol and NHL was observed, changing with length of follow-up (Lim *et al.*, 2007a) but total or non-HDL cholesterol didn't affect risk. Type 2 diabetes mellitus is a reported risk factor for NHL (Chao & Page 2008).

Autoimmune disorders. A bidirectional association between NHL and rheumatoid arthritis, systemic lupus erythematosus, Sjogren disease and autoimmune related thyroid disease has been reported (Ehrenfeld *et al.*, 2001). Sjogren disease was associated with risk of MALT lymphoma and celiac disease with risk of small bowel lymphoma (Smedby *et al.*, 2006). Sjogren syndrome and lupus were associated with salivary gland and marginal zone NHL (Engels *et al.*, 2005) and evaluating the role of altered immunity in NHL etiology has been suggested (Grulich *et al.*, 2007). Allergies (excluding drug allergies) decreased risk of all NHL, including DLBCL and follicular lymphoma. Hay fever had a similar effect but eczema was associated with increased risk of follicular lymphoma. Being asthmatic did not affect NHL risk but exposure to pesticides increased NHL risk in asthmatics compared to nonasthmatics (Lee *et al.*, 2004, 2006).

Agricultural risk factors. Studies evaluating agricultural practice and NHL risk are summarized in Table 1. Men who farmed (Cantor *et al.*, 1992; Richardson *et al.* 2008) were at greater risk of developing NHL. Farming and the use of phenoxyacetic acid herbicides, such as 2,4-D were associated with NHL risk (Blair & Zahm, 1991). The herbicide 2,4-D is used to kill broadleaf weeds in farm fields and lawns. Farming and the use of dieldrin, toxaphene, lindane, atrazine and fungicides were associated with an increased risk of t(14;18)-positive NHL (Schroeder *et al.*, 2001). NHL risk was increased in Spanish farmers working exclusively as crop or animal farmers and exposed to non-arsenic pesticides and in women who had worked for at least ten years on a farm where pesticides were used (Kato *et al.*, 2004). A Kansas study reported farm herbicide use increased risk of NHL (Hoar *et al.*, 1986) and many pesticides, including atrazine, have been associated with NHL risk (Zahm *et al.*, 1993a). Rusiecki *et al.* (2004) reported an association between NHL and organophosphates, carbamates and chlorinated hydrocarbons but not atrazine. NHL risk was reportedly greater in counties where more than 20% of the wells were contaminated by nitrate (>10 ppm) and in counties with intense fertilizer use (Weisenburger, 1990).

Increased exposure to any pesticide, especially those other than herbicides was associated with NHL risk (Fritschi *et al.*, 2005) and MCPA (4-chloro-2-methyl phenoxyacetic acid) was associated with significant risk (Hardell & Eriksson, 1999) as was the use of organophosphate insecticides coumaphos, diazinon and fonofos, chlordane, dieldrin and copper acetoarsenite, sodium chlorate, glyphosate and atrazine (De Roos *et al.*, 2003). NHL risk in women was associated with personally handling organophosphate and chlorinated hydrocarbon insecticides, especially among those with family history of cancer. NHL risk increased in subjects with lymphatic or hematopoietic cancer among first degree relatives; however no association was found between insecticide or herbicide use on the farm and NHL (Zahm *et al.*, 1993b). A positive association between Hodgkin lymphoma and multiple myeloma and pesticides has been reported but there was no association between NHL and organochlorine, organophosphate, carbamate or triazine pesticides (Orsi *et al.*, 2009).

Elevated nitrate concentrations in drinking water are primarily a direct result of leaching nitrogen-based fertilizer, runoff from feedlots, and sewage. Nitrate in drinking water was associated with increased risk of NHL in Nebraska (Ward *et al.*, 1996) but not in Iowa women

Study	Author (Year)	Risk (Odds Ratio)
NITRATE		
Counties with greater than 20% of wells contaminated with > 10 ppm nitrate	Weisenburger (1990)	2.0
Nitrate in drinking water	Ward *et al.* (1996)	2.0
	Ward *et al.* (2006)	1.2 NA*
	Freedman *et al.* (2000)	NA
	Weyer *et al.* (2001)	NA
PESTICIDES/FARMING		
Ever used pesticide (Livestock insecticides; Crop insecticides; Herbicides; Fungicides)	Cantor *et al.* (1992)	1.2 (1.1; 1.2; 1.3; 1.3)
Farm Herbicides (> 20 days; mixers/applicators)	Hoar *et al.* (1986)	1.6 (6.0; 8.0)
Phenoxyacetic acids	Hardell *et al.* (1981)	4.8
2,4-D (> 20 days per year) **Insecticides** (organophosphates; carbamates; chlorinated hydrocarbons)	Weisenburger (1990)	1.5 (3.3) (1.9; 1.8; 1.4)
Herbicides (phenoxyacetic acids; MCPA) **Fungicides**	Hardell and Eriksson (1999)	1.6 (1.5; 2.7) 3.7
Atrazine	Zahm *et al.* (1993a)	1.2 NA
	Rusiecki *et al.* (2004)	1.61 NA
Insecticides (organophosphates; chlorinated; hydrocarbons) **Dairy Cattle** **Herbicides**	Zahm *et al.* (1993b)	1.3 (4.5; 1.6) 3.0 1.2
Farming; Dieldrin; Toxaphene; Lindane; Atrazine; Fungicides	Schroeder *et al.* (2001)	1.4; 3.7; 3.0; 2.3; 1.7; 1.8
Non-arsenic pesticides; Farming	Balen *et al.* (2006)	1.8; NA
Animal Insecticides; Crop insecticides; Herbicides; Fumigants	Chiu *et al.* (2006)	2.6; 3.0; 2.9; 5.0
Pesticides (family history)	Chiu *et al.* (2004)	NA
Organochlorine pesticides	Cocco *et al.* (2008)	NA
Pesticide use and farming	Kato *et al.* (2004)	2.12
Asthma and pesticide exposure (crop insecticides; chlordane; lindane; fonofos)	Lee *et al.* (2004) (Lee *et al.* 2006 confirmed results)	1.0 NA (1.8; 2.7; 2.4; 3.7)
Pesticides (organochlorine and organophosphate insecticides; carbamate fungicides and triazine herbicides)	Orsi *et al.* (2009)	NA
Any pesticide	Fritschi *et al.* (2005)	3.09

Organophosphate insecticides, coumaphos, diazinon and fonofos, chlordane, dieldrin, copper acetoarsenite, atrazine, glyphosate and sodium chlorate	De Roos *et al.* (2003)	≥1.3
FARMING OCCUPATION		
Agricultural workers; Farmers	Richardson *et al.* (2008)	2.46; 1.98
Farming	Bofetta and de Vocht (2007)	1.11
Cattle; Pigs	Tranah *et al.* (2008)	1.6; 1.8
Agricultural workers (crops)	Zheng *et al.* (2002)	1.6 (1.9)

*NA-no association

Nitrite-plus-nitrate concentrations are based on elemental nitrogen and in this paper are referred to as "nitrate" because the nitrite contribution is negligible in groundwater.

Table 1: Epidemiological studies evaluating agricultural exposures and risk of NHL.

(Weyer *et al.*, 2001), or in a Minnesota case control study (Freedman *et al.*, 2000). The discrepancy in these findings suggests that methodology to determine exposure differs between studies or the exposure data may be unreliable.

2.2   Nitrosamine Exposure and Carcinogenesis

Drinking nitrate-contaminated water has been associated with many types of cancer (Gulis *et al.*, 2002) including NHL (Ward *et al.*, 1996) and it is hypothesized that this is due to carcinogenic nitrosamine formation *in vivo*. When the nitrate concentration in drinking water is low, the primary source of nitrate intake is from vegetables although many vegetables contain ascorbic acid or other inhibitors of endogenous nitrosation. However, endogenous formation of nitrosamines may increase when drinking water containing nitrate (Mirvish, 1986). Endogenous exposure is estimated to account for 45-75% of the total exposure to *N*-nitroso compounds (Tricker, 1997). Nitrosamines form a large group of chemical carcinogens that occur in the environment and are formed in mammalian systems. Over 300 *N*-nitroso compounds are reportedly carcinogenic to one or more animal species (Pruessman & Stewart, 1984). Organ specificity is dependent on the chemical structure of the nitrosamine (Magee, 1989). Chronic nitrosamine administration has been shown to be more effective in tumor induction than administration of one large dose. The size of the molecule can influence the type of tumor and aliphatic nitrosamines behave differently than cyclic nitrosamines in tumorigenesis (Lijinsky, 1977). *In vivo* formation of nitrosamines can be catalyzed by acidic conditions, via bacterial nitrosation or nitric oxide formation due to an inflammatory process (Krull *et al.*, 1980; Cova *et al.*, 1993, 1996; Mirvish, 1995). NNAT readily forms in aqueous solution at pH 2-4, comparable to that of the human stomach, and in soil at pH 5 or below (Wei *et al.*, 2011).

Although the mechanism of action for NNAT is not known, the pathway most frequently attributed to nitrosamine toxicity requires metabolic activation by the cytochrome P450 (CYP450) enzymes, most commonly CYP450 2E1. In this reaction, an intermediate radical is generated and subsequently hydroxylated at the alpha carbon to produce a hydroxyalkyl nitrosamine (Figure 1). These α-hydroxy derivatives lose aldehydes to form alkylnitrosamines and aldehydes. Alkylnitrosamines are unstable and can decompose to an alkyldiazonium ion, an aggressive alkylating agent of DNA bases, especially N-7 and O-6 of guanine and O-4 of thymine. Initiation of cancer is thought to occur when the O-6-alkylguanine pairs with thymine rather than cytosine, producing G:C-A:T mutations (Mirvish, 1975; Mirvish, 1995; Liteplo and Meek, 2002).

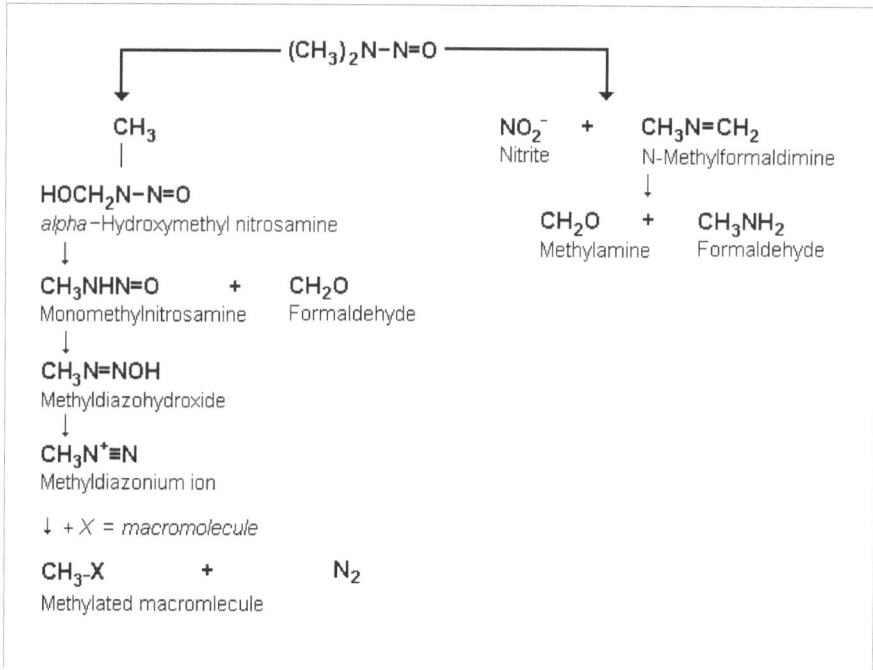

Figure 1: Activation and decomposition of nitrosamines by Cytochrome P450 enzymes (Liteplo & Meek, 2002).

Many nitrosamines will denitrosate with time, exposure to light or under acidic conditions (pH < 2.5). The atrazine molecule has two sites available for nitrosation (Figure 2a) to produce mono-NNAT and di-NNAT. Nitrosation is most favorable at the *N*-ethyl moiety because weakly basic amine groups are nitrosated more easily and the *N*-ethyl moiety is a weaker base than the *N*-isopropyl (Mirvish *et al.*, 1991). Di-NNAT is unstable, rapidly degrading to mono-NNAT and finally atrazine. In this chapter, NNAT refers to mono-NNAT (the NO group is located at the ethylamine moiety of the atrazine molecule). NNAT is quite stable in water at pH greater than 4 with no degradation observed after several weeks (Wolfe *et al.*, 1976; Mirvish *et al.*, 1991).

Nitrosation is influenced by pH and depends on the relative concentrations of substrates, catalysts and inhibitors. Endogenously, nitrate is reduced to nitrite which is converted to nitrous acid (HNO_2) under acidic conditions. Nitrous acid is then converted to an active nitrosating agent such as dinitrogen trioxide (N_2O_3), nitrosyl thiocyanate (ON-NCS), nitrosyl halide (NOX), or nitrous acidium ion ($H_2NO_2^+$) (Mirvish, 1975). Nitrosation by bacteria occurs at neutral pH and is most likely to take place in the achlorhydric stomach. Chronic use of antacids may contribute to nitrosation if pH in the stomach increases after taking these medications.

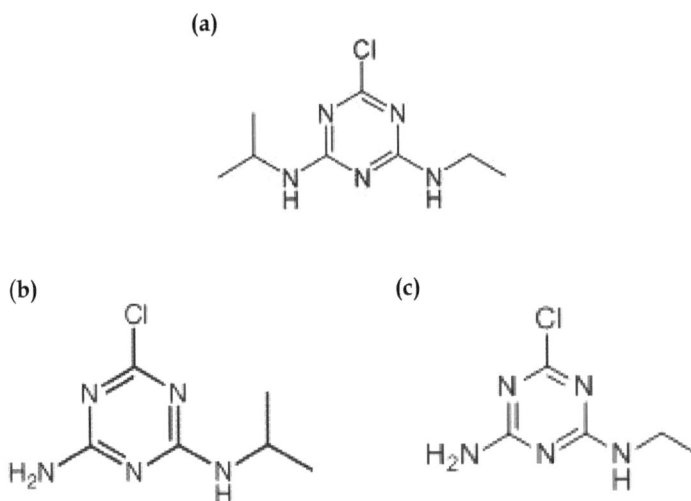

Figure 2: Atrazine (a), deethylatrazine (b), and deisopropylatrazine (c).

Nitrite is a precursor for the formation of nitrosamines in the stomach. Gastric nitrite is a result of nitrate intake followed by absorption in the digestive system. Approximately 5% of total nitrate intake is secreted in the saliva where it is reduced to nitrite and then swallowed (Spiegelhalder *et al.*, 1976; Tannenbaum *et al.*, 1976). This might partially account for the observation that age is associated with NHL risk since salivary nitrate/nitrite is increased in older people, especially men (Mirvish *et al.*, 2000). Nebraskans with high concentrations of nitrate in their drinking water had increased salivary nitrate and nitrite concentrations (Mirvish *et al.* 1992). Nitric oxide synthase (NOS) enzymes regulate nitric oxide (NO) concentration in cells. When the ω-nitrogen of arginine is oxidized, NO is released. Dissolved oxygen reacts with NO to produce N_2O_3 and N_2O_4. During inflammation, NO production increases and NO is oxidized to nitrite and then nitrate. This results in increased salivary nitrate which increases nitrite concentrations in the stomach and the potential for formation of *N*-nitroso compounds during digestion (Mirvish, 1975). A 4:1 ratio of nitrite:secondary amine is required for nitrosation to occur (Mirvish *et al.*, 1991). Drinking water supplies containing both nitrate and atrazine typically have nitrate concentrations 100 – 1000 times higher than atrazine. It is biologically plausible for NNAT to form in the acidic environment of the stomach, enter the bloodstream and denitrosate, increasing cellular NO which would alter the activation/inhibition of NOSs.

2.3 *N*-Nitrosoatrazine Toxicity

Exposing human lymphocyte cultures to 0.1 *u*g NNAT/L resulted in significant increases in chromosome breakage, as well as an increase in the mitotic index. This is a 1,000- to 10,0000-fold smaller concentration than nitrate, nitrite, and/or atrazine producing comparable damage (Meisner *et al.*, 1993). If NNAT enters the blood stream after formation in the stomach, it may be mitogenic and a strong correlation exists between mitogenesis, mutagenesis and carcinogenesis (Ames & Gold, 1990). In our laboratory (Joshi *et al.*, 2013) NNAT produced embryotoxicity in chicken embryos, suggesting that NNAT is genotoxic. In a mammalian urine study, rats excreted approximately 37% of atrazine administered but only about 2% of the NNAT administered (Meli *et al.*, 1992), suggesting metabolism differs between atrazine and NNAT. In the Ames assay, NNAT was weakly mutagenic but NNAT was a potent mutagen in the Chinese hamster V-79 assay (Weisenburger *et al.*, 1987). In Swiss mice and Wistar rats, carcinogenicity tests for NNAT were negative (Weisenburger *et al.*, 1990).

3   Nitrate and Atrazine in Nebraska's Drinking Water: Regulation, Monitoring, and the Use of Historical Water Quality Data in Epidemiological Studies

Nebraska's most precious natural resource is groundwater and, largely due to the High Plains Aquifer, has more groundwater than any other state in the country (NNRD, 2004). Trends in water quality data over several decades show pesticide and nitrate contamination is threatening Nebraska's drinking water supply (NNRD, 2004). Pesticide and/or nitrate exposure from drinking water has been associated with increased risk for developing several cancer types, especially NHL. Associating diseases such as cancer, many of which have long latency periods, to environmental exposures using historical data, such as drinking water data, is difficult. Quantifying subject-specific exposure is challenging when the subject's source of domestic drinking water exists as a connection in a complex public water supply infrastructure. Historically, epidemiology studies have collected substantial data, but when calculating exposure may not have accounted for such variables as the subject's residential contribution from water sources (wells) with different contaminant concentrations within each public water system (PWS) (Ward *et al.*, 2005).

The U.S. Public Health Service (1962) issued an advisory statement warning that nitrate (NO_3-N) concentrations greater than 10 mg/L could result in methemoglobinemia in infants under six months of age (Comley, 1945). Nitrite-plus-nitrate concentrations are based on elemental nitrogen and in this report are referred to as "nitrate" because the nitrite contribution is negligible in groundwater. The Safe Drinking Water Act (SDWA) was established in 1974 to protect public health by regulating the nation's public drinking water supply. This law requires the Environmental Protection Agency (EPA) to determine what concentrations of contaminants in drinking water are safe and to develop maximum contaminant level (MCL) goals. These are unenforceable goals based on potential health risks and lifetime exposure. The Phase II rule (regulation of nitrate) became effective in 1992, making the MCL of 10 mg/L for nitrate an enforceable standard for public drinking water in the U.S.

Compulsory nitrate monitoring began for municipalities and other public water suppliers (PWSs) in 1974 when the SDWA went into effect. Monitoring for nitrate is performed annually unless the concentration is ≥ 5 mg/L. If ≥ 5 mg/L, monitoring must be performed quarterly until the concentration drops below 5 mg/L. Amendments were made to the law in 1986 and 1996. Monitoring for metals and synthetic organic compounds (SOCs), which includes pesticides, was part of the 1986 amendments. SOC monitoring is required every three years. If an SOC is detected, the point of entry (POE) into the system must be monitored quarterly for at least a year. If concentrations remain below the MCL over that year, the POE will be placed on annual monitoring as long as detections occur and are below the MCL. An MCL of 3 μg/L for atrazine was promulgated by the EPA in 1992 (USEPA). Sample collection from the distribution system may not be representative of all services connected to the PWS and since 1993 monitoring has been performed at the POE for atrazine and nitrate. Monitoring is not required for domestic water supplies because private wells are not regulated by the SDWA.

3.1 Nitrate in Nebraska Groundwater

Increasing concentrations of nitrate in groundwater have heightened concern about nitrate in drinking water and is likely to continue to be a significant issue to communities. Groundwater is the source of drinking water for more than half of the U.S. population (Solley *et al.*, 1993) and the sole source in many areas. No state is immune to nitrate contamination of groundwater, but vulnerability to and extent of contamination varies. Several United States Geological Survey (USGS) researchers indicate a nitrate concentration greater than 2-3 mg/L is indicative of contamination by human activity (Bachman, 1984; Panno *et al.*, 1997; Nolan & Stoner, 2000). Major nonpoint nitrate contamination occurs in intensely farmed areas of the U.S., including the central grain-belt and irrigated agricultural regions of California and Texas. Point sources of groundwater nitrate occur in the northern states, where intensive livestock operations are interspersed with relatively dense rural populations (Hallberg, 1989) and where commercial fertilizers are applied to rangeland, lawns, and golf courses (Tinker, 1991; Puckett, 1994) or where animal and human manure is spread, injected, or spray irrigated onto crop or range land (Nolan *et al.*, 1997). Additional point sources of groundwater nitrate include septic systems, leaking sewers, spills at fertilizer distribution sites and manufacturing plants, explosives used in mining operations, munitions, and animal waste lagoons. In Nebraska, extensive cropland has had an adverse impact on nitrate concentrations in groundwater with the overriding source of contamination identified as leaching of commercial fertilizer (Gormly & Spalding 1979; Exner & Spalding 1994), exacerbated by irrigation (Spalding & Exner, 1993). The more than 202,000 contiguous hectares underlain by nitrate-contaminated groundwater in the Central Platte region are the largest areal expanse of nitrate-contaminated groundwater in Nebraska (Figure 3), where concentrations doubled between 1974 and 1984 (Exner *et al.*, 2010, Exner *et al.*, 2014).

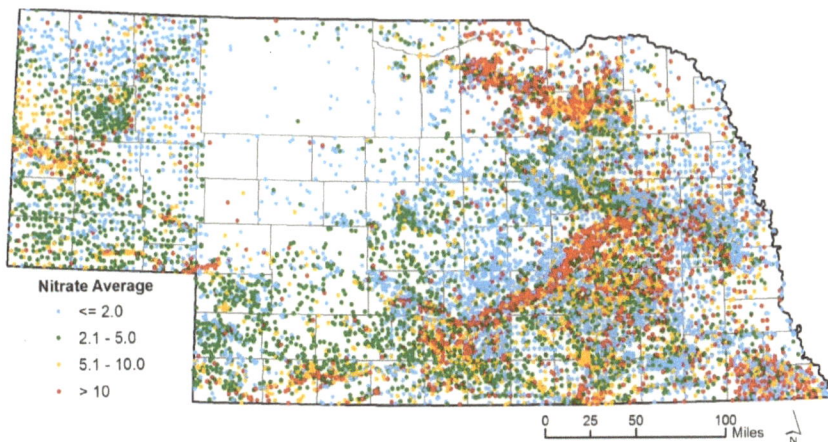

Figure 3. Average nitrate concentrations (mg/L) in wells sampled 1978-1998 (Source: Quality-Assessed Agrichemical Contaminant Database for Nebraska Groundwater-UNL. Website: http://dnrdata.dnr.ne.gov/clearninghouse. Query completed by Les Howard).

Public water supplies must be sampled annually for nitrate. A public water system (PWS) is defined as a system that supplies drinking water to 25 or more people or supplies 15 or more service connections for more than 60 days each year. There are three types of public water systems (Figure 4). Community water systems have a minimum of 15 service connections which are used by year-round residents of the area served by the system or regularly serve at least 25 year-round residents. Included in community water systems are mobile home parks, rural water districts, sanitary improvement districts and municipalities. Non-transient, non-community water systems regularly serve at least 25 of the same individuals over six months of the year. Examples include a business or small school with its own well. Transient non-community water systems are smaller than non-transient, non-community systems and do not regularly serve at least 25 of the same persons over six months per year. A highway café having its own well and restrooms in state parks and interstate rest areas are examples of transient non-community water systems (NHHS, 2007). The case-control study described later in this chapter includes only community water systems. The distribution of participants among these community water systems is shown in Table 2.

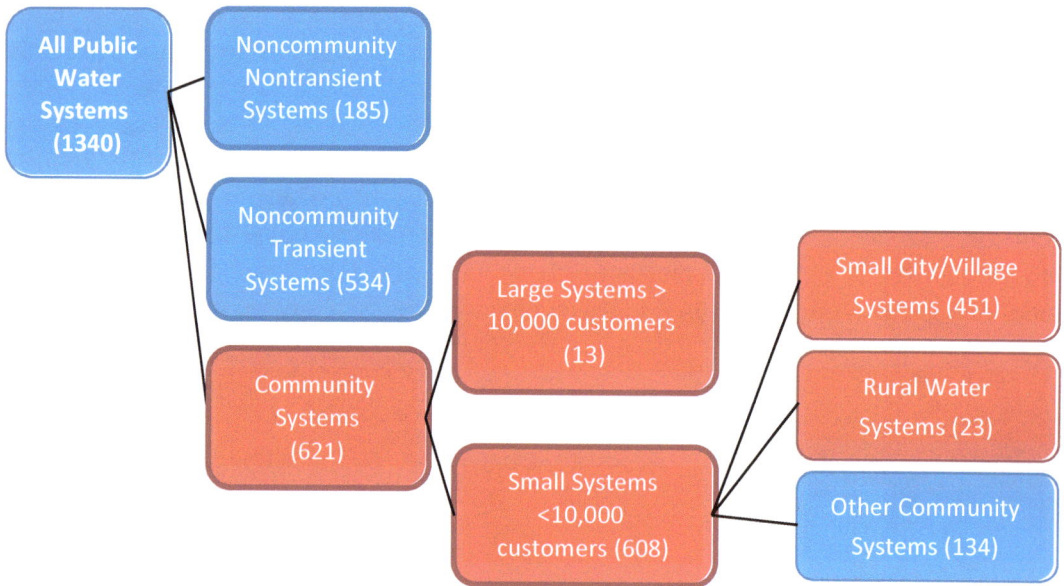

Figure 4: Public water systems in Nebraska (NHHS, 2007).

	Cases	Controls
Public Water System	134 (96%)	180 (94%)
Small system (<10,000)	47 (33%)	45 (23%)
Large system (≥10,000)	87 (62%)	128 (67%)
Rural Water System	1 (<1%)	7 (4%)
Bottled Water	4 (3%)	7 (4%)
Purified Water	2 (1%)	4 (2%)
Total	141 (100%)	191 (100%)

Table 2: Reported drinking water source among cases and controls (1978-1998).

Public supply well sampling requirements are based on contaminant concentration. These requirements give rise to municipal data describing the quantity of groundwater contaminant data available for this study. If the concentration is greater than 5 mg/L, the PWS must sample quarterly. If a PWS has a concentration greater than 10 mg/L, a confirmation sample is taken and the average of the two analyses calculated. If the average is greater than 10.5 mg/L a nitrate violation is issued (NHHS, 2007). Consequently, PWSs with nitrate concentrations ≤ 5 mg/L have less data.

In 1980, a Nebraska Department of Health and Human Services assessment of 451 community water systems found 18 systems exceeded the MCL for nitrate. The Nebraska Department of Environmental Quality (NDEQ) reported in 2003 that 152 of 570 groundwater-based community water systems were required to perform quarterly sampling for nitrate (NDEQ, 2003). Of 83 communities requesting technical assistance through the NDEQ's Nebraska Mandates Management Initiative between May 1995 and January 1998, more than half identified nitrate as a significant issue. Between January 1981 and February 1998, 16 of these communities had received an administrative order (AO) to take action on a nitrate problem. Nitrate problems accounted for nearly half (34/69) of the water quality AOs issued by NHHS from 1991 through 1997. The 2009 record showed 40 AOs issued for nitrate since 1991. Of these, 36 PWSs qualified for our case-control study (Figure 5). There were 19 active AOs in 2004 and 14 at the end of 2009, indicating that the problem is not worsening, probably due to better agricultural management practices and municipalities taking steps to avoid nitrate contamination in their wells (NHHS, 2009).

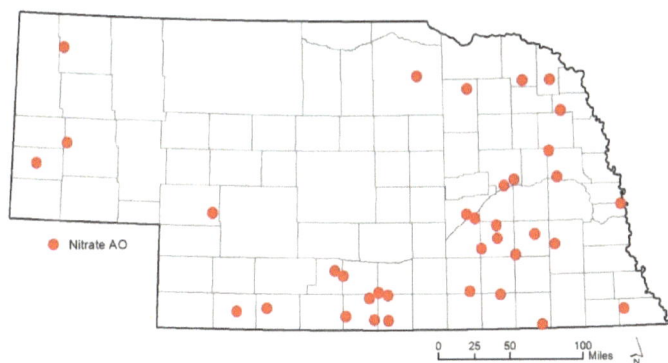

Figure 5: Administrative orders issued to community water systems 1991-2009 (NHHS, 2009).

3.2   Atrazine in Nebraska Groundwater

Nebraska is a chiefly agricultural state which has grown in production of corn and soybeans over the past 50 years, leading to more irrigation and agrichemical application. In addition to nitrate, pesticides are leaching into PWSs. With advancements in analytical capabilities over the past 20-30 years, pesticides and their degradation products are now detectable at nanogram per liter or lower concentrations. Some pesticides are persistent in groundwater and degradation products can remain in groundwater for extended periods. Examples include the atrazine degradation products, deethylatrazine (DEA) (Figure 2b) and deisopropylatrazine (DIA) (Figure 2c).

Atrazine is the most commonly detected pesticide in Nebraska groundwater (Figure 6), consistent with its usage and relatively high mobility (Spalding *et al.*, 1980, 2003). In a 1997 Nebraska study, Gosselin and associates (1997) reported that atrazine was the most commonly detected pesticide in 70 domestic wells with detectable pesticide concentrations. If concentrations of DEA and DIA, both of which are nitrosatable, are included, total atrazine residues in groundwater may be 2-5 times the concentration of atrazine alone (Ribaudo and Bousahaer, 1994; Spalding *et al.*, 2003). Calculating the ratio of DIA + DEA to atrazine from the Clearinghouse (UNL, 2000) Management Systems Evaluation Area data 1991-1997, the total atrazine residue is 2.1 times that of atrazine. Atrazine and DEA were detected in 99.9% and 100%, respectively, of 7,848 samples from the unconfined aquifer beneath a 54-hectare (2.47 acre) research demonstration site in the Central Platte Valley of Nebraska, while DIA was detected in 86.4% of the samples (Spalding *et al.*, 2003). Atrazine concentrations were at or above their reporting limit in all samples but remained below the 3 µg L^{-1} MCL set by the EPA (USEPA). Spalding *et al.* (2003) also reported that during the five-year investigation period, atrazine and DEA concentrations remained relatively constant in older, deeper groundwater (>7 years old and >6 meters below the water table).

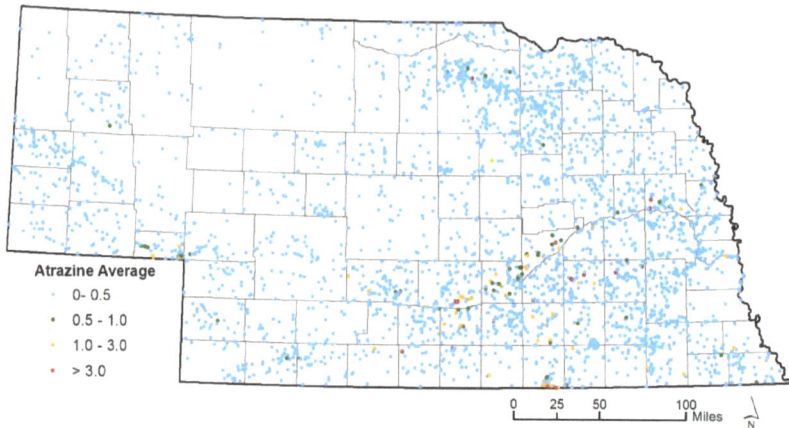

Figure 6. Average atrazine concentrations (µg/L) in wells sampled 1978-1998 (Source: Quality-Assessed Agrichemical Contaminant Database for Nebraska Groundwater-UNL. Website: http://dnrdata.dnr.ne.gov/clearinghouse. Query completed by Les Howard).

Initially, when atrazine was commercially available to producers in the early 1960s, application rates in Nebraska averaged 1.35 pounds (lb) active ingredient/acre, peaked at 1.48 lb/acre in 1980 and by 1993 was 1.09 lb/acre. Between 1952 and 1976, corn acreage treated with herbicides increased from 11% to 90%. The major increase occurred between 1971 and 1976 and required a 68% increase in state-wide atrazine application (Farm and Ranch Irrigation Survey, 2003). In 1982, of the 49 million acres within Nebraska, approximately 7.4 million acres were planted to corn with 5.9 million acres (79%) treated with atrazine at 1.88 lb/acre. Sorghum was planted on 1.86 million acres and atrazine was applied to 1.3 million acres (72%) at 1.43 lb/acre (Johnson & Kamble, 1984). In 1992, application rates averaged 1.06 lb/acre and 1.02 lb/acre in 2003 (NASS). Irrigated land in Nebraska has risen from 3.3 million acres in 1967 to 8.6 million acres in 2007. Forty years ago, just a little over 40% of all corn harvested was irrigated compared to 67% in 2007 (NASS 1969-2007). Most irrigation wells are not metered but estimates were made of water applied for irrigation purposes. Of the 7.4 million acres of corn planted in Nebraska in 1982, 5 million acres were irrigated at rates higher than the U.S. average of 1.8 acre feet (596,307 gallons per acre). However, in 2003, it was estimated that only 1.12 acre feet of water was applied to irrigated cropland in Nebraska (Farm and Ranch Irrigation Survey, 2003). Spalding and associates (2003) studied the influence of improved water management practices on groundwater pesticide contamination and reported lower atrazine concentrations in groundwater beneath sprinkler irrigated fields than groundwater below fields utilizing furrow irrigation. This was attributed to sprinkler irrigation applying water with much greater uniformity than furrow irrigation, where pooling of water on the soil surface promotes leaching. Atrazine was also reported to enter the groundwater at surface pooling areas on the edge of the field and within the field after heavy spring rains. Mandatory atrazine monitoring of PWS wells began in the early 1990s, but with the application and irrigation trends noted above, it would be reasonable to assume that where leaching occurred before monitoring began, shallow groundwater atrazine concentrations would have been greater (Figure 7). Therefore, the period of highest exposure would fall into the latency period for NHL, believed to be 10-20 years before contracting the disease (Hardell & Eriksson, 1999, 2003). Currently there are 73 PWS wells required to sample annually for the EPA SW-846 525 scan which includes atrazine. No detections have been found that exceed the 3 μg/L MCL. To date, no AOs have been issued for violation of the atrazine MCL.

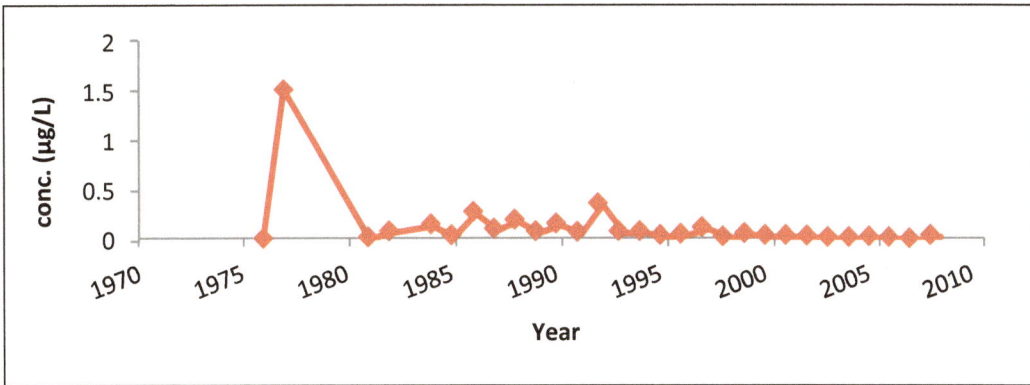

Figure 7. Average atrazine concentrations for Nebraska, 1976-2008 excluding monitoring wells (Source: Quality-Assessed Agrichemical Contaminant Database for Nebraska Groundwater-UNL. Website; http://dnrdata.dnr.ne.gov/clearninghouse Query completed by Colleen Steele).

3.3   Nitrate, Atrazine, non-Hodgkin Lymphoma and Nebraska Drinking Water

In recent years, the incidence of NHL has increased more rapidly in rural areas (Devesa & Fears, 1992; NCI; CDC) and is consistently higher in Nebraska than for the U.S. as a whole. The NHL age-adjusted incidence rate for Nebraska males in 2000 was 22.2 (per 100,000), compared to 21.6 for the U.S. (3% difference) and for Nebraska females was 18.4, compared to 15.4 for the U.S. (18% difference) (USCS, 2003). A 2005 Surveillance, Epidemiology and End Results update reported a 2002 NHL incidence rate of 25.6 in Nebraska males and 22.0 in males in the

U.S., an approximately 15% difference. The incidence for females was 16.3 and 15.5 in Nebraska and the U.S., respectively, after adjusting for age (USCS, 2005).

Individuals exposed to triazine herbicides (such as atrazine) are reportedly at increased risk of NHL (Zahm *et al.*, 1993a) as are those exposed to nitrate in drinking water in Nebraska (Ward *et al.*, 1996). Since these studies were completed, additional relevant data have been collected, better water quality records are maintained, and new data are more well-specific. Rhoades (2010) conducted a study to: replicate earlier findings that exposure to nitrate in drinking water is associated with NHL, evaluate NHL risk in association with exposure to atrazine in drinking water, and evaluate NHL risk associated with the interaction of nitrate and atrazine in drinking water.

The amount of water applied from irrigation coupled with the application of atrazine and the relatively shallow water table under corn-growing areas increases the rate of leaching to groundwater in more susceptible areas of Nebraska. The heavier application rates of water and atrazine during the 1970s and 1980s exacerbated contaminant leaching and increased risk of exposure to nitrate- and atrazine-contaminated drinking water in Nebraska. This coincides with this study's expected latency period of NHL, from 1970 to 1989. Epidemiologic evidence showing a link between nitrate concentrations in drinking water and NHL has been inconsistent (Ward *et al.*, 1996, 2006), and literature documenting the possible association of NHL incidence with drinking water contaminated with atrazine or both nitrate and atrazine is limited. With the recent push for more continuous corn farming to accommodate demand for food and biofuel production, coupled with EPA consideration of revising the MCL, it is timely to revisit and analyze atrazine and/or nitrate in drinking water as risk factors for NHL.

4   Water Containing Nitrate/Atrazine and Non-Hodgkin Lymphoma Risk in Nebraska, USA: A Bayesian Analysis

With the considerable interest in disease mapping over the past decade, there has been greater use of spatial statistical tools to examine the geographical distribution of disease. Initially, a spatial model was used to examine groundwater atrazine and nitrate concentration in association with NHL incidence in Nebraska (Rhoades, 2010). Standard morbidity ratios (SMRs) were determined for each county, followed by the application of a Bayesian spatial conditional autoregressive (CAR) model to analyze the geographical distribution of NHL in relation to atrazine and nitrate concentration and establish relative risk estimates. One desirable feature of the Bayesian application is that it provides a way to borrow strength (provide soft data to fill in missing data) from the full data set. Bayesian spatial CAR modeling is widely used in the field of disease mapping to generate hypotheses related to disease risk and environmental exposures (Mollie & Richardson, 1991; Cowles *et al.*, 1999; Meza, 2003; Kousa *et al.*, 2004; Molitor *et al.*, 2006). The Bayesian statistical approach reports high density regions (HDR) which are similar to the more commonly used confidence interval (CI) used for frequentist methods. A CI is constructed from random sampling within a population and the HDR indicates the probability that a range of values contains the true mean.

4.1 Methods

NHL cases were identified through the Nebraska Cancer Registry. From January 1, 1990 to December 31, 1998, 2708 cases of NHL were reported in Nebraska. NHL incidence data were combined into one dataset for analysis by county. Three counties (Banner, Grant and McPherson) had no observed cases of NHL during this period.

Atrazine and nitrate data for municipal water systems were obtained from the Nebraska Department of Health and Human Services and from the Quality-Assessed Agrichemical Contaminant Database for Nebraska Groundwater (UNL, 2000) for domestic, monitoring, irrigation, commercial and livestock wells. Nebraska Health and Human Services System collected most of the domestic well data during 1985-1989 using stratified randomized sampling to assess groundwater quality with respect to drinking water quality. Most of the irrigation well data were collected by the Natural Resources Districts (NRDs) as part of their groundwater monitoring program. All 93 Nebraska counties were represented in the 44,297 nitrate and 15,867 atrazine samples reported from 1978 through 1998, capturing water quality data that includes the expected latency period of 10-20 years. Table 3 shows the distribution of analyses by well type. The spatial distribution of the sampled wells is shown in Figure 3 for nitrate and Figure 6 for atrazine.

Well Type	Nitrate	Atrazine
Public	6436	1608
Domestic	8088	3501
Livestock	658	27
Irrigation	15,666	981
Commercial	68	24
Monitoring	13,381	9726
Total	44,297	15,867

Table 3: Nitrate and atrazine water quality analyses by type of well for which samples were obtained.

Because risk for NHL is associated with age and sex, the standardized morbidity ratio (SMR) was used to adjust for differences in age and gender distributions among counties. The SMR, an estimate of relative risk, is the ratio of observed cases (O_i) to expected cases (E_i) within a geographic region (i.e. the odds of being in the disease group rather than in the background group). The SMR used in this analysis accounts for age and gender distribution in the county and the national age-specific incidence rate. An SMR greater than 1 indicates that the age-gender-adjusted incidence rate for that county is higher than for the nation as a whole.

A supraregional rate was used for the expected number of cases because the Nebraska rate was not available. The national age- and gender-specific rates for 1996-2000 from SEER Table XVIII-2 (USCS) for each of 19 age groups (<1, 1-4, 5-9, 10-14, 15-19, 20-24, 25-29, 30-34, 35-39, 40-44, 45-49, 50-54, 55-59, 60-64, 65-69, 70-74, 75-79, 80-84, and 85 and older) were used. This risk profile was utilized to establish a Nebraska SMR for 1990-1998, with the assumption that it would not vary significantly from 1990-1995. Census data from 1990-2000 were used to determine the number of males and females in each age group for each county (SEER). The number of expected cases in each county i (E_i, $i=1, …, 93$) is the product of the number of individuals in each age-gender group (n_{ijk}) and the age-gender specific rate (r_{jk}), summed over all age groups and genders and is given by:

$$E_i = \sum_{k=1}^{2} \sum_{j=1}^{19} n_{ijk} r_{jk},$$

for gender k ($k=1,2$) and age group j ($j=1,...,19$).

The SMR is a commonly used measure of the relative risk of disease, but it has limitations. The variance of the SMR is the inverse of the expected value and thus the variance of the SMR is large for a region in which the expected value is small (i.e., counties with small populations). This can lead to difficulties in interpreting the SMR. For example, an SMR of 1 is obtained when the expected and observed number of cases is each 500 or when they are each 5. In addition, when there are no observed cases in a county, the SMR is 0, regardless of the population size (Meza, 2003). These SMRs are not valid measures and some adjustment should be applied. Due to the difficulties in interpreting the SMR, statistical methods have focused on borrowing information from other geographic areas and/or covariates using empirical Bayes and Bayesian methods which borrow strength from the full data set, thus reducing the variance of the estimates and "shrinking" individual SMR estimates toward the mean SMR for the collection of regions. Estimates from areas with less valid SMRs due to small populations are shrunk more than areas with larger populations (Cowles *et al.*, 1999).

NHL incidence rates vary geographically. Many statistical models that focus on geographically dependent correlations can be extended to examine the covariate associations. A random-effects Poisson model to account for spatial conditional modeling using the intrinsic CAR model of Besag *et al.* (1991) was used to examine the association between groundwater atrazine and nitrate concentrations and the risk of NHL. In this method, the SMRs are smoothed toward the mean of the adjacent neighboring counties. The model is given by:

$$Oi \sim Poisson\ (\mu_i)$$
$$\log(\mu_i) = \log(E_i) + \alpha_0 + \alpha_1 X_1 + \alpha_2 X_2 + b_i$$

where α_0 is the intercept term and represents the baseline log relative risk of disease, X_1 is the covariate representing atrazine concentration (X_2 is the covariate representing nitrate concentration) for county I ($i=1, ...,93$) with regression coefficient α_1 (and α_2), and b_i is an area-specific random effect measuring the unexplained log relative risk of disease in county i.

Two models were examined. First, atrazine and nitrate exposure was modeled by the proportion of sampled wells in the county testing positive. If one or more detections were reported in a well during the time period specified for this study, the well was categorized as positive. Then atrazine and nitrate exposure was modeled using the mean concentration of all the sampled wells in each county. If a well was sampled more than once during the study period, the mean concentration was used. Concentrations below the reporting limit were censored to half the reporting limit. High censored concentrations were excluded because they resulted from point sources or high reporting limits (1.1 µg L^{-1} for atrazine). The reporting limit for nitrate was 0.1 mg/ L^{-1}. For each model, results were compared with and without data from monitoring wells.

The analysis was conducted with WinBUGS (Lawson *et al.*, 2003), which uses Markov chain Monte Carlo techniques (Spiegelhalter *et al.*, 2003). A total of 20,000 iterations with 5,000 burn-ins were used. Posterior joint and marginal distributions of the parameters were used. The variability of the estimates was examined using the highest density regions (HDRs).

4.2   Results

The SMR for Nebraska is 0.93. Crude SMRs were > 1.5 in five counties, between 1.26 and 1.5 in ten counties, 1 to 1.25 in 29 counties, < 1.0 in 49 (about 53%) counties (Figure 8).

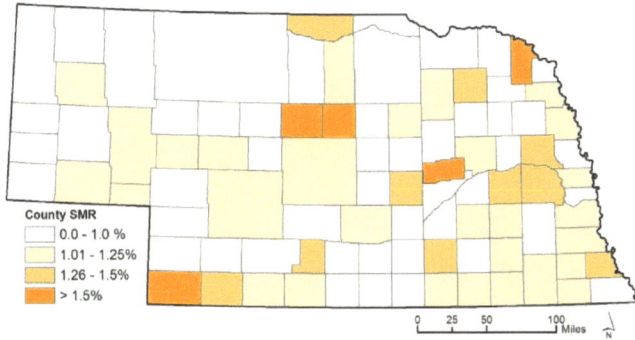

Figure 8: Nebraska standard morbidity ratios by county before adjustment.

Figure 9 displays the smoothed SMRs (CAR model) with atrazine modeled as the mean concentration and monitoring wells excluded. All five counties with SMRs > 1.5 prior to application of CAR had a smoothed SMR <1.0. The posterior mean for α_1 was 2.99 (HDR 0.014-5.80). Nuckolls County had an SMR of 1.27 (SMR 1.15 prior to CAR modeling). Dodge, Douglas and Merrick Counties had SMRs slightly > 1 (Table 4). The results were similar when monitoring wells were included in the model, though the SMR for Nuckolls County was slightly lower at 1.12 and for Merrick County was below 1. In addition to the four counties at risk in the model without monitoring wells, Buffalo, Fillmore and York Counties had SMRs greater than 1. However, when atrazine was modeled as percent positive, atrazine was not associated with risk of NHL.

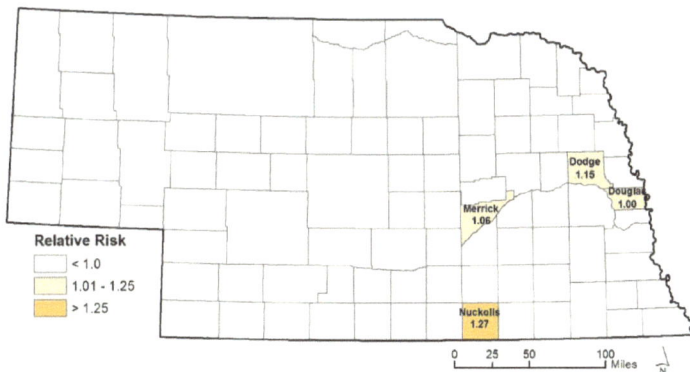

Figure 9: Relative risk of NHL due to mean atrazine concentration without monitoring wells afterconditional autoregression.

County	Crude SMR	Smoothed SMR w/o monitoring wells	Smoothed SMR with monitoring wells
Nuckolls	1.16	1.27	1.12
Dodge	1.27	1.15	1.09
Douglas	1.03	1.00	1.01
Merrick	0.91	1.06	0.99

Table 4: Increased SMRs associated with mean atrazine concentration by county, before and after autoregression, with and without monitoring wells.

Mean nitrate concentration was associated with increased risk of NHL (HDR: -0.018-0.226) both with and without monitoring wells included (Figure 10). When including the mean concentration of nitrate, atrazine was not associated with increased risk (HDR: -0.475-3.18 and -0.098-0.181 for atrazine and nitrate, respectively). Risk of NHL increased slightly when nitrate was modeled as the percent of wells testing positive (excluding monitoring wells) in 11 counties (α_1 0.080; HDR 0.011-0.151) and the results were similar when monitoring wells were included (α_1 0.090; HDR 0.019-0.157) (Figure 11). A comparison between crude and adjusted SMRs, with and without monitoring wells, is summarized in Table 5. When nitrate percent positive was modeled with atrazine percent positive for all wells, there was an association between risk of NHL and percent positive nitrate wells (α_1=0.083; HDR: 0.008-0.149).

4.3   Conclusion

Mortality from NHL increased markedly in the U.S. over the last five decades before leveling off in the last few years and geographic variation in lymphoma rates suggests environmental effects are important (Hartge & Wang, 2004). Some of the areas of high mortality rates are heavily agricultural, suggesting a possible agrichemical effect and/or other farm-related exposure.

This study showed a slight association of risk for NHL due to atrazine in drinking water (SMR 1.27 in Nuckolls County). Some authors indicate that a nitrate concentration greater than background (2-3 mg/L) is indicative of contamination by human activity (Bachman, 1984; Panno *et al.*, 1997; Nolan & Stoner, 2000) and accept these values as background concentrations. SMRs were unchanged when nitrate concentrations less than or equal to 1.5 mg were excluded from the analysis. Excluding data values that were 2 or less would have excluded counties from the study due to concentrations less than 2 mg/L for the entire study period.

Monitoring wells are used to define source area plumes and delineate high concentrations of contaminants. Monitoring wells have much shorter screen lengths than domestic and irrigation wells and therefore draw groundwater from discrete zones that may have elevated concentrations. Excluding monitoring well data from the analysis reduced exposure misclassification due to well type. Conversely, livestock, irrigation and commercial wells could be drinking water sources. In this analysis, inclusion of monitoring wells decreased the SMR.

Evidence from several epidemiologic studies suggests that associations between risk factors and NHL histologic subtypes may be stronger than associations between the same risk factors and NHL in aggregate. In Nuckolls County, there were 17 NHL cases. Of these, two (12%) were unclassified, six (35%) classified as DLBCL, six (35%) as follicular lymphoma and three (18%) as other. When assessing risk of NHL by histological type, Zahm *et al.* (1993a) re

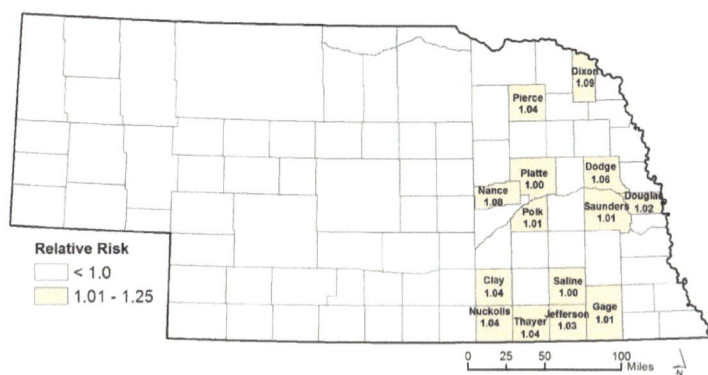

Figure 10: Relative risk of NHL due to mean nitrate concentration for all wells after conditional autoregression.

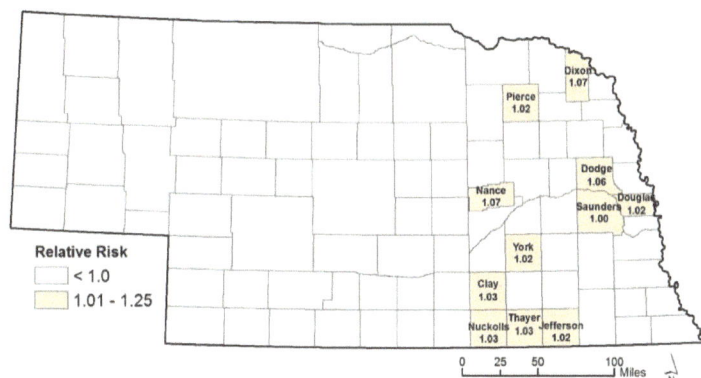

Figure 11. Relative risk of NHL due to percent of nitrate positive wells, excluding monitoring wells, after conditional autoregression.

County	Crude SMR	Smoothed SMR w/o monitoring wells	Smoothed SMR with monitoring wells
Clay	1.38	1.03	1.04
Dixon	1.42	1.07	1.09
Dodge	1.27	1.06	1.06
Douglas	1.03	1.02	1.02
Jefferson	0.95	1.02	1.03
Nance	1.67	1.07	1.08
Nuckolls	1.16	1.03	1.04
Pierce	1.36	1.02	1.04
Saunders	1.17	1.00	1.01
Thayer	1.07	1.03	1.04
York	0.99	1.02	0.91

Table 5: Increased SMRs associated with percent of wells testing positive for nitrate by county, before and after autoregression, with and without monitoring wells.

ported DLBCL to be most strongly associated with atrazine use. We did not include histology in the analysis because it would have decreased sample size and therefore statistical power.

This study did not control for dietary nitrate. Diet in the Midwest is fairly homogeneous and relatively stable across time and community. Dietary intake of red meat and nitrite preserved meat has been shown to be important in the formation of fecal nitroso-compounds, a result of sodium nitrite used as a preservative (Mirvish *et al.*, 2003) and heme has been associated with nitrosation (Cross *et al.*, 2003). Epidemiological studies have reported no association or an inverse association between dietary nitrate and several cancers, including NHL (Ward *et al.*, 1996, 2005; Aschebrook-Kilfoy *et al.*, 2013), probably because many of the nitrate-containing foods are vegetables which also contain nitrosation inhibitors such as vitamin C and other antioxidants. Nitrosamine formation due to nitrate consumption is suggested to be mainly due to drinking water nitrate (Mirvish, 1986).

This spatial analysis suggests an association between atrazine-contaminated drinking water and NHL risk in Nebraska but has limitations. NHL has a latency period of 10-20 years (Hardell & Eriksson, 1999, 2003) and participants may have been non-differentially misclassified by residence and could have been exposed to more or less nitrate/atrazine in their drinking water. Wells were not sampled randomly across the state. Some counties had very few wells sampled relative to area compared with other counties (Figures 3 and 6). Because of the sparse population, there may not be wells in these areas. The number of analyses conducted varied from year to year (Figure 12). Atrazine data from 1970-1988 would provide more accurate groundwater concentrations during the NHL latency period but atrazine data is limited for these years. Finally, not having data for family history of NHL, other routes of exposure to agrichemicals, and other groundwater contaminants are additional limitations.

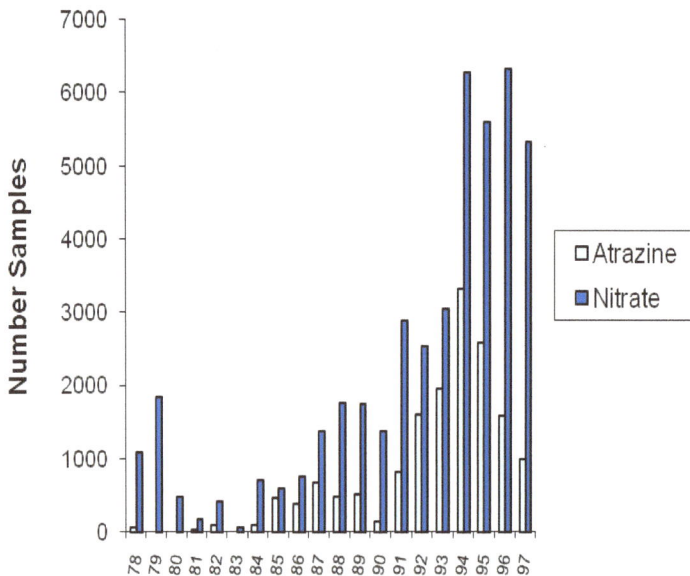

Figure 12: Atrazine and nitrate samples taken annually.

5   Non-Hodgkin Lymphoma Risk and Exposure to Nitrate and Atrazine in Public Drinking Water Supplies in Nebraska: A Case-Control Study

To further investigate the risk of NHL in association with drinking water contaminated with atrazine and nitrate, we conducted a case-control study. Ecological studies such as the one previously discussed are particularly useful for generating hypotheses because they can use existing data sets and rapidly test the hypothesis. However, ecological studies are susceptible to bias because disease incidence and exposure data are analyzed at the level of the group rather than the level of the individual.

Previous studies evaluating NHL risk due to drinking nitrate-contaminated water and pesticide exposure are inconsistent in their findings. Discrepancies may be due to differences in study design, methodology used to determine exposure, analytical techniques, confounding from other drinking water contaminants, uncontrolled confounding from other causes or exposure misclassification. Many study participants consume water from a complex PWS infrastructure. Our Nebraska study (Rhoades, 2010; Rhoades *et al.*, 2013) evaluated the association of NHL and drinking water contaminated with nitrate, atrazine and the combination of atrazine and nitrate after estimating each subject's residential contribution from water sources (wells), with different contaminant concentrations within each PWS.

Based on the pathways of nitrosamine formation, metabolism and subsequent carcinogenicity, we hypothesized that exposure to both atrazine and nitrate in drinking water would increase risk of NHL. Associations between risk factors and NHL histological subtypes are reportedly stronger than associations between the same risk factors and NHL in aggregate (Vose *et al.*, 2002). Therefore, we further hypothesized that differences would be observed based on NHL subtype (aggressive B-cell, indolent B-cell and T-cell). The aims of this case-control study were to estimate each subject's exposure to atrazine and nitrate from municipal wells that directly contribute to a subject's exposure from his/her drinking water supply, evaluate the association between NHL and drinking water contaminated with atrazine and/or nitrate and, assess the association of exposure to nitrate- and/or atrazine-contaminated drinking water by NHL subtype.

5.1   Methods

The sample of participants for this analysis was selected from a population-based sample of 389 NHL cases and 535 controls recruited between January, 1999 and December, 2002 (Chiu *et al.*, 2005, 2007a,b). Cases were identified using a rapid-reporting system through the Nebraska Lymphoma Registry and Tissue Bank. Controls were identified by two-stage random-digit dialing. Cases and controls were residents in one of 66 counties in eastern Nebraska. Eligibility criteria are described elsewhere (Rhoades, 2010). All tumor cases were classified according to the NHL classification system of the World Health Organization (Mauch *et al.*, 2004).

Information on basic demographics, tobacco use and family history of cancer was obtained as well as city and state of residence between 1970 and the interview date, the number of years lived at each residence, and past sources of drinking water (Chiu *et al.*, 2005; Rhoades, 2010). Exact addresses were collected for the most recent residence but previous residences included only city and state. To identify the associated water source(s) it was imperative that the exact location of all residences be known. From the original study, a subgroup of partici-pants was included in the analysis. This subgroup included those subjects who reported one residence between 1978 and recruitment. Tumor classes were categorized as aggressive B-cell lymphoma, indolent B-cell lymphoma and T-cell lymphoma. The protocol for use of human subjects in this research was approved by the Institutional Review Board at the University of Nebraska Medical Center (IRB# 318-05-EP).

For each PWS represented in this study, the manager was contacted to confirm that the address of interest was connected to the PWS during the time period of interest. The 59 partic-ipants listing private well as their water supply were excluded for lack of well water quality data. Private wells are not subject to mandatory testing under the SDWA. Eligible to partici-pate in this study were 140 cases and 192 controls, representing 98 PWSs.

Archived records of nitrate and pesticide concentrations were obtained from the Ne-braska Department of Health and Human Services and PWS managers. Data included the date the well went into service, annual well production during the time period of interest, contami-nant concentrations and geographical location of residence respective to the well(s) or storage reservoir of interest for 1967 through 1998. Not all wells contribute an equal amount of water to the PWS. Pumping volumes for PWS wells are calculated and reported annually. From the-se data, we calculated yearly exposure concentrations for each contaminant for each study subject. For each subject, total annual production of each well contributing to the subject's res-idence was multiplied by the average contaminant concentration for that well and then weighted based on the percentage of that well's contribution relative to the total contribution of all wells pumping into the distribution system for the residence of interest. These annual exposure concentrations were then averaged to give a final exposure concentration of each contaminant for each participant (Rhoades, 2010). For those listing purified or bottled water as water supply, concentrations were entered as 0, as were PWS values reported as "no detect" or "<MDL" (less than method detection limit). All nitrate and pesticide analyses were performed at the State of Nebraska Department of Public Health Environmental Laboratory in Lincoln. The analytical method used for the majority of pesticide analyses was USEPA 525 (GC-MS) and nitrate was analyzed using automated cadmium reduction. MDLs are determined on an annual basis. Reporting limits are determined from MDLs and are 3-5 times greater than the MDL. We elected not to use censored data because reporting limits varied slightly from year to year. Therefore the use of 0 for nondetects simplified the methodology.

Atrazine and nitrate were the primary contaminants of interest. To eliminate confound-ing from exposure to other pesticides in drinking water we also obtained information on methoxychlor, 2,4-D, simazine and alachlor. As previously noted, based on groundwater mon-itoring reports and research conducted in Nebraska evaluating atrazine application and irriga-tion trends, an assumption was made that the period of greatest exposure would occur during the latency period for NHL, believed to be 10-20 years before contracting the disease (Spalding et al., 1980, Spalding et al., 2003, Rhoades, 2010). If this assumption results in misclassification, it would likely underestimate exposure and bias the study toward the null hypothesis that there is no association between NHL risk and exposure to nitrate and atrazine in drinking wa-ter.

To estimate "lifetime exposure dose" for each subject, data generated from a 1989 report was used to estimate total tap water intake based on age and gender (Ershow & Cantor, 1989). The average yearly contaminant exposure for each participant was then multiplied by their total tap water intake and the yearly exposures summed for a lifetime dose.

The primary outcomes of interest were all NHL cases and three subtypes of NHL: aggressive B-cell (mantle cell, diffuse large cell, Burkett, other B-cell and other), indolent B-cell (chronic lymphocytic/small lymphocytic, marginal zone and follicular), and T-cell (peripheral T-cell and other T-cell). Covariates assessed included adult body mass index (BMI), years of education, gender, ethnicity, family history of cancer, age, marital status, smoking history and water supply. Six participants in the subgroup and 43 participants in the original study group reported their drinking water source as "other" which we were able to classify as PWS or bottled water. Agrichemical covariates assessed were methoxychlor, 2,4-D, simazine, alachlor, nitrate and atrazine. The agrichemicals were evaluated initially as individual compounds and then as mixtures. Analyses were conducted using SPSS (Statistical Package for Social Sciences version 17.0, IBM, Chicago, IL). Because we were analyzing a subset of the original sample, we examined whether restricting the analysis to those with only one residence might have selected for those at greater risk of NHL. Descriptive statistics were used to summarize participant characteristics. Covariates and exposures to nitrate, atrazine, methoxychlor, 2,4-D, simazine and alachlor in cases and controls were compared using the odds ratio (OR) and 95% confidence intervals (CI) from univariate logistic regression models. Multivariable logistic regression was conducted and covariates identified in the univariate analysis shown to be associated with case-control status and associated with the contaminant of interest were used to adjust the logistic regression model. For pesticides, exposed was defined as the pesticide ever being detected in the drinking water supply at a concentration above the MDL. For nitrate, participants were dichotomized as either exposed to ≤2 mg nitrate/L or >2 mg/L. Multivariable models were then reduced using manual backward regression. To test the interaction of atrazine and nitrate in drinking water in association with increased risk of NHL, the effects of atrazine, nitrate and the interaction of atrazine and nitrate were calculated using multivariable logistic regression. Adjusted ORs and CIs were calculated maintaining only those confounders and interaction terms with a two-sided p-value ≤ 0.05.

5.2   Results

Subgroup cases and controls tend to be older than original study participants (Rhoades *et al.*, 2013). Participants in the original study group were slightly more educated than the subgroup. There was no association between the number of residences and disease status, water supply, gender, race or marital status. The subgroup included 78 controls and 101 cases reporting a family history of cancer. In the univariate analysis, family history of cancer was not associated with increased risk of developing NHL and risk of NHL was not associated with BMI, smoking history or education. There was no association between NHL risk and nitrate or atrazine and no increased risk of developing NHL associated with methoxychlor, 2,4-D, simazine, or alachlor exposure (Rhoades *et al.*, 2013).

Thirty-six percent of Nebraska's population resides in the two major cities, Lincoln and Omaha, and in this analysis 51% (n=163) of participants listed Omaha or Lincoln as their city of residence. To ensure that our results were not biased towards residing in these cities we excluded participants from Lincoln and Omaha and repeated the analysis. NHL risk associated with nitrate exposure was unchanged. The same sample showed risk of NHL in those exposed to atrazine as slightly elevated (OR, 1.3; CI, 0.9-1.9) but not significantly (p=0.20).

Multivariable logistic regression showed the relationship between the log odds and atrazine increased by 0.916 (SE=0.48) when nitrate exposure was greater than 2 mg/L as opposed to nitrate exposure of 2 mg/L or less. After transforming into odds, our statistical model resulted in the odds of developing NHL to be 2.9 times greater when subjects were exposed to both nitrate- and atrazine-contaminated drinking water (OR, 2.9; CI, 1.1-7.4) (p=0.025) compared to only atrazine or nitrate being present. After adjusting for age by adding age as an additional continuous independent variable in the model, the risk of developing NHL remained elevated (OR, 2.5; CI, 1.0-6.2) (p=0.047) (Table 6).

	No. of Controls*	No. of Cases†	Univariate OR (95% CI)	Multivariable OR (95% CI)
Nitrate	**192**	**140**		
Never	135	102	1.0*	1.0 referent
Ever	57	38	0.9 (0.5-1.4)	0.6 (0.3-1.1)
Atrazine	**190**	**138**		
Never	93	58	1.0*	1.0 referent
Ever	97	80	1.2 (0.8-1.7)	1.0(0.7-1.4)
Atrazine+Nitrate	**190**	**138**		
Never	174	120		
Ever				
NHL in aggregate	16	18		2.5 (1.0-6.2)
Indolent B-cell NHL	16	7		3.5 (1.0-11.6)
Aggressive B-cell NHL	16	11		1.9 (0.6-5.6)

*Controls may not sum to 192 due to missing data
†Cases may not sum to 140 due to missing data

Table 6: Age adjusted odds ratios (ORs) and 95% confidence intervals (CI) from univariate and multivariable main effects and interaction models of nitrate, atrazine, and the interaction of nitrate and atrazine in assessing risk for NHL in Nebraska.

We investigated the association of nitrate and atrazine with risk of NHL by subtype. After adjusting for age, the risk of indolent B-cell lymphoma (n=64) was significantly greater (OR, 3.5; CI, 1.0-11.6) (p=0.04) for those exposed to drinking water containing both nitrate and atrazine than those not exposed. There was also an elevated, but nonsignificant risk (OR, 1.9; CI, 0.6-5.6, p=0.26) for aggressive B-cell lymphoma (n=68). Analysis by subtype strongly suggests that those exposed to nitrate- and atrazine-contaminated drinking water may be at greater risk for indolent B-cell lymphoma than aggressive B-cell lymphoma. The number of T-cell lymphoma cases was small (n=8) and therefore not included in this analysis.

Approximately 30% of controls and 27% of cases were exposed to average nitrate concentrations greater than 2 mg/L but did not show an association with increased risk of NHL in the univariate analysis. Similarly, no associated risk of NHL was found when cutoff values were lowered to 1 mg/L or 0 mg/L modeled as binary variables. Atrazine exposure occurred in 51% of controls and 57% of cases but NHL risk was not associated with drinking water contaminated with atrazine. There was no difference in mean nitrate exposure or mean atrazine exposure over time between cases and controls. When mean nitrate and mean atrazine exposures were multiplied, the resulting median exposure is eight times greater for cases than controls (0.42 for cases and 0.05 for controls).

5.3 Discussion

For many years, the risk of developing NHL has been postulated to be associated with exposure to pesticides, one of which is the commonly used herbicide atrazine, and to nitrate-contaminated drinking water, but studies have been inconsistent in confirming this association (Weisenburger, 1990; Zahm *et al.*, 1993a; Ward *et al.*, 1996). To our knowledge, this is the first case-control study to examine the risk of NHL associated with exposure to both nitrate and atrazine in drinking water. NHL risk associated with drinking water containing nitrate or atrazine alone was not observed; however our analysis suggests increased NHL risk for subjects exposed to drinking water containing both nitrate and atrazine. We hypothesize that endogenous formation and subsequent metabolism of NNAT is responsible for carcinogenesis. Mono-NNAT is stable when stored at 0°C in an amber vial. NNAT forms readily in aqueous solution at pH 2-4, comparable to that of the human stomach, and in soil at pH ≤5 (Wei *et al.*, 2011). No di-NNAT was detected in these experiments. Di-nitrosated atrazine is much less stable and readily decomposes to mono-NNAT (Kearney *et al.*, 1977). Both nitrosamines may be forming during digestion and di-NNAT could be more toxic than mono-NNAT.

Studies have shown that nitrosamines act differently depending on chemical structure and physicochemical properties, and metabolism can vary among nitrosamines (Graves & Swann, 1993; Eisenbrand & Janzowski, 1994). Contamination of groundwater with atrazine and nitrate can be chronic and nitrosamines are reportedly more effective in tumor induction when administered chronically than as a single large dose (Kearney *et al.*, 1977). Although the topic is controversial, researchers have concluded that neither nitrate nor atrazine are mutagenic or carcinogenic (WHO 50, Gammon *et al.*, 2005; WHO 2010; Lubo & Howd, 2011; Freeman *et al.*, 2011; Simpkins *et al.*, 2011) and the results of our study are consistent with those reports.

In the present study, subjects exposed to both nitrate and atrazine were exposed to nitrate at a concentration nearly 1000-fold greater than atrazine. Approximately 5% of ingested nitrate is converted to nitrite in saliva (Mirvish, 1975). Simultaneous exposure to 1 mg of nitrate and 1 µg of atrazine in 1 L of drinking water would yield a nitrite concentration 50 times greater than atrazine which is more than adequate for nitrosation.

When conducting epidemiology studies assessing disease risk due to drinking water exposure, the contribution of water supply infrastructure must be considered to limit misclassification. The Nebraska study (Ward *et al.*, 1996) included all well and distribution data and could have led to exposure misclassification, producing a false positive finding (type I error). Many active PWS wells do not provide drinking water but are not decommissioned. These wells remain available for fire protection, irrigation or use other than for human consumption and are routinely sampled. Data from these wells are entered into the Nebraska Health and Human Services drinking water database because they are classified as active wells. Unless a well is formally decommissioned and capped, quarterly monitoring is required under the SDWA. These wells may have higher nitrate concentrations or detectable levels of atrazine, biasing results away from the null hypothesis of no association between exposure to nitrate and atrazine in drinking water and the risk of developing NHL. To reduce misclassification we investigated the PWS infrastructure and only included wells contributing to the subject's residence. Furthermore, sampling from the distribution system occurs at random locations within the PWS and contaminant concentrations can differ depending on where the sample was obtained. Since 1993, sampling must be performed where the water enters the distribution system. This point of entry (POE) may be a treatment plant, reservoir, or well. Data in the current study were from samples obtained at the POE and water source inclusion/exclusion criteria were based on contribution to the location of interest. Finally, more water quality data have been compiled since the previous Nebraska study, resulting in a more exact assessment of individual-specific drinking water exposures. Although excluding participants not living at the same residence for the entire time period of interest reduced sample size, it more importantly eliminated exposure misclassification due to differences in drinking water quality between residence locations and exposure duration.

Consideration should be given to the limitations of the study. Transcription of large amounts of water data is not likely to be error-free and could result in misclassification. This is likely to be nondifferential, random error, moving the association towards the null hypothesis. Second, most environmental epidemiological datasets have missing exposure data for many, if not all participants. There is a concern that participants with greater amounts of missing data are "different" than those with less missing data. In this study, missing water data are generally due to data being destroyed (PWSs are required to maintain water quality records for 10 years), frequency of monitoring, which can depend on previous concentrations (monitoring of nitrate is required only yearly if the concentration is less than or equal to 5 mg/L and pesticide monitoring is required every three years if no detection), and when the PWS implemented the SDWA (PWSs were allowed a few years to bring the system into compliance). We generally assume that missing data alters the results of the analysis and makes findings less meaningful. In this study there was no change in the results after imputation of missing data, either by carrying the first observed value forward to the next observed value or by imputing the last observed value backward to the next observed value. In the future, the amount of water quality data will increase and the quality of the data will improve. Record keeping continues to improve with technological advances in computer software and, more documentation of the infrastructure characteristics is being done which should result in less missing data. Third, pesticide exposure history and occupational history, not available for this secondary analysis, could be confounding the results. The original study found that farmers using insecticides had a weak elevated risk of NHL (OR, 1.2; CI, 0.9-1.6) as did farmers who used herbicides (OR, 1.1; CI, 0.8-1.5), compared with non-farmers. Family history of hematopoietic cancer among first-degree relatives was significantly associated with increased risk of NHL (OR, 1.5; CI, 1.0-2.5) in the original study but not in this study. Diet (information not provided for this study) may be confounding our results. When the highest quartile of intake was compared with the lowest, the original study group had increased risk of NHL associated with total fat (OR, 1.6; CI, 0.8-3.0) (Chiu et al., 2005). In a followup study, red meat consumption was associated with elevated risk and findings suggested that meat fat and meat-related mutagens impact NHL subtype risk differently (Aschebrook-Kilfoy et al., 2012). Also, a higher intake of cruciferous vegetables and green leafy vegetables may lower NHL risk, particularly follicular and DLBCL (Chiu et al., 2011).

Farmers may live in areas where water has higher nitrate and atrazine concentrations and because of their occupation also had other modes of pesticide exposures. Alternatively, one could assume that most farmers live in rural areas and use private wells. This study only included subjects who used public water systems and lived at one residence during the latency period (1978-1998). It is expected, however, that small town residents would have increased exposure from application due to their residence being closer to farm fields. Water quality may be a surrogate for some other environmental factor such as exposure to farm animals (Tranah et al., 2008), another drinking water contaminant such as arsenic, uranium or another agrichemical, or exposure to nitrosamines produced from drinking water disinfection treatments (Zhao *et al.*, 2008). The data were not sufficient to evaluate NHL risk associated with alachlor combined with nitrate (3 cases, 3 controls) or simazine combined with nitrate (1 case, 3 controls). Simazine is a nitrosatable pesticide as is glyphosate (Young & Khan, 1978) which was not included in this study.

Finally, increased risk of NHL associated with nitrate- and atrazine-contaminated drinking water was only shown when nitrate and atrazine were modeled as binary variables. When categorizing variables, cutoffs may not be optimally placed. There is increased power of detecting a true association when variables are modeled as continuous variables. No association was shown between risk of NHL and atrazine- and nitrate- contaminated drinking water when atrazine and nitrate were modeled as continuous variables. Hence, the question arises of whether the positive association between risk of NHL and drinking water contaminated with nitrate and atrazine is real. The distribution of the data may contribute to the lack of association seen when running the model with atrazine and nitrate as continuous variables. The nitrate data have a positively skewed distribution and transformation did not correct the data to a normal distribution (Rhoades, 2010). Mean nitrate exposure concentrations range from 0.00 to 8.08 mg/L with a median concentration of 0.94 mg/L (Figure 13). The atrazine data have a bimodal distribution and are zero-inflated, with mean exposure concentrations ranging from 0.00 to 0.80 µg/L and a median exposure concentration of 0.08 µg/L (Figure 14). The second highest quartile of atrazine exposure showed an association between exposure and risk of NHL (OR, 4.8; CI, 1.2-19.9; p=0.03; n=56 cases and 64 controls) but the association was less strong for the highest atrazine exposure quartile and NHL risk (OR, 3.3; CI, 1.0-11.1; p=0.06; n=16 cases and 28 controls). To evaluate the quantitative dose-response relationship regarding the interaction of atrazine and nitrate, we fit the logistic regression and found that the relationship between log odds and atrazine increased as nitrate dose increased, although not significantly (p=0.168).

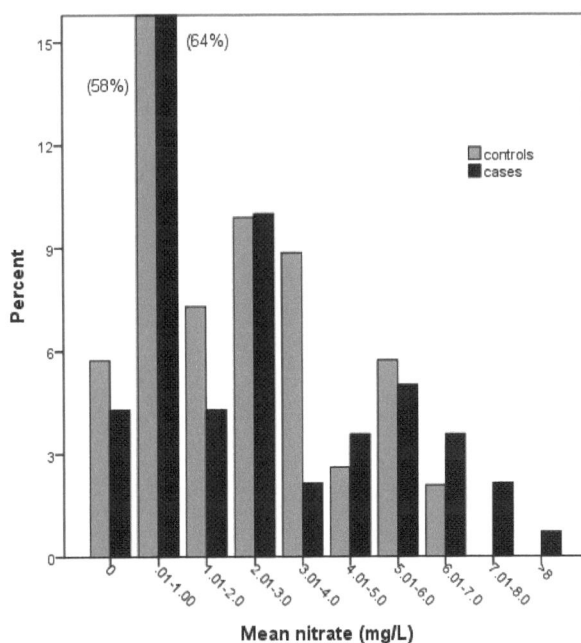

Figure 13: Mean nitrate exposure for cases and controls.

Confounding due to t(14;18) translocation typically seen in NHL patients with indolent B-cell lymphoma could be a limiting factor (Chiu *et al.* 2008). A study evaluating the occurrence of t(14;18) in cases versus controls and exposure to nitrate and atrazine in drinking water is underway. An additional limitation is subject-specific water consumption information. We could only estimate tap water intake based on a 1989 report in which the investigators evaluated total water and tap water intake in the United States by age and gender (Ershow & Cantor, 1989). Incorporating these data into the analysis did not elicit a discrepancy with our original findings. With just over 8% of controls exposed to nitrate and atrazine, this study has a post-hoc power of 79% to detect a true difference in risk of NHL in aggregate and 97% power to detect a difference in risk of indolent B-cell NHL between subjects exposed and subjects not exposed to nitrate and atrazine in drinking water. We recognize that dichotomization is less efficient for statistical analysis and decreases power but the finding of an increased risk of NHL in association with exposure to nitrate and atrazine in drinking water warrants further investigation.

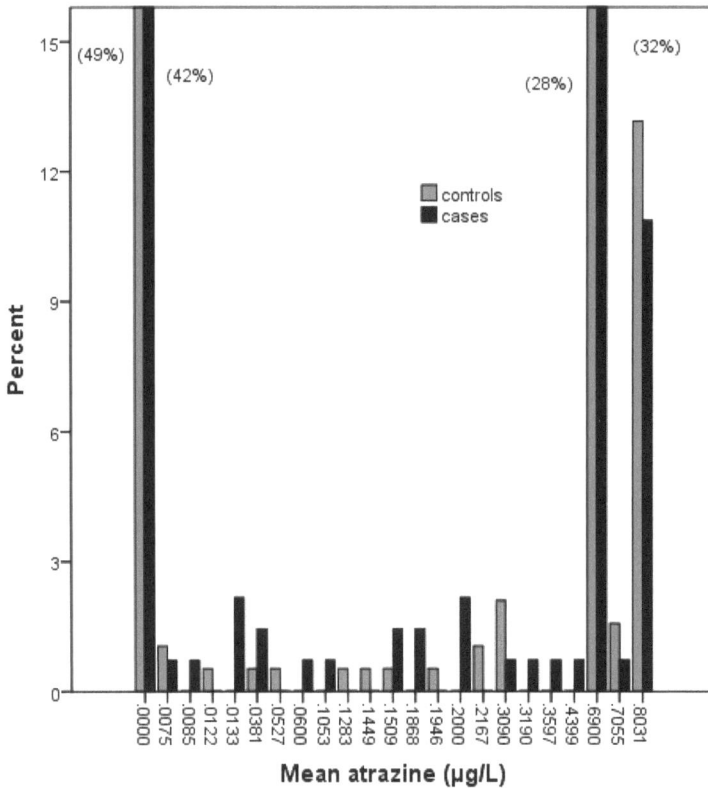

Figure 14: Mean atrazine exposure for cases and controls.

6   Recommendations for Future Research

To increase confidence in generalizing the results to individuals chronically exposed to these two drinking water contaminants, our findings should be confirmed in a larger study and should include pesticide exposure history and occupational history. This could be accomplished with a historical cohort study. Using water quality data from several agricultural regions, subjects would be stratified according to the occurrence of nitrate, atrazine and the combination of nitrate and atrazine. Then incidence of NHL would be compared between the groups: high nitrate:low nitrate; nitrate+atrazine:nitrate; nitrate+atrazine:atrazine; atrazine:no atrazine. Alternatively, a case control study could be repeated with a larger number of participants to increase the power of the findings. A crucial element to epidemiology studies evaluating cancer risk in association with environmental exposures such as drinking water contaminants is the longevity at a residence. Most cancers have latency periods of 10-20 years. Therefore to eliminate exposure misclassification, an investigator must be able to estimate exposure retrospectively over a long time period. A prospective cohort study would be the optimal follow-up study. Subjects would be enrolled and their drinking water sampled annually for 20 years. Statistical analysis would then be conducted to evaluate if those exposed to nitrate, atrazine or nitrate+atrazine were more likely to develop NHL than those not exposed, controlling for other reported risk factors and confounders. A cohort study would offer subject-specific water data to determine exposure rather than estimating exposure as is the practice for retrospective studies. Analysis also could be performed for drinking water contaminants not regulated under the SDWA, such as the two nitrosatable atrazine degradation products, deethylatrazine and deisopropylatrazine. Atrazine, deethylatrazine and nitrate, are the most prevalent contaminants occurring as mixtures in public drinking water supplies (Squillace *et al.*, 2002). A literature search produced no studies evaluating the toxicity of nitrosated atrazine degradation products. Prospective cohort studies elicit the most reliable information but, these studies are very expensive and time-consuming.

Our findings illustrate the potential significance of evaluating mixtures of compounds for toxicity. Future studies addressing nitrate in drinking water as a risk factor for NHL should evaluate concurrent exposure to atrazine and also NHL subtype. When exposed to a mixture of contaminants in drinking water, there is potential for *in vivo* formation of a more toxic compound. This is of particular concern when biological plausibility exists, as in the case of exposure to nitrate and secondary amines, many of which will nitrosate under conditions similar to that of the human stomach to form cancer-causing nitrosamines. The importance of evaluating mixtures when assessing risk has been underscored by the EPA, National Research Council and the USGS (National Research Council, 2009; Toccalino *et al.*, 2012).

More epidemiological research should be conducted to assess the association of exposure to nitrate and other nitrosatable compounds with NHL as well as other cancer types. Nitrosamines are organ-specific in carcinogenesis; different nitrosamines cause cancer in different organs. Not only are compounds with secondary amine moieties nitrosatable but tertiary amines can break down into a more reactive secondary amine during the water treatment process and then be released into drinking water supplies (Mitch & Schreiber, 2008). Many medications are nitrosatable and have been shown to readily nitrosate in conditions similar to that of the human digestive system (Brambilla *et al.*, 1985, 2009; Brambilla & Martelli, 2007). These nitrosated medications should be evaluated for toxicity and their association with disease processes.

The mechanism for toxicity of nitrosamines should be further investigated. NO mediates physiological responses in the immune system and is important to lymphatic vessel function. NO donors were shown to induce proliferation and/or survival of cultured lymphatic endothelial cells (Lahdenranta *et al.*, 2009) and nitroso-compounds have been reported to release NO (Bai *et al.* 2007). It is possible that NO is released from nitrosamines, causing disruption in NOS activity and subsequent disturbance of NO homeostasis, the result of which may be tumor formation. Additionally, it is possible that NOS activity is inhibited because the NO group on the nitrosamine is detected by these enzymes as free NO. The Meisner (1993) study should be repeated to identify the chromosomal abnormalities in lymphocytes after exposure to NNAT. CYP2E1 expression in NNAT-treated lymphocytes should be compared to untreated lymphocytes. The impact of NNAT on *bcl-2* proliferation should be studied in population and laboratory studies. In an experiment using fertilized chicken eggs, we observed significant malformations in embryos treated with NNAT after five days of incubation, suggesting that NNAT causes alterations in embryonic development (Joshi *et al.*, 2013). Developmental abnormalities and carcinogenesis frequently share mechanistic pathways.

Fumigant applicators reportedly had a significant increase in double-strand DNA breaks at chromosomes 18q21 and 14q32, the same regions as t(14;18) (Garry *et al.*, 1992, 1996). A wide range of types of pesticides show varying effect sizes between t(14;18) and NHL generally and by subtype, perhaps due to patterns of pesticide use in the community that represents the probability of being exposed to nitrate and atrazine. Associations of a number of different pesticides to NHL in those who are t(14;18) positive might be a surrogate for contaminants such as atrazine and nitrate in the drinking water supply. This needs to be ruled out before any conclusions can be drawn about the association between pesticides and NHL risk. Stronger mechanistic evidence exists for NNAT and NHL than for pesticides. The t(14;18) aberration has been found at very low frequency in healthy individuals (Meijerink, 1997) and in future studies t(14;18) assays should be performed in the control group.

The centralized repository for data on agrichemicals in groundwater is an asset to Nebraska and the study of disease as it relates to drinking water (UNL, 2000). Large amounts of data are collected in Nebraska by local natural resources districts, state and federal agencies, pesticide manufacturers, and university researchers. The Clearinghouse collects and organizes these data and currently has over 400,000 entries. This is an open access database and an excellent source of water data for conducting ecological studies to correlate groundwater contamination with the occurrence of disease.

Acknowledgments

The authors are grateful to the study participants who made this research possible and the public water supply managers for their assistance in collecting and analyzing the water data. We also thank Kent Eskridge, University of Nebraska-Lincoln for his statistical advice, Brian Chiu, University of Chicago for providing the case-control data, and Les Howard and Colleen Steele for the Database queries and creation of the maps.

Authors

Martha G. Rhoades
School of Natural Resources, University of Nebraska-Lincoln, USA

Jane L. Meza
Department of Biostatistics, University of Nebraska Medical Center, USA

Cheryl L. Beseler
Department of Psychology, Colorado State University, USA

Patrick J. Shea
School of Natural Resources, University of Nebraska-Lincoln, USA

Andy Kahle
Nebraska Department of Health and Human Services, State of Nebraska, USA

Julie M. Vose
Division of Hematology/Oncology, University of Nebraska Medical Center, USA

Mary E. Exner
School of Natural Resources, University of Nebraska-Lincoln, USA

Roy F. Spalding
Department of Agronomy and Horticulture, University of Nebraska-Lincoln, USA

References

Abeloff MD, Armitage JO, Niederhuber JE, Kastan MV, McKenna WG. 2004. Clinical Oncology. 3rd and 4th Editions. Elsevier, Churchill Livingstone. Copyright 2004 and 2008, Elsevier Inc.)

Ames BN, Gold LS. 1990. Too many rodent carcinogens: Mitogenesis increases mutagenesis. Science 249: 970-971.

Anderson JR, Armitage JO, Weisenburger DD. 1998. Epidemiology of the non-Hodgkin's lymphomas: Distributions of the major subtypes differ by geographic locations. Annals of Oncology 9:717-720.

Aschebrook-Kilfoy B, Ward MH, Dave BJ, Smith SM, Weisenburger DD, Chiu BCH. 2013. Dietary nitrate and nitrite intake and risk of non-Hodgkin lymphoma. Leukemia and Lymphoma 54(5): 945-950.

Aschebrook-Kilfoy B, Ollberding NJ, Kolar C, Lawson TA, Smith SM, Weisenburger DD, Chiu BCH. 2012. Meat intake and risk of non-Hodgkin lymphoma. Cancer Causes control 23: 1681-1692

Bachman J. 1984. Department of Natural Resources Maryland. Geological Survey. Report of Investigations No.40: The Columbia aquifer of the eastern short of Maryland. Hydrogeology, selected water well records, chemical analyses, water level measurements, lithologic logs and geophysical logs.

Bai P, Hegedűs C, Erdelyi K, Szabó E, Bakondi E, Gergely S, Szabó C, Virág L. 2007. Protein tyrosine nitration and poly-(ADP-ribose) polymerase activation in N-methyl-N-nitro-N-nitrosoguanidine-treated thymocytes: implication for cytotoxicity. Toxicology Letters 170: 203-213.

Besag JE, York J, Mollie A. 1991. Bayesian image restoration with two applications in spatial statistics (with discussion). Annals of the Institute of Statistical Mathematics 43:1-59.

Blair A, Zahm SH. 1991. Cancer among farmers. Occupational Medicine: State of the Art Reviews 6(3): 335-354

Boffetta P, de Vocht F. 2007. Occupation and the risk of NHL. Cancer Epidemiology, Biomarkers and Prevention 16(3): 369-372.

Bracci PM, Dalvi TB, Holly EA. 2006. Residential history, family characteristics, and NHL, a population based case-control study in the San Francisco Bay area. Cancer Epidemiology, Biomarkers and Prevention 15(7): 1287-1294.

Brambilla G, Cajelli E, Finollo R, Maura A, Pino A, Robbiano L. 1985. Formation of DNA-damaging nitroso compounds by interaction of drugs with nitrite. A preliminary screening for detecting potentially hazardous drugs. Journal of Toxicology and Environmental Health 15: 1-24.

Brambilla G, Martelli A. 2007. Genotoxic and carcinogenic risk to humans of drug-nitrite interaction products. Mutation Research 635: 17-52.

Brambilla G, Mattioli F, Martelli A. 2009. *Genotoxic and carcinogenic effects of antipsychotics and antidepressants.* Toxicology 261: 77-88.

Cantor KP, Blair A, Everett G, Gibson R, Burmeister LF, Brown LM, Schuman L, Dick FR. 1992. *Pesticides and other agricultural risk factors for non-Hodgkin's lymphoma among men in Iowa and Minnesota.* Cancer Research H52: 2447-2455

Cerhan JR, Anderson KE, Janney CA, Vachon CM, Witzig TE, Habermann TM. 2003. *Association of aspirin and other non-steroidal anti-inflammatory drug use with incidence of NHL.* International Journal of Cancer 106: 784-788.

Chang ET, Balter KM, Torrang A, Smedby KE, Melbye M, Sundstrom C, Glimelius B, Adami H. 2006. *Nutrient intake and risk of non-Hodgkin's Lymphoma.* American Journal of Epidemiology 164(12): 1222-1232.

Chang ET, Smedby KE, Hjalgrim H, Schollkopf C, Porwit-MacDonald A, Sundstrom C, Tani E, d'Amore F, Melbye M, Adami H, Glimelius B. 2005. *Medication use and risk of non-Hodgkin's lymphoma.* American Journal of Epidemiology 162: 965-974.

Chao C, Page JH. 2008. *Type 2 diabetes mellitus and risk of NHL: A systemic review and meta analysis.* American Journal of Epidemiology 168: 471-480.

Chiu BCH, Dave BJ, Blair A, Gapstur SM, Zahm SH, Weisenburger DD. 2006. *Agricultural pesticide use and risk of t(14;18)-defined subtypes of NHL.* Blood 108(4): 1363-1369.

Chiu BC, Dave BJ, Ward MH, Fought AJ, Hou L, Jain S, Gapstur S, Evens AM, Zahm SH, Blair A, Weisenburger DD. 2008. *Dietary factors and risk of t(14;18)-defined subgroups of NHL.* Cancer Causes and Control 19: 859-867.

Chiu BC-H, Dave BJ, Blair A, Gapstur SM, Chmiel JS, Fought AJ, Zahm SH, Weisenburger DD. 2007a. *Cigarette smoking, familial hematopoietic cancer, hair dye use and risk of t(14;18)defined subtypes of NHL.* American Journal of Epidemiology 165 (6): 652-659.

Chiu BC, Soni L, Gapstur SM, Fought AJ, Evens AM, Weisenburger DD. 2007b. *Obesity and risk of NHL (United States) Cancer Causes Control 18: 677-685.*

Chiu BC-H, Kolar C, Gapstur SM, Lawson TA, Anderson JR, Weisenburger DD. 2005. *Association of NAT and GST polymorphisms with non-Hodgkin lymphoma: a population-based case-control study.* British Journal of Haematology 128:610-615.

Chiu BC-H, Weisenburger DD, Zahm SH, Cantor KP, Gapstur SM, Holmes F, Burmeister LF, Blair A. 2004. *Agricultural pesticide use, familial cancer, and risk of NHL.* Cancer Epidemiology, Biomarkers and Prevention 13(4): 525-531.

Chiu BCH, Kwon S, Evens AM, Surawicz T, Smith SM, Weisenburger DD. 2011. *Dietary intake of fruit and vegetables and risk of non-Hodgkin lymphoma.* Cancer Causes control 22: 1183-1195

Cocco P, Brennan P, Ibba A, Llongeras SS, Maynadie M, Nieters A, Becker N, Ennas MG, Tocco MG, Boffetta P. 2008. *Plasma polychlorobiphenl and organochlorine pesticide level and risk of major lymphoma subtypes.* Occupational and Environmental Medicine 65: 132-140

Colt JS, Davis S, Severson RK, Lynch CF, Cozen W, Camann D, Engels EA, Blair A, Hartge P. 2006. *Residential insecticide use and risk of non-Hodgkin's lymphoma.* Cancer Epidemiology, Biomarkers and Prevention 15(2):251-257.

Colt JS, Rothman N, Severson RK, Hartge P, Cerhan JR, Chatterje N, Cozen W, Mortin LM, De Roos AJ, Davis S, Chanock S, Wang SS. 2009. *Organochlorine exposure, immune gene variation and risk of NHL.* Blood 113: 1899-1905.

Comley HH. 1945. *Cyanosis in infants caused by nitrates in well water.* Journal of American Medical Association 129(2): 112-116.

Cova D., Perego R., Nebuloni C., Arnoldi A., Trevisan M., Ghebbioni C 1993. *In vitro formation of N-Nitroso triazines in water/soil systems and human gastric juice.* In: Del Re A.A.M., Capri E., Evans S.P., Natali P., Trevsian M. (ed.) Atti del IX Symposium Pesticide Chemistry "Degradation and mobility of Xenobiotics". Piacenza, 11-13 403-410. Edizioni Biagini, Lucca.

Cova, D, Nebuloni, C, Arnoldi, A, Bassoli, A, Trevisan, M, Del Re A AM. 1996. *N-Nitrosation of Triazines in Human Gastric Juice.* Journal of Agriculture and Food Chemistry 44: 2852-2855

Cowles MK, Anderson J, Mueller KJ, Ullrich F. 1999. *Prostate cancer incidence rates by county in Nebraska 1990-1991.* Nebraska Health Data Reporter 2 (4):1-9

Cozen W, Cerhan JR, Martinez-Maza O, Ward MH, Linet M, Colt JS, Davis S, Severson RK, Hartge P, Bernstein L. 2007. *The effect of atopy, childhood crowding and other immune-related factors on NHL risk.* Cancer Causes Control 18:821-831.

Cross AJ, Pollock JRA, Bingham SA. 2003. *Haem, not protein or inorganic iron is responsible for endogenous intestinal N-nitrosation arising from red meat. Cancer research 63: 2358-2360.*

Cross AJ, Ward MH, Schenk MJ, Kulidorff M, Cozen W, Davis S, Colt JS, Hartge P, Cerhan JR, Sinha R. 2006. *Meat and meat mutagen intake and risk of NHL: Results from a NCI-SEER case-control study. Carcinogenesis 27(2): 293-297*

De Roos AJ, Hartge P, Lubin JH, Colt JS, Davis S, Cerhan JR, Severson RK, Cozen W, Patterson DG Jr., Needham LL, Rothman N. 2005. *Persistent organochlorine chemicals in plasma and risk of non-Hodgkin's lymphoma. Cancer Research 65(23): 11214-11226.*

De Roos AJ, Zahm SH, Cantor KP, Weisenburger DD, Holmes FF, Burmeister LF, Blair A. 2003. *Integrative assessment of multiple pesticides as risk factors for non-Hodgkin's lymphoma among men. Occupational and Environmental Medicine;60:e11 downloaded at www.occenvmed.com/cgi/content/full/60/9/e11.*

Devesa SS, Fears T. 1992. *Non-Hodgkin's lymphoma time trends: United States and international data. Cancer Research 52(suppl): 5432S-5440S.*

Ehrenfeld M, Abu-Shakra M, Buskila D, Shoenfeld Y. 2001. *The dual association between lymphoma and autoimmunity. Blood Cells, Molecules and Diseases 27(4): 750-756.*

Eisenbrand G, Janzowski C. 1994 (s.l). *Found in Nitrosamines and Related N-nitroso Compounds. Chapter 15. Potential mechanism of action of nitrosamines with hydroxyl, oxo or carboxy groups. pages 179-194 In: Michejda CJ, Loeppky RN, eds.*

Engel LS, Laden F, Andersen A, Strickland PT, Blair A, Needham LL, Barr DB, Wolff MS, Helzlsouer K, Hunter DJ, Lan Q, Cantor KP, Comstock GW, Brock JW, Bush D, Hoofer RN, Rothman N. 2007a. *Polychlorinated biphenyl levels in peripheral blood and non-Hodgkin's lymphoma: a report from three cohorts. Cancer Research 67(11): 5545-5552.*

Engel LS, Lan Q, Rothman N. 2007b. *Polychlorinated biphenyls and NHL. Cancer Epidemiology, Biomarkers and Prevention 16(3): 373-376*

Engels EA, Cerhan JR, Linet MS, Cozen W, Colt JS, Davis S, Gridley G, Severeson RK, Hartge P. 2005. *Immune-related conditions and immune-modulating medications as risk factors for non-Hodgkin's lymphoma: a case-control study. American Journal of Epidemiology 162: 1153-1161.*

Engels EA. 2007. *Infectious agents as causes of NHL. Cancer Epidemiology, Biomarkers and Prevention 16(3): 401-404.*

Ershow AG, Cantor KP. 1989. *Total water and tapwaer intake in the United States: Population based estimates of quantities and sources. Report prepared under NCI order #263-MD-810264*

Exner ME, Hirsh AJ, Spalding RF. 2014. *Nebraska's groundwater legacy: Nitrate contamination beneath irrigated cropland. Water Resources Research 50, doi:10.1002/2013WRO15073.*

Exner ME, Spalding RF. 1994. *N-15 identification of nonpoint sources of nitrate contamination beneath cropland in the Nebraska Panhandle: two case studies. Applied Geochemistry 9:73-81.*

Exner ME, Perea-Estrada H, Spalding RF. 2010. *Long-term response of groundwater nitrate concentrations to management regulations in Nebraska's central Platte valley. The Scientific World Journal 10:286-297*

Exner ME, Spalding RF. 1990. *Occurrence of pesticides and nitrate in Nebraska's ground water. Water Center Publication1. Institute of Agriculture and Natural Resources. University of Nebraska-Lincoln.*

Farm and Ranch Irrigation Survey. 2003. *Volume 3, special studies. Available at www.nass.usda.gov/census*

Flick, ED, Chan KA, Bracci PM, Holly A 2006. *Use of nonsteroidal anti-inflammatory drugs and NHL: A population-based case-control study. American Journal of Epidemiology 164: 497-504.*

Freedman DM, Cantor KP, Ward MH, Helzlsouer KJ. 2000. *A case-control study of nitrate in drinking water and non-Hodgkin's lymphoma in Minnesota. Archives of Environmental Health 55(5): 326-329.*

Freeman LEB, Rusiecki JA, Hoppin JA, Lubin JH, Koutros S, Andreotti G, Zahm SH, Hines CJ, Coble JB, Barone-Adesi F, Sloan J, Sandler DP, Blair A, Alavanja MCR. 2011. *Atrazine and cancer incidence among pesticide applicators in the agricultural health study (1994-2007). Environmental Health Perspectives 119(9):1253-1259.*

Freeman MD, Kohles SS. 2012. *Plasma levels of polychlorinated biphenyls, non-Hodgkin lymphoma and causation. Journal of Environmental and Public Health. vol. 2012, Article ID 258981, 15 pages, 2012. doi:10.1155/2012/258981*

Fritschi L, Benke G, Hughes AM, Kricker A, Turner J, Vajdic CM, Grulich A, Milliden S, Kaldor J, Armstrong BK. 2005. *Occupational exposure to pesticides and risk of non-Hodgkin's lymphoma. American Journal of Epidemiology 162:849-857.*

Gaikwad NW, Yang L, Weisenburger DD, Vose J, Beseler C, Rogan EG, Cavalieri EL. 2009. *Urinary biomarkers suggest that estrogen-DNA adducts may play a role in the aetiology of non-Hodgkin lymphoma. Biomarkers 14 (7): 502-512.*

Gammon DW, Aldous CN, Wesley CC, Sanborn JR, Pfeifer KF. 2005. *A risk assessment of atrazine use in California: Human health and ecological aspects. Pest Management Science 61:331-355.*

Garry VF, Danzl TJ, Tarone R, Griffith J, Cervenka J, Krueger L, Whorton EB, Nelson RL. 1992, *Chromosome rearrangements in fumigant appliers: Possible relationship to non-Hodgkin's lymphoma risk. Cancer Epidemiology, Biomarkers and Prevention 1: 287-291.*

Garry VF, Tarone RE, Long L, Griffith J, Kelly JT, Burrough B. 1996. *Pesticide appliers with mixed pesticide exposure: G-banded analysis and possible relationship to non-Hodgkin's lymphoma.. Cancer Epidemiology, Biomarkers and Prevention 5: 11-16.*

Gillom RJ, Barbash JE, Crawford CG, Hamilton PA, Martin JD, Nakagaki N, Nowell LH, Scott JC, Stackelberg PE, Thelin GP, Wolock DM. 2006. *The Quality of Our Nation's Waters – Pesticides in the Nation's Streams and Ground Water. 1992-2001. Circular 1291, Reston, VA: U.S. Geological Survey. 172 p.*

Gormly JR, Spalding RF. 1979. *Sources and concentrations of nitrate nitrogen in ground water of the central Platte region, Nebraska. Ground Water 17:291-301.*

Gosselin D, Headrick CJ, Tremblay V, Chen X, Summerside S. 1997. *Domestic Well Water Quality in Rural Nebraska: Focus on Nitrateitrogen, Pesticides, and Coliform Bacteria. Ground Water Monitoring and Remediation 17(2): 77-87.*

Graves RJ, Swann PF. 1993 *Clearance of N-nitrosodimethylamine and N-nitrosodiethylamine by the perfused rat liver. Relationship to the K_m and V_{max} for nitrosamine metabolism. Biochemical Pharmacology 45(5): 983-989.*

Grulich AE, Vajdic CM, Cozen W. 2007. *Altered immunity as a risk factor for NHL Cancer Epidemiology, Biomarkers and Prevention 16(3): 405-408.*

Gulis G, Czompolyova M, Cerhan JR. 2002. *An ecologic study of nitrate in municipal drinking water and cancer incidence on Trnava distric Slovakia. Environmental Research Section A 88: 182-187.*

Hallberg GR. 1989. *Nitrate in ground water in the United States. Chapter 3:35-74. In Nitrogen Management and Groundwater Protection. Ed: RF. Follett. Elsevier Science Publishers. B.V. Amsterdam. Printed in the Netherlands.*

Hardell L, Eriksson M. 1999. *A case-control study of non-Hodgkin lymphoma and exposure to pesticides. Cancer 85(6): 1353-1360.*

Hardell L, Eriksson M. 2003. *Is the decline of the increasing incidence of non-Hodgkin lymphoma in Sweden and other countries a result of cancer preventive measures? Environmental Health Perspectives 111(14): 1704-1706.*

Hardell L, Eriksson M, Lenner P, Lundgren E. 1981. *Malignant lymphoma and exposure to chemicals, especially organic solvents, chlorophenols and phenoxy acids: A case-control study. British Journal of Cancer 43: 169-172.*

Hartge P, Wang SS. 2004. *Overview of the etiology and epidemiology of lymphoma. In: Mauch PM, Armitage JO, Coiffier B, Dalla-Favera R, Harris NL (ed.) Non-Hodgkin's Lymphomas, Lippincott Williams and Wilkins, Philadelphia: 711-727.*

Hoar SK, Blair A, Holmes FF, Boysen KD, Robel RJ, Hoover R, Fraumeni JF Jr. 1986. *Agricultural herbicide use and risk of lymphoma and soft tissue sarcoma. Journal of American Medical Association 256: 1141-1147.*

Hoeft B, Becker N, Deeg E, Beckmann L, Nieters A. 2008. *Joint effect between regular use of nonsteroidal anti-inflammatory drugs, variants in inflammatory genes and risk of lymphoma. Cancer Causes and Control 19:163-173.*

Johnson, BB, Kamble, S.T. 1984. *Pesticide use on major crops in Nebraska-1982. Department of Agricultural Economics, University of Nebraska-Lincoln. Dept. rpt. No.10. 29 pp.*

Joshi N, Rhoades MG, Bennett GD, Wells SM, Mirvish SS, Breitbach MJ, Shea PJ. 2013. *Developmental abnormalities in chicken embryos exposed to N-nitrosoatrazine. Journal of Toxicology and Environmental Health, Part A: Current Issues 76(17): 1015-1022*

Karipidis K, Benke G, Sim M, Fritschi L, Yost M, Armstrong B, Hughes AM, Grulich A, Vajdic CM, Kaldor JM, Kricker A. 2007. *Occupational exposure to power frequency magnetic fields and risk of NHL. Occupational and Environmental Medicine. 64: 25-29.*

Kato I, Koenig KL, Watanabe-Meserve H, Baptiste MS, Lillquist PP, Frizzera G, Burke JS, Moseson M, Shore RE. 2005. *Personal and occupational exposure to organic solvents and risk of non-Hodgkin's lymphoma in women (United States). Cancer Causes and Control 16: 1215-1224.*

Kato I, Watanabe-Meserve H, Koenig KL, Baptiste MS, Lillquist PP, Frizzera G, Burke JS, Moseson M, Shore RE. 2004. Pesticide product use and risk of NHL in women. *Environmental Health Perspectives* 112(13): 1275-1281.

Kearney PC, Olifer JE, Helling CS, Isensee AR, Kontson A. 1977. Distribution, movement, persistence and metabolism of N-nitrosoatrazine in soils and a model aquatic ecosystem. *Journal of Agriculture and Food Chemistry* 25(5):1177-1181.

Kousa A, Moltchanova E, Viik-Kajander M, Rytkonen M, Tuomilehto J, Tarvainen T and Karvonen M. 2004. Geochemistry of ground water and the incidence of acute myocardial infarction in Finland. *Journal of Epidemiology and Community Health* 58:136-139.

Koutros SA, Zhant Y, Zhu Y, Mayne ST, Zahm SH, Holford TR, Leaderer BP, Boyle P, Zheng T. 2008. Nutrients contributing to one-carbon metabolism and risk of NHL subtypes. *American Journal of Epidemiology* 167(3):287-294.

Krull IS, Mills K, Hoffman G, Fine DH. 1980. The analysis of N-nitrosoatrazine and N-nitrosocarbaryl in whole mice. *Journal of Analytical Toxicology* 4: 260-262.

Lahdenranta J, Hagendoorn J, Pader TP, Hoshida T, Nelson G, Kashiwagi, Jain RK, Fudumura D. 2009. Endothelial nitric oxide synthase mediates lymphangiogenesis and lymphatic metastasis. *Cancer Research* 69(7): 2801-2808

Lan Q, Zheng T, Chanock S, Zhant Y, Shen M, Wang SS, Berndt SI, Zahm SH, Holford TR, Leaderer B, Yeager M, Welch R, Hosgood D, Boyle P, Rothman N. 2007. Genetic variants in caspase genes and susceptibility to NHL. *Carcinogenesis* 10 (4): 823-827.

Lawson AB, Vidal-Rodeiro CL, Browne WB. 2003. Disease mapping basics. *Disease Mapping with WinBUGS and MlwiN. John Wiley &Sons. Ltd.*: 1-15.

Lee JS, Bracci PM, Holly EA. 2008. NHL in women: Reproductive factors and exogenous hormone use. *American Journal of Epidemiology* 168: 278-288.

Lee WJ, Cantor KP, Berzofsky JA, Zahm SH, Blair A. 2004. Non-Hodgkin's lymphoma among asthmatics exposed to pesticides. *International Journal of Cancer:* 111 298-302.

Lee WJ, Purdue MP, Steward P, Schenk M, De Roos AJ, Cerhan JR, Severson RK, Cozen W, Hartge P, Blair A. 2006. Asthma history, occupational exposure to pesticides and the risk of non-Hodgkin's lymphoma. *International Journal of Cancer* 118: 3174-3176.

Lightfoot TJ, Skibola CF, Willett EV, Skibola DR, Allan JM, Coppede F, Adamson PJ, Morgin GJ, Roman E, Smith MT. 2005. Risk of non-Hodgkin lymphoma associated with polymorphisms in folate-metabolizing genes. *Cancer Epidemiology Biomarkers and Prevention* 14(12): 2999-3003.

Lim U, Schenk M, Kelemen LE, Davis S, Cozen W, Hartge P, Ward MH, Stolzenberg-Solomon R. 2005. Dietary determinants of one-carbon metabolism and the risk of non-Hodgkin's lymphoma: NCI-SEER case-control study, 1998-2000. *American Journal of Epidemiology* 162: 953-964.

Lim U, Weinstein S, Albanes D, Pietinen P, Teerenhovi L, Taylor PR, Virtamo J, Stolzenberg-Solomon R. 2006. Dietary factors of one-carbon metabolism in relation to non-Hodgkin lymphoma and multiple myeloma in a cohort of male smokers. *Cancer Epidemiology, Biomarkers and Prevention* 15(6): 1109-1114.

Lim U, Gayles T, Katki HA, Stolzenberg-Solomon R. 2007a. Serum high density lipoprotein cholesterol and risk of non-Hodgkin lymphoma. *Cancer Research* 67(11): 5569-5574.

Lim U, Morton LM, Subar AF, Baris D, Stolzenberg-Solomon R, Leitzmann M, Kipnis V, Mouw T, Carroll L, Schatzkin A, Hartge P. 2007b. Alcohol, smoking and body size in relation to incident Hodgkin's and non-Hodgkin's lymphoma risk. *American Journal of Epidemiology* 166(6): 697-708.

Lijinsky W. 1977. How nitrosamines cause cancer. *New Scientist* 73 (1036) : 216-217.

Lijinsky, W. 1986. The significance of N-nitroso compounds as environmental carcinogens. *Journal of Environmental Science and Health Part C: Environmental Carcinogenesis Reviews*: 1-45.

Liteplo RG, Meek ME, Windle W. United Nations Environment Programme, International Labour Organization, and the World Health Organization. N-nitrosodimethylamine Concise International chemical Assessment Document 38. Available at: http://www.inchem.org/documents/cicads/cicads/cicad38.htm.

Lubow J, Howd R. 2011. Should atrazine and related chlorotriazines be considered carcinogenic for human health risk assessment? *Journal of Environmental Science and Health: Part C* 29(2): 99-144

Magee PN. 1989. The experimental basis for the role of nitrosamines in human cancer. *Cancer Surveys* 8: 207–239.

Mandel JH, Kelsh MA, Mink PH, Alexander DD, Kalmes RM, Weingart M, Yost L, Goodman M. 2006. *Occupational trichloroethylene exposure and non-Hodgkin's lymphoma: a meta-analysis and review. Occupational and Environmental Medicine 63(9): 597–607.*

Mauch PM, Armitage JO, Coiffier B, Dalla-Favera R, Harris NL. 2004. *Non-Hodgkin's Lymphomas. Lippincott Williams and Wilkins, Philadelphia, PA.*

Meijerink, JPP. 1997. *t(14;18): A journey to eternity. Leukemia 11: 2175-2187.*

Meisner LF, Roloff BD, Belluck DA. 1993. *In Vitro effects of N-nitrosoatrazine on chromosome breakage. Archives of Environmental Contamination and Toxicology 24: 108-112.*

Meli G, Bagnati R, Fanelli R, Benfenati E, Airoldi L. 1992. *Metabolic profile of atrazine and N-Nitrosoatrazine in rat urine. Bulletin of Environmental Contamination and Toxicology 48:701–708.*

Mensah FK, Willett EV, Ansell P, Adamson PJ, Roman E. 2007. *Non-Hodgkin's lymphoma and family history of hematologic malignancy. American Journal of Epidemiology 165: 126-133.*

Meza JL. 2003. *Empirical Bayes estimation smoothing of relative risks in disease mapping. Journal of Statistical Planning and Inference 112: 43-62.*

Mitch WA, Schreiber IM. 2008. *Degradation of tertiary alkylamines during chlorination/chloramination: Implications for formation of aldehydes, nitriles, halonitroalkanes and nitrosamines. 2008 Environmental Science and Technology 42(13): 4811-4816.*

Mirvish SS, Gannett P, Babcook DM, Williamson D, Chen SC, Weisenburger DD. 1991. *N-nitrosoatrazine: synthesis, kinetics of formation and nuclear magnetic resonance spectra and other properties. Journal of Agricultural and Food Chemistry 39:1205-1210.*

Mirvish, SS. 1975. *Formation of N-nitroso compounds: chemistry, kinetics and in vivo occurrence. Toxicology and Applied Pharmacology. 31:325-351.*

Mirvish SS, Haorah J, Zhou L, Hartman M, Morris CR, Clapper ML. 2003 *N-nitroso compounds in the gastrointestinal tract of rats and in the feces of mice with induced colitis or fed hot dogs or beef. Carcinogenesis 24(3): 595-603.*

Mirvish SS, Grandjean AC, Moller H, Fike S, Maynard T, Jones L, Rosinsky S, Nie G. 1992. *N-nitrosoproline excretion by rural Nebraskans drinking water of varied nitrate content. Cancer Epidemiology Biomarkers and Prevention 1:455–461.*

Mirvish SS. 1995. *Role of N-nitroso compounds (NOC) and N-nitrosation in etiology of gastric, esophageal, nasopharyngeal and bladder cancer and contribution to cancer of known exposures to NOC. Cancer Letters 93:17-48.*

Mirvish SS. 1986. *Effects of vitamins C and E on N-nitroso compound formation, carcinogenesis, and cancer. Cancer 58 (S8): 1842-1850.*

Mirvish SS, Reimers KJ, Kutler B, Chen SC, Haorah J, Morris CR, Grandjean AC, Lyden ER. 2000. *Nitrate and nitrite concentrations in human saliva for men and women at different ages and times of the day and their consistent over time. European Journal of Cancer Prevention 9:335-342.*

Molitor J, Molitor NT, Jerrett M, McConnell R, Gauderman J, Berhane K, Thomas D. 2006. *Bayesian modeling of air pollution health effects with missing exposure data. American Journal of Epidemiology 164(1):69-76.*

Mollie A, Richardson S. 1991. *Empirical Bayes estimates of cancer mortality rates using spatial models. Statistical in Medicine 10: 95-112.*

Morton LM, Bernstein L, Want SS, Hein DW, Rothman N, Colt JS, Davis S, Cerhan JR, Severson RK, Welch R, Hartge P, Zahm SH. 2001. *Hair dye use, genetic variation in N-acetyltransferase 1 (NAT1) and 2 (NAT2) and risk of NHL. Carcinogenesis 28 (8): 1759-1764.*

(NASS) National Agricultural Statistics Service, Nebraska Department of Agriculture, Division of Agricultural Statistics, Lincoln, NE. *Available at http://www.nass.usda.gov/census (accessed 04/30/14)*

NCI National Cancer Institute. *Available at http://www.cancer.gov/cancertopics/wyntk/non-hodgkin-lymphoma/page4*

National Research Council. 2009 *Committee on Improving Risk Analysis Approaches Used by the U.S. EPA, National Research Council. Science and Decisions: Advancing Risk Assessment. Washington, DC: National Acadamies Press.*

(NDEQ) Nebraska Department of Environmental Quality. *Nebraska Groundwater Quality Monitoring Report. 2003, 2005, 2006, 2007 Available at www.deq.state.ne.us*

Negri Eva, Talamini R, Montella M, Maso LD, Crispo A, Spina M, Veccia CL, Franceschi S. 2006. *Family history of hemolymphopoietic and other cancers and risk of non-Hodgkin's lymphoma. Cancer Epidemiology, Biomarkers and Prevention* 15(2): 245-250.

(NHHS) Nebraska Department of Health and Human Services. 2007. *Nebraska's Public Water System Program 2007 Annual Report.* Available at http://www.dhhs.ne.gov/enh/pwsindex.htm

(NNRD) Nebraska's Natural Resources Districts. 2004. *Cornhusker Press. Hastings, NE 68901*

Nolan BT, Stoner JD. 2000. *Nutrients in groundwaters of the conterminous United States, 1992-1995. Environmental Science and Technology* 34: 1156-1165.

Nolan BT, Ruddy BC, Hitt KJ, Helsel DR. 1997. *Risk of Nitrate in groundwaters of the United States -A national perspective. Environmental Science and Technology* 31:2229-2236.

Norgaard M, Poulsen AH, Pedersen L, Gregersen H, Frils S, Ewertz M, Johnsen HE, Sorensen HT 2006. *Use of postmenopausal hormone replacement therapy and risk of non-Hodgkin's lymphoma: a Danish population-based cohort study. British Journal of Cancer* 94: 1339-1341.

Novak AJ, Slager SL, Fredericksen ZS, Wang AH, Manske MM, Ziesmer S, Liebow M, Macon WR, Dillon SR, Witzig TE, Cerhan JR, Ansell SM. 2009. *Genetic variation in B-cell-activating factor is associated with an increased risk of developing B-cell NHL. Cancer Research* 69(10): 4217-4224.

Novik KL, Spinelli JJ, MacArthur AC, Shumanski K, Sipahimalani P, Leach S, Lai A, Connors JM, Gascoyne RD, Gallagher RP, Brooks-Wilson AR. 2007. *Genetic Variation in H2AFX contributes to risk of NHL. Cancer Epidemiology, Biomarkers and Prevention* 16(6): 1098-1106.

Orsi L, Delabre L, Monnereau A, Delval P, Berthou C, Fenaux P, Marit G, Soubeyran P, Huguet F, Milpied N, Leporrier M, Hemon D, Troussard X, Clavel J. 2009. *Occupational exposure to pesticides and lymphoid neoplasms among men: results of a French case-control study. Occupational and Environmental Medicine* 66: 291-298.

Pan SY, Mao Y, Ugnat A. 2005. *Physical activity, obesity, energy intake and the risk of non-Hodgkin's lymphoma: A population based case-control study. American Journal of Epidemiology* 162: 1162-1173.

Panno SV, Weibel CP, Krapac IG. 1997. *Differences in groundwater contamination of a shallow karst aquifer in Illinois; sinkhole plain relative to sinkhole density. Program with Abstracts. Geological Society of America* 29: 288 (Abstract).

Preussmann R., Stewart BW. 1984. *N-nitroso carcinogens. Ed: Searle, C.E.. In Chemical Carcinogens, ACS Monograph 182, Vol.2, American Chemical Society. Washington, D.C.* Pages 643-868.

Puckett LJ. 1994. *Nonpoint and point sources of Nitrogen in major watersheds of the United States; U.S. Geological Survey: Reston, VA: Water Resources Investigations Report 94-4001.*

Purdue MP, Hartge P, Davis S, Cerhan JR, Colt JS, Cozen W, Severson RK, Li Y, Chanock SJ, Rothman N, Wang SS. 2007a. *Sun exposure, vitamin D receptor gene polymorphisms and risk of NHL. Sun exposure, vitamin D receptor gene polymorphisms and risk of NHL. Cancer Causes Control* 18: 989-999.

Purdue MP, Lan Q, Kricker A, Grulish AE, Vajdic CM, Turner J, Whitby D, Chanock S, Rothman N, Armstrong BK. 2007b. *Polymorphisms in immune function genes and risk of NHL: findings from the new South Wales NHL study. Carcinogenesis* 28(3): 704-712.

Ribaudo MO, Bouzahaer A. 1994. *Atrazine: environmental characteristics and economics of management. Economic Research Services, U.S. Department of Agriculture. Agricultural Economic Report No. 699.*

Rhoades MG. 2010 *Risk of non-Hodgkin Lymphoma and Drinking Water in Nebraska:Atrazine and Nitrate. Omaha, NE. University of Nebraska Medical Center.*

Rhoades MG, Meza JL, Beseler CL, Shea PJ, Kahle A, Vose JM, Eskridge KM, Spalding RF. 2013. *Atrazine and nitrate in public drinking water supplies and non-Hodgkin lymphoma in Nebraska, USA. Environmental Health Insights* 7: 15-27.

Richardson DB, Terschuren C and Hoffman W. 2008. *Occupational risk factors for non-Hodgkin's lymphoma: A population based case-control study in Northern Germany. American Journal of Industrial Medicine* 51: 258-268.

Rusiecki JA, De Ross A, Lee WJ, Dosemeci M, Lubin JH, Hoppin JA, Blair A, Alavanga MC. 2004. *Cancer incidence among pesticide applicators exposed to atrazine in the agricultural health study. Journal of the National Cancer Institute* 96 (18): 1375-1832.

Sass JB, Colangelo JD. 2006. *European Union bans atrazine, while the United States Negotiates continued use. International Journal of Occupational and Environmental Health* 12:260-267.

Sanjose SD, Benavente Y, Nieters A, Foretova L, Maynadie M, Cocco PL, Staines A, Vornanen M, Boffetta P, Becker N, Alvaro T, Brennan P. 2006. Association between personal use of hair dyes and lymphoid neoplasms in Europe. American Journal of Epidemiology 164: 47-55.

Schenk M, Purdue MP, Colt JS, Hartge P, Blair A, Steward P, Cerhan JR, De Roos AJ, Cozen W, Severson RK. 2009. Occupation/industry and risk of non-Hodgkin's lymphoma in the United States. Occupational and Environmental Medicine 6: 23-31.

Schroeder JC, Olshan AF, Baric R, Dent GA, Weinberg CR, Yount B, Cerhan JR, Lynch CF, Schuman LM, Tolbert PE, Rothman N, Cantor KP, Blair A. 2001. Agricultural risk factors for t(14;18) subtypes of non-Hodgkin's lymphoma. Epidemiology 12(6): 701-709.

Simpkins JW, Swenberg JA, Weiss N, Brusick D, Eldridge JC, Stevens JT, Handa RJ, Hovey RC, Plant TM, Pastoor TP, Breckenridge CB. 2011. Atrazine and breast cancer: A framework assessment of the toxicological and epidemiological evidence. Toxicological Science. Toxicological Sciences 123(2): 441-459.

Smedby KE, Baecklund E, Askling J. 2006. Malignant lymphomas in autoimmunity and inflammation: a review of risks, risk factors and lymphoma characteristics. Cancer Epidemiology, Biomarkers and Prevention 15(11): 2069-2077.

Smedby KE, Hjalgrim H, Chang ET, Rostgaard K, Glimelius B, Adami H, Melbye M. 2007. Childhood social environment and risk of NHL in adults. Cancer Research 67(22): 11074-11082.

Smith MT, Jones RM, Smith AH. 2007. Benzene exposure and risk of NHL. Cancer Epidemiology, Biomarkers and Prevention 16(3): 385-391.

Solley WB, Pierce RR, Perlman HA. 1993. Circular 1081. Estimated Use of Water in the United States in 1990. U.S. Geological Survey: Reston, VA.

Spalding RF, Exner ME. 1993. Occurrence of nitrate in groundwater-a review. Journal of Environmental Quality 22(3): 392-402.

Spalding RF, Exner ME, Snow DD, Cassada DA, Burbach ME, Monson SJ. 2003. Herbicides in ground water beneath Nebraska's Management Systems Evaluation Area. Journal of Environmental Quality 32: 92-99.

Spalding RF, Junk GA, Richard JJ. 1980. Water: Pesticides in ground water beneath irrigated farmland in Nebraska August 1978. Pesticide Monitoring Journal 14(2): 70-73.

Spiegelhalder B, Eisenbrand G, Preussmann R. 1976. Influence of dietary nitrate on nitrite content of the human saliva: possible relevance to in vivo formation of N-nitroso compounds. Food and Cosmetics Toxicology 14:545-548.

Spiegelhalter DJ, Thomas A, Best NG, Lunn D. 2003. WinBUGS-- Version 1.4 User Manual, January 2003, MRC Biostatistics Unit.

Squillace PJ, Scott JC, Moran MJ, Nolan BG, Kolpin DW. 2002. VOCs, pesticides, nitrate and their mixtures in groundwater used for drinking water in the United States. Environmental Science and Technology 36: 1923-1930.

Steinmaus C, Smith AH, Jones RM, Smith MT. 2008. Meta-analysis of benzene exposure and NHL: Biases could mask an important association. Occupational and Environmental Medicine 65: 371-378.

Tannenbaum SR, Weisman M, Fett D. 1976. The effect of nitrate intake on nitrite formation in human saliva. Food and Cosmetics Toxicology 14: 549–552.

Tinker, J.R. 1991. An analysis of nitrateitrogen in ground-water beneath unsewered subdivisions. Groundwater Monitoring and Remediation. 11(1):141-150.

Toccalino PL, Norman JE, Scott JC. 2012. Chemical mixtures in untreated water from public-supply wells in the U. S. - Occurrence, composition, and potential toxicity. Science of the Total Environment 431:262-270.

Tranah GJ, Bracci PM, Holly EA. 2008. Domestic and farm animal exposures and risk of non-Hodgkin's lymphoma in a population based study in the San Francisco Bay area. Cancer Epidemiology, Biomarkers and Prevention 7(9): 2382-2387.

Tricker AR. 1997. N-nitroso compounds and man: sources of exposure, endogenous formation and occurrence in body fluids. European Journal of Cancer Prevention 6:226-268.

(USCS) U.S. Cancer Statistics Working Group. 2000, 2002, 2003, 2005. United States Cancer Statistics: 2002 Incidence and Mortality. Atlanta (GA):Department of Health and Human Services, Centers for Disease Control and Prevention and National Cancer Institute; 2003. Available at www.cdc.gov/cancer/npcr/uscs

(UNL) University of Nebraska-Lincoln. 2000. Quality-assessed Agrichemical Contaminant Database for Nebraska Ground Water. A cooperative project of the Nebraska Departments of Agriculture, Environmental Quality, and Natural Resources and the University of Nebraska -Lincoln. On-line at http://dnrdata.dnr.state.ne.us/clearinghouse/index.asp

(USEPA) United States Environmental Protection Agency. Available at http://www.epa.gov/safewater/contaminants/basicinformation/atrazine.html (accessed 2/16/10)

Vajdic CM, Grulich AE, Kaldor JM, Fritschi L, Benke G, Hughes AM, Kricker A, Turner JJ, Milliken S, Armstrong BK. 2006. Specific infections, infection-related behavior and risk of NHL in adults. Cancer Epidemiology, Biomarkers and Prevention 15(6): 1102-1108.

Vineis P, Miligi L, Costantini AS. 2007. Exposure to solvents and risk of NHL: Cclues on putative mechanisms. Cancer Epidemiology, Biomarkers and Prevention 16(3): 381-384.

Vose JM, Chiu BCH, Cheson BD, Dancey J, Wright J. 2002. Update on epidemiology and therapeutics for non-Hodgkin's lymphoma. Hematology 2002; 241-262 for the American Society of Hematology.

Wang SS, Davis S, Cerhan JR, Hartge P, Severson RK, Cozen W, Lan Q, Welch R, Chanock SJ, Rothman N. 2006. Polymorphisms in oxidative stress genes and risk for NHL. Carcinogenesis 27(9): 1828-1834.

Wang SS, Slater SL, Brennan P, Holly EA, Sanjose SD, Bernstein L et al. 2007a. Family history of hematopoietic malignancies and risk of NHL: a pooled analysis of 10,211 cases and 11,905 controls from the International Lymphoma Epidemiology Consortium (Interlymph). Blood 109(8): 3479-3488.

Wang SS, Cozen W, Cerhan JR, Colt JS, Mortin LM, Engels EA, Davis S, Severson RK, Rothman N, Chanock SJ, Hartge P. 2007b. Immune mechanisms in NHL: joint effects of the TNF G308A and IL10 T3575A polymorphisms with NHL risk factors. Cancer Research 67(10): 5042-5054.

Ward MH, Cerhan JR, Colt JS, Hartge. 2006. Risk of non-Hodgkin lymphoma and nitrate and nitrite from drinking water and diet. Epidemiology 17(4): 375-382.

Ward, MH, deKok TM, Levallois P, Brender J, Gulis G, Nolan BT, VanDerslice J. 2005. Workgroup report: drinking-water nitrate and health – recent findings and research needs. Environmental Health Perspectives 113 (11): 1607-1614.

Ward MH, Mark SD, Cantor KP, Weisenburger DD, Villasenor AC, Zahm SH. 1996. Drinking water nitrate and the risk of non-Hodgkin's lymphoma. Epidemiology 7(5): 465-470.

Ward MH, Zahm SH, Weisenburger DD, Gridley G, Cantor KP, Saal RC, Blair A. 1994. Dietary factors and non-Hodgkin's lymphoma in Nebraska. Cancer Causes and Control 5(5): 422-432.

Wei HR, Rhoades MG, Shea PJ. 2011. Formation, adsorption, and stability of N-nitrosoatrazine in water and soil. Vol. ACS Symposium Series 1086, in It's All in the Water: Studies of Materials and Conditions in Fresh and Salt Water Bodies, edited by Roberts-Kirchohoff ES, Murray MN, Garshott DM Benvenuto MA, 3-19. Washington, DC.: American Chemical Society.

Weisenburger DD. 1990. Environmental epidemiology of non-Hodgkin's lymphoma in eastern Nebraska. American Journal of Industrial Medicine 18:303-305.

Weisenburger, DD 1992. Pathological classification of non-Hodgkin's lymphoma for epidemiological studies. Cancer Research (Suppl) 52: 5456s-5464s.

Weisenberger DD, Hickman TI, Patil KD, Lawson TA, and Mirvish SS. 1990. Carcinogenesis tests of atrazine and N-nitrosoatrazine compounds of special interest to the Midwest. Proceedings of the American Association for Cancer Research 31: 102.

Weisenburger DD, Joshi SS, Hickman TI, Babcock DM, Walker BA, and Mirvish SS. 1987. N-nitrosoatrazine (NNAT). Synthesis, chemical properties, acute toxicity and mutagenicity. Proceedings of the American Association for Cancer Research 28: 103.

Weyer PJ, Cerhan JR, Kross BC, Hallberg GR, Kantamneni J, Breuer G, Jones MP, Zheng W, Lynch CF. 2001. Municipal drinking water nitrate level and cancer risk in older women: the Iowa women's health study. Epidemiology 11(3): 327-338.

Wolfe NL, Zepp RG, Gordon JA, Fincher RC. 1976. N-nitrosamine formation from Atrazine. Bulletin of Environmental Contamination and Toxicology 15(3): 342-347.

World Health Organization: WHO food additives series: 50 Nitrate (and potential endogenous formation of N-nitroso compounds) http://www.inchem.org/documents/jecfa/jecmono/v50je06.htm

World Health Organization: WHO/HSE/WSH/10.01/11 Atrazine and its metabolism in drinking water. Background document for development of WHO Guidelines for Drinking-water Quality. World Health Organization 2010.

Young JC, Khan SU. 1978. Kinetics of nitrosation of the herbicide glyphosate. Journal of Environmental Science and Health Part B: Pesticides, Food Contaminants and Agricultural Waste 13(1): 59-72.

Zahm SH, Weisenburger DD, Cantor KP, Holmes FF, Blair A. 1993a. Role of the herbicide atrazine in the development of non-Hodgkin's lymphoma. Scandinavian Journal of Work and Environmental Health 19:108-114.

Zahm SH, Weisenburger DD, Saal RC, Vaught JB, Babbitt PA, Blair A. 1993b. The role of agricultural pesticide use in the development of non-Hodgkin's lymphoma in women. Archives of Environmental Health 48(5): 353-358.

Zhang S, Hunter DJ, Rosner BA, Colditz GA, Fuchs CS, Speizer FE, Willett WC. 1999. Dietary fat and protein in relation to risk of non-Hodgkin's lymphoma among women. Journal of the National Cancer Institute 91(20): 1751-1758.

Zhang Y, Holford TR, Leaderer B, Boyle P, Zahm SH, Flynn S, Tallini G, Owens PH, Zheng T. 2004. Hair-coloring product use and risk of non-Hodgkin's lymphoma: a population based case-control study in Connecticut. American Journal of Epidemiology 159: 148-154.

Zhang Y, Holford TR, Leaderer, Boyle P, Zahm SH, Flynn S, Tallini G, Owens PH, Zheng T. 2007. UV radiation exposure and risk of non-Hodgkin's lymphoma. American Journal of Epidemiology 165: 255-1264.

Zhang Y, Sanjose SD, Bracci PM, Morton LM, Wang R, Brennan P, Hartge P, Boffetta P, Becker N, Maynaidie M, Foretova L, Cocco P, Staines A, Holford T, Holly EA, Nieters A, Benavente Y, Bernstein L, Zahm SH, Zheng T. 2008. Personal use of hair dye and the risk of certain subtypes of NHL. American Journal of Epidemiology 167: 1321-1331.

Zhao Y, Boyd JM, Woodbeck M, Andrews RC, Qin F, Hrudey SE, Li X. 2008. Formation of N-nitrosamines from eleven disinfection treatments of seven different surface waters. Journal of Environmental Science and Technology 42:4857-4862.

Comparative Effectiveness of Fluoropyrimidine-based Chemotherapy in Elderly Medicare Patients Diagnosed with Metastatic Colorectal Cancer

Sacha Satram-Hoang, Carolina Reyes, Edward McKenna, Khang Q. Hoang

1 Introduction

Colorectal cancer (CRC) is the third most frequently diagnosed cancer as well as the third leading cause of cancer mortality in men and women in the United States (US) (Siegel, Naishadham, & Jemal, 2012). Incidence increases with age, with about 70% of patients diagnosed over the age of 65; 40% are 75 years or older (Howlader *et al.*, 2011). Roughly 20% of CRC patients present with metastatic disease and have a 5-year survival rate of 12% (Howlader *et al.*, 2011).

Treatment of patients with advanced or metatstatic CRC (mCRC) is palliative and mostly consists of systemic chemotherapy. For several decades, the mainstay of systemic treatment was fluoropyrimidines (FP) administered as monotherapy or in combination with leucovorin (LV) or newer agents such as irinotecan (IFL) and oxaliplatin (Douillard, Bennouna, & Senellart, 2008; Koukourakis *et al.*, 2008). Clinical trials and meta-analyses demonstrate that 5-fluorouracil (5-FU) and LV (5-FU/LV) improve response rates (RR) and survival among patients with mCRC (Douillard *et al.*, 2008; Thirion *et al.*, 2004). Randomized controlled trials have also established the efficacy of 5-FU/LV plus oxaliplatin (FOLFOX) with significant improvements in RR and progression-free survival (PFS) when administered as first-line therapy for patients with advanced CRC (Goldberg *et al.*, 2006).

Capecitabine (CAP) is an oral fluoropyrimidine that is converted to 5-FU. Two randomized, non-blinded phase 3 trials compared single-agent CAP with 5-FU/LV as first-line therapy of patients with mCRC and established that CAP was at least as active as 5-FU/LV in achieving an objective tumor RR, (Braun *et al.*, 2004; Van Cutsem *et al.*, 2001) and PFS and OS were equivalent between treatment arms in a prospective pooled analysis of 2 similarly designed phase 3 trials (Van Cutsem *et al.*, 2004). CAP plus oxaliplatin (CAPOX) have demonstrated clinical activity in multiple clinical trials as first-line treatment for patients with mCRC (J. Cassidy, Clarke, & Diaz-Rubio, 2006; Comella, Massidda, *et al.*, 2005; Comella, Natale, *et al.*, 2005; Diaz-Rubio *et al.*, 2007; Ducreux *et al.*; Goldberg *et al.*, 2004; Porschen *et al.*, 2007; Welles L, 2004) and provide comparable clinical outcomes to FOLFOX (J. Cassidy *et al.*, 2011; Ducreux *et al.*) and infusional 5-FU/oxaliplatin (Arkenau *et al.*, 2008).

Historically, elderly patients have been underrepresented in clinical trials with only one-quarter to one-third of potentially eligible older patients enrolled in cancer clinical trials (Hutchins, Unger, Crowley, Coltman, & Albain, 1999; Murthy, Krumholz, & Gross, 2004; Townsley, Selby, & Siu, 2005). This presents a significant challenge to efforts to evaluate treatment efficacy and safety in elderly patients (Townsley *et al.*, 2005). Furthermore, there is limited knowledge about the use of recommended newer agents for the treatment of mCRC in community settings, particularly for older and demographically diverse patient populations (Chagpar *et al.*, 2012). However, there is evidence to suggest variations in the management of patients with all stages of CRC with several studies reporting lower rates of chemotherapy for older patients (Ayanian *et al.*, 2003; Chagpar *et al.*, 2012; Kahn *et al.*, 2010; O'Grady *et al.*, 2011; Schrag, Cramer, Bach, & Begg, 2001) and almost 30% of stage III and IV patients were less likely to receive guideline-recommended therapies (O'Grady *et al.*, 2011). An analysis of patients in the National Cancer Data Base who were treated for CRC from 2003 to 2007 revealed that 25.9% of patients with stage IV disease received no chemotherapy and older patients with pre-existing comorbid conditions were at increased risk of under-treatment (Chagpar *et al.*, 2012). Comorbid health conditions and older age appear to influence physicians' choice of treatment regimen for all stages of CRC with older patients more likely to receive shorter chemotherapy regimens with less toxicity (Ayanian *et al.*, 2003; Chagpar *et al.*, 2012; Kahn *et al.*, 2010; O'Grady *et al.*, 2011; Schrag, Cramer, *et al.*, 2001).

With an increasingly aging population, the number of patients presenting with CRC over the age of 70 is expected to rise. In light of this as well as the need for comparative effectiveness research in this area, it is important to understand the benefits of these newer therapeutic agents in the real-world setting. The objectives of this study were to evaluate treatment patterns, OS, and frequency of complications requiring medical resource utilization in older, demographically diverse patients undergoing treatment for mCRC.

2   Methods

2.1   Data Sources

Population-based claims data from the Surveillance, Epidemiology, and End Results (SEER)–Medicare linked database were utilized. The SEER-Medicare database is a collaborative effort of the National Cancer Institute, the SEER registries, and the Centers for Medicare & Medicaid Services (CMS). As detailed elsewhere (Warren, Klabunde, Schrag, Bach, & Riley, 2002), this database provides information on Medicare patients included in SEER, a collection of 18 population-based cancer registries of incident cases from diverse geographic areas representative of approximately 28% of the US population. All incident cancer patients reported to SEER registries are cross-matched with a master file of Medicare enrollment (Potosky, Riley, Lubitz, Mentnech, & Kessler, 1993). Approximately 97% of persons 65 years or older are eligible for Medicare with all beneficiaries eligible for Part A coverage including inpatient care, skilled nursing, home healthcare and hospice care. Approximately 95% of beneficiaries also subscribe to Part B, which covers physician services and outpatient care. The SEER-Medicare linkage includes all Medicare-eligible persons in the SEER database through 2007 and their Medicare claims for Part A (inpatient care) and Part B (outpatient and physician services) through 2009.

Institutional review board approval for this study was waived because the SEER-Medicare database does not include personal identifiers.

2.2 Study Design

This was an observational retrospective cohort analysis of incident CRC cases receiving treatment in routine clinical oncology practice.

2.3 Study Population

Eligibility criteria for study inclusion included: (1) a first primary diagnosis of stage IIIB, IIIC, or IV CRC from January 1, 2000 through December 31, 2007, (2) age ≥ 66 years, (3) treatment with any oral or infused chemotherapy after diagnosis, and (4) survival time ≥ 60 days following the date of first-line chemotherapy initiation. Patients were eliminated whose survival was less than 60 days to minimize the introduction of immortal-time bias into the analyses. (Suissa, 2008) Patients were also excluded if their date of death was recorded prior to or in the same month as diagnosis, enrollment in Medicare Parts A and B for less than 12 months before the diagnosis date, enrollment in a health maintenance organization (HMO) for any period of the 12 months prior to diagnosis (because data were unavailable for this time), 2 or more claims for chemotherapy prior to diagnosis (to ensure that the cases were previously untreated) and finally, cases were excluded if they underwent primary resection of the tumor prior to initiating chemotherapy (to eliminate potential adjuvant cases). Of the patients receiving treatment with 5-FU/LV, FOLFOX, CAP and CAPOX in the final cohort, 1,681 were excluded due to having surgery prior to initiating chemotherapy, and of these 908 had stage IV disease. The final analytical cohort contained 4250 patients who received treatment with 5-FU/LV (n=2213), FOLFOX (n=1298), CAP (n=617), and CAPOX (n=122). See Figure 1 for schematic of inclusion/exclusion process.

2.4 Study Variables

2.4.1 Demographic Characteristics

The SEER program routinely collects data on patient demographics including age, race/ethnicity, residence, and socioeconomic status (income and education). Patient age at diagnosis was stratified into four groups: 66 - 70; 71 - 75; 76 - 80; and >80. Race/ethnicity was defined using the SEER recoded race variable and categorized into three mutually exclusive groups White, non-White, and Other/Unknown. Median annual household income at the census tract level and percentage of the adult population who completed specific levels of education at the zip code level were used as a proxy for socioeconomic status.

2.4.2 Clinical Characteristics

The SEER program also collects data on primary tumor site, tumor morphology, and disease stage. SEER site codes identified colon (18.0 to 18.9) and rectum (19.9 and 20.9) cancer cases. The American Joint Committee on Cancer (AJCC) classification scheme encompasses all aspects of cancer distribution in terms of primary tumor size and invasiveness (T), regional lymph nodes involvement (N) and if distant metastasis is present (M). The AJCC classification scheme uses a combination of pathologic and clinical information to derive best stage and include all information available through completion of surgery. Patients were classified into the following categories for metastatic disease: IIIB, IIIC, and IV. Stage IIIB and IIIC cases noted here reflect patients who underwent definitive locoregional treatment after initial treatment with chemotherapy.

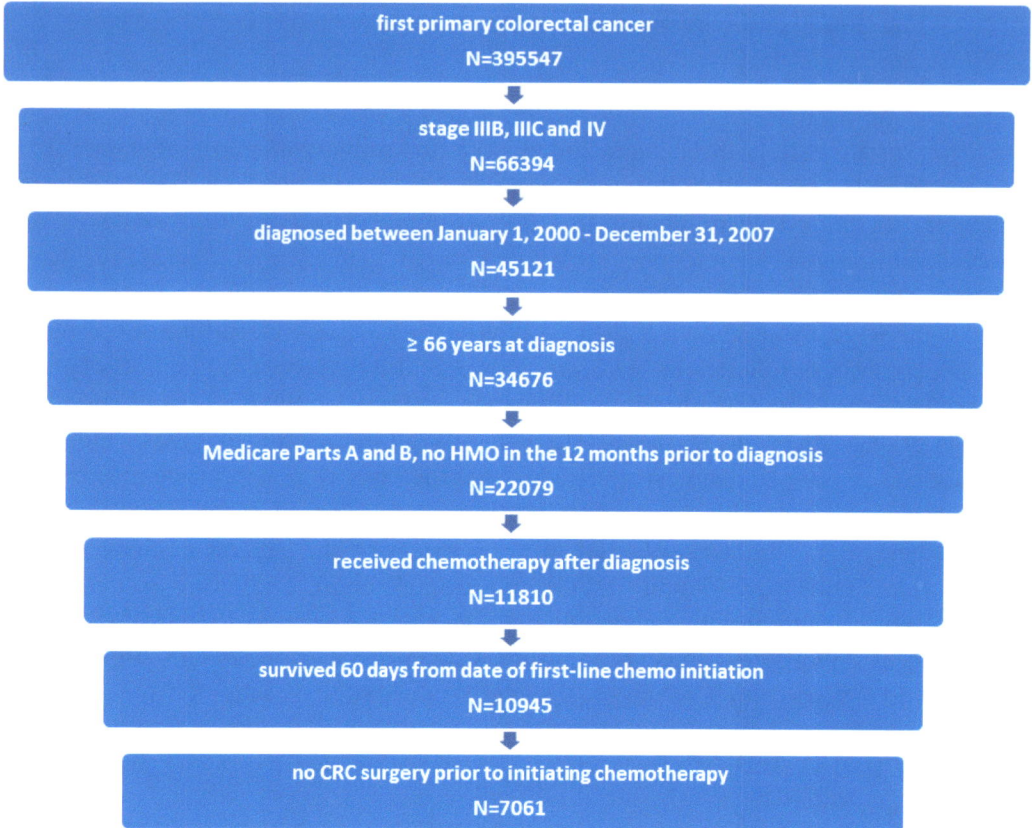

first primary colorectal cancer
N=395547

stage IIIB, IIIC and IV
N=66394

diagnosed between January 1, 2000 - December 31, 2007
N=45121

≥ 66 years at diagnosis
N=34676

Medicare Parts A and B, no HMO in the 12 months prior to diagnosis
N=22079

received chemotherapy after diagnosis
N=11810

survived 60 days from date of first-line chemo initiation
N=10945

no CRC surgery prior to initiating chemotherapy
N=7061

Figure 1: Schematic of Inclusion/Exclusion Process.

The National Cancer Institute (NCI) comorbidity index (Klabunde, Legler, Warren, Baldwin, & Schrag, 2007) was calculated for each patient using diagnosis and procedure codes in the Medicare Parts A (inpatient) and B (physician/outpatient) claims files to identify the 15 non-cancer comorbidities from the Charlson Comorbidity Index (CCI). (Charlson, Pompei, Ales, & MacKenzie, 1987) A weight is assigned to each condition based on its potential influence on 2-year mortality, and the weights are summed to obtain a comorbidity index for each patient. The NCI comorbidity index accounts for the number and severity of the conditions with higher scores indicating a greater burden of comorbid disease.

2.4.3   Treatment

Medicare claims identified patients who underwent primary resection of the tumor prior to initiating chemotherapy. Surgical procedures included hemicolectomy, subtotal colectomy, and total colectomy. To identify claims for chemotherapy administration, (Warren, Harlan, *et al.*, 2002) data were abstracted from 4 merged SEER-Medicare claims files including (1) Medicare provider analysis and review (MEDPAR), (2) carrier claims from the National Claims History (NCH), (3) outpatient claims (OUTSAF), and (4) durable medical equipment (DME). Claims for oral equivalents of intravenous chemotherapies (ie, capecitabine) were identified in the DME file. Chemotherapy agents were characterized and quantified using International Classification of Disease (ICD) diagnosis codes, ICD procedural codes, Current Procedural Terminology (CPT) codes, Healthcare Common Procedural Coding System (HCPCS) codes, and revenue center codes. Chemotherapy claims were searched for specific drug codes to identify the type of chemotherapy used. The absence of these claims indicated lack of treatment. The first chemotherapy claim following diagnosis indicated the start of therapy. Patients were classified into 1 of 4 treatment groups (5-FU/LV, CAP, FOLFOX, and CAPOX) based on all chemotherapy administered during the first 60 days after treatment initiation. Duration of first-line treatment was defined as time from date of first chemotherapy claim to 30 days following last administration of first-line agent, or to the day prior to second-line treatment initiation or 30 days following last administration of first-line agent if gap in therapy is >90 days. A second-line therapy occurred when a new agent not given in the first-line regimen begins, or if there was a gap of >90days between successive chemotherapy claims.

2.4.4   Treatment Complications

The incidence of specific treatment-related complications (anemia, neutropenia, nausea/vomiting, diarrhea, and dehydration) requiring medical resource utilization (were assessed 180 days following treatment initiation. This 180-day period was selected as appropriate based on the National Comprehensive Cancer Network (NCCN) guidelines that recommend 6 months of adjuvant treatment for stage II and III CRC or for stage IV stable disease (NCCN, 2012). Anemia was defined by the condition specific ICD-9 diagnosis codes, a revenue center code or HCPCS code for a red blood cell transfusion, or a revenue center code or J-code for an erythropoiesis stimulating agent. Other treatment complications were defined using the condition specific ICD-9 codes in both inpatient and outpatient Medicare claims records.

2.4.5   Mortality and Censoring

The date of death was determined by using the Medicare date or the SEER date of death if the Medicare date was missing. All other patients were assumed to be alive at the end of the follow-up period on December 31, 2009, although they may have been censored earlier for other reasons such as development of a second primary cancer or Medicare claims no longer available.

2.5   Statistical Analysis

All statistical analyses were performed using SAS software, version 9.1.3 (SAS Institute Inc., Cary, North Carolina). Statistical comparisons were made between 5-FU/LV vs. CAP, and FOLFOX vs. CAPOX. Descriptive statistics were calculated for demographic and clinical variables, and treatment patterns. Differences between treatment groups were evaluated with chi-square tests for categorical variables and analysis of variance or t-test for continuous variables. A p-value < 0.05 was considered statistically significant.

Kaplan-Meier survival curves and corresponding log-rank tests were generated to determine unadjusted OS by treatment type. In the multivariate survival models to assess overall risk of death, two approaches were used as a sensitivity exercise: (1) multivariate Cox proportional hazards regression and (2) propensity score-weighted Cox proportional hazards regression. In the first model, adjustment for confounders that were selected from demographic and clinical characteristics using the backward elimination strategy-a stepwise removal of covariates in the full model until only the significant variables remain (Greenland, 1998). In the second model, multinomial logistic regression was used to calculate a propensity score for each individual. The propensity score is the conditional probability of each patient receiving a specific treatment based on baseline characteristics (Kurth *et al.*, 2006). The effect of the propensity score weights was to balance the groups to reduce potential bias associated with treatment selection. A propensity score-weighted Cox proportional hazards regression model was fitted to compare overall survival between treatment groups. Follow-up was calculated beginning on the date of treatment initiation up until the first occurrence of a censoring event: date of death, development of a second primary tumor, last date for which Medicare claims were available, or last date of the follow-up period (December 31, 2009).

3   Results

3.1   Treatment Patterns

Of the 7,061 patients who met all study inclusion criteria, 2213 were treated with 5-FU/LV, 1298 received FOLFOX, 617 were administered CAP, and 122 received CAPOX. Of the remaining 2,811 patients, about 28% received irinotecan-based therapy, 57% received other types of chemotherapy, and 15% received an unknown type of chemotherapy. Use of CAP, CAPOX, and FOLFOX increased over time while treatment with 5-FU/LV decreased during the same time period.

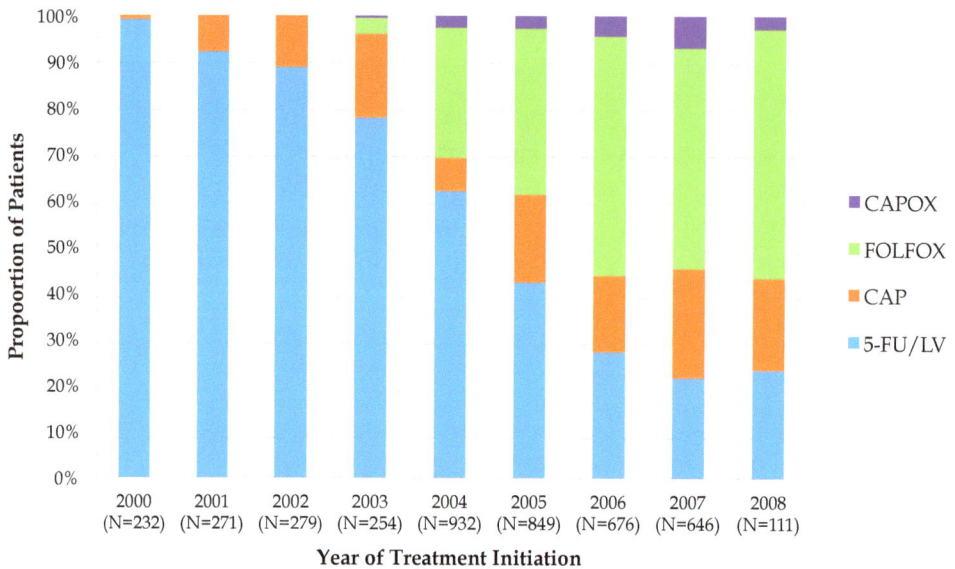

Figure 2: Distribution of Therapy by Year of Initiation.

The mean time to initiation of chemotherapy following diagnosis was slightly longer for patient receiving CAP (mean 81 days after diagnosis) compared to patients receiving 5FU/LV (74 days after diagnosis) and similar between patient receiving CAPOX and FOLFOX (mean 77-78 days after diagnosis) (Table 1).

Treatment	N	Time to Treatment [1], days				P-value
		Mean	SD	Median	Range	
CAP	545	80.68	34.93	74	7 - 179	<0.0001
5FU/LV	2117	73.80	29.63	69	1 - 177	
CAPOX	120	77.11	33.68	72	15 - 175	0.8811
FOLFOX	1255	77.53	29.18	72	14 - 175	

Table 1: Time to first-line treatment.

The mean duration of treatment (Table 2) was longer for those administered 5-FU/LV (147 days) compared with 128 days for the CAP group ($p < 0.0001$) while there was no significant difference in duration of treatment with CAPOX (143 days) and FOLFOX (151 days; $p = 0.2335$).

Treatment	N	Duration of Treatment [2], days				P-value
		Mean	SD	Median	Range	
CAP	603	128.41	76.91	118	30 - 357	<0.0001
5FU/LV	2140	147.48	75.01	143	30 - 365	
CAPOX	119	143.43	64.45	141	31 - 300	0.2335
FOLFOX	1285	150.93	65.78	157	30 - 360	

Table 2: Duration of first-line treatment.

3.2 Demographic and Socioeconomic Characteristics

Overall, 44% of the cohort were older than 75 years, the majority were female (54%), white (84%) and residing in the southern part of the U.S. (Table 3). In general, older patients were more likely to receive CAP (mean age: 78 years) and 5-FU/LV (mean age: 76 years) while patients receiving CAPOX (74 years) and FOLFOX (73 years) were slightly younger. Sixty-two percent of patients receiving CAP were over the age of 75 compared to 48% of 5-FU/LV patients, while 40% of those receiving treatment with CAPOX were over 75 compared to 30% in the FOLFOX group. A higher proportion of females were receiving treatment with CAP compared to 5-FU/LV. Higher rates of treatment with CAP and CAPOX were evident for patients

---

[1] Time to treatment initiation defined as "time from diagnosis" to "date of first chemotherapy claim".

[2] Duration of treatment defined as time from date of first chemotherapy claim to 30 days following last administration of first-line agent, or to the day prior to second-line treatment initiation or 30 days following last administration of first-line agent if gap in therapy is >90 days.

residing in the West and those with higher levels of income and education compared with patients administered 5-FU/LV and FOLFOX, respectively.

Char.	TOTAL (N = 4250) n (%)	CAP (N = 617) n (%)	5-FU/LV (N = 2,213) n (%)	P-value	CAPOX (N = 122) n (%)	FOLFOX (N = 1,298) n (%)	P-value
Age							
66-70	1137 (26.8)	96 (15.6)	503 (22.7)	<.0001	43 (35.2)	495 (38.1)	0.0924
71-75	1227 (28.9)	137 (22.2)	641 (29.0)		30 (24.6)	419 (32.3)	
76-80	1085 (25.5)	160 (25.9)	591 (26.7)		38 (31.1)	296 (22.8)	
> 80	801 (18.8)	224 (36.3)	478 (21.6)		11 (9.0)	88 (6.8)	
Sex							
Male	1960 (46.1)	243 (39.4)	1029 (46.5)	0.0017	56 (45.9)	632 (48.7)	0.5557
Female	2290 (53.9)	374 (60.6)	1184 (53.5)		66 (54.1)	666 (51.3)	
Race / ethnicity							
White	3583 (84.3)	499 (80.9)	1850 (83.6)	0.1115	104 (85.2)	1130 (87.1)	0.5708
Non-White	667 (15.7)	118 (19.1)	363 (16.4)		18 (14.8)	168 (12.9)	
Geographic region							
Midwest	519 (12.2)	81 (13.1)	261 (11.8)	0.0001	17 (13.9)[3]	170 (13.1)	<.0001
Northeast	274 (6.4)	34 (5.5)	145 (6.6)			85 (6.5)	
South	1950 (45.9)	251 (40.7)	1102 (49.8)		30 (24.6)	567 (43.7)	
West	1507 (35.5)	251 (40.7)	705 (31.9)		75 (61.5)	476 (36.7)	
Median income quartiles							
1-Low	1059 (24.9)	130 (21.1)	576 (26.0)	0.0002	21 (17.2)	334 (25.7)	0.1633
2	1060 (24.9)	145 (23.5)	559 (25.3)		35 (28.7)	319 (24.6)	
3	1059 (24.9)	146 (23.7)	557 (25.2)		30 (24.6)	325 (25.0)	
4-High	1057 (24.9)	195 (31.6)	509 (23.0)		36 (29.5)	318 (24.5)	
Education							
	Mean (95% CI)	Mean (95% CI)	Mean (95% CI)	P-value	Mean (95% CI)	Mean (95% CI)	P-value
Less than high school, %	19.3 (18.9-19.6)	18.7 (17.7 - 19.8)	20.0 (19.5 - 20.5)	0.0298	17.1 (14.8 - 19.4)	18.5 (17.9 - 19.2)	0.1966
High school only, %	28.1 (27.8 - 28.3)	26.7 (25.9 - 27.4)	28.7 (28.3 - 29.1)	<.0001	23.1 (21.4 - 24.9)	28.1 (27.5 - 28.6)	<.0001
Some colleges, %	27.5 (27.3 -27.7)	27.5 (26.9 - 28.0)	27.1 (26.9 - 27.4)	0.3359	28.6 (27.3 - 29.9)	28.0 (27.7 - 28.4)	0.4058
At least a college degree, %	25.2 (24.7 - 25.6)	27.1 (25.8 - 28.5)	24.2 (23.6 - 4.8)	<.0001	31.2 (28.0 - 34.4)	25.4 (24.5 - 26.3)	0.0002

Table 3: Baseline demographic and socioeconomic characteristics.

3.3 Clinical Characteristics

Compared with patients administered 5-FU/LV, patients treated with CAP were diagnosed with stage IIIB/C disease, higher number of positive lymph nodes and higher tumor grade. A higher proportion of patients treated with CAPOX had stage IV disease compared with those treated with FOLFOX (Table 4).

---

[3] Cells with counts of less than 11 are combined in compliance with the National Cancer Institute data use agreement for small cell sizes.

Char.	TOTAL (N = 4250) n (%)	CAP (N = 617) n (%)	5-FU/LV (N = 2,213) n (%)	P-value	CAPOX (N = 122) n (%)	FOLFOX (N = 1,298) n (%)	P-value
Stage							
Stage IIIB/C	2449 (57.6)	381 (61.8)	1027 (46.4)	<.0001	79 (64.8)	962 (74.1)	0.0254
Stage IV	1801 (42.4)	236 (38.2)	1186 (53.6)		43 (35.2)	336 (25.9)	
Positive lymph nodes							
0	348 (8.2)	46 (7.5)	232 (10.5)	0.0348	66 (54.1) [4]	66 (5.1)	0.6125
1-3	2091 (49.2)	310 (50.2)	1052 (47.5)			667 (51.4)	
≥ 4	1599 (23.7)	239 (38.7)	785 (35.4)		56 (45.8) [4]	521 (40.1)	
Unknown	212 (13.9)	22 (3.6)	144 (6.5)			44 (3.4)	
Tumor grade							
Grade 1	205 (4.8)	33 (5.3)	96 (4.3)	0.0145	81 (66.4) [4]	69 (5.3)	0.9117
Grade 2	2612 (61.5)	351 (56.9)	1397 (63.1)			790 (60.9)	
Grade 3	1215 (28.6)	189 (30.6)	617 (27.9)			373 (28.7)	
Grade 4	79 (1.9)	18 (2.9)	33 (1.5)		41 (33.6) [4]	27 (2.1)	
Unknown	139 (3.3)	26 (4.2)	70 (3.2)			39 (3.0)	
NCI comorbidity score							
0	2529 (59.5)	338 (54.8)	1307 (59.1)	0.1999	78 (63.9)	806 (62.1)	0.9469
1	1109 (26.1)	173 (28.0)	562 (25.4)		32 (26.2)	342 (26.3)	
2	378 (8.9)	60 (9.7)	213 (9.6)		12 (9.9) [4]	97 (7.5)	
≥ 3	234 (5.5)	46 (7.5)	131 (5.9)			53 (4.1)	

Table 4: Baseline clinical characteristics.

Complications	CAP (N = 617) n	%	5-FU/LV (N = 2,213) n	%	p-value	CAPOX (N = 122) n	%	FOLFOX (N = 1,298) n	%	p-value
None	511	82.8	1012	45.7	< 0.0001	53	43.4	326	25.1	< 0.0001
Anemia	80	13.0	879	39.7	<.0001	38	31.1	699	53.9	<.0001
Nausea/vomiting	24	3.9	453	20.5	<.0001	36	29.5	494	38.1	<.0001
Diarrhea	18	2.9	157	7.1	<.0001	-4	-4	89	6.9	<.0001
Neutropenia	-4	-4	13	0.6	0.0013	-4	-4	121	9.3	<.0001
Thrombocytopenia	-4	-4	13	0.6	0.0013	-4	-4	42	3.2	<.0001
Dehydration	-4	-4	52	2.3	<.0001	-4	-4	108	8.3	<.0001

Table 5: Incidence of Medical Resource Utilization Related Treatment Complications Requiring Intervention (Hospitalization or Treatment) within 180 Days after Initiation of Treatment.

---

[4] Cells with counts of less than 11 are combined in compliance with the National Cancer Institute data use agreement for small cell sizes.

3.4   Complications Requiring Medical Resource Utilization

Table 5 shows the overall rate of complications requiring medical resource utilization within 180 days after treatment initiation were higher for patients treated with 5-FU/LV (54.3%) and FOLFOX (74.9%) compared with CAP (17.2%) and CAPOX (56.6%), respectively ($P < 0.0001$ for both comparisons). The three most frequent complications requiring medical resource utilization were anemia, nausea/vomiting, and diarrhea with significantly higher rates for 5-FU/LV vs. CAP and FOLFOX vs. CAPOX ($P < 0.0001$ for all comparisons).

3.5   Overall Survival

The median survival time was 32.6 months (95% CI, 28.1-38.8) in the CAP group and 31.9 months (95% CI, 29.1-34.9) in the 5-FU/LV group (log rank $p = 0.6683$).

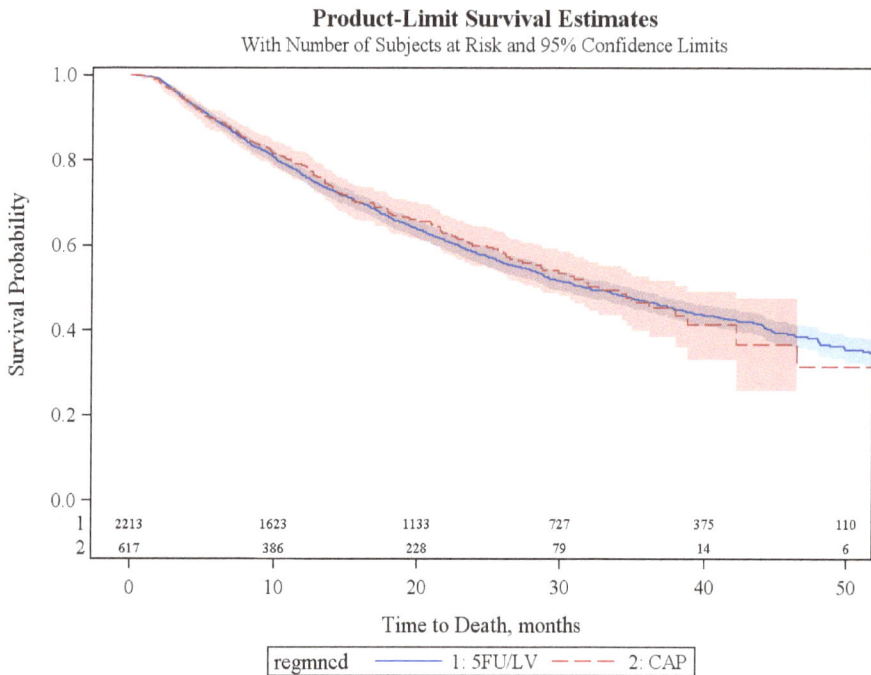

Figure 3: Kaplan Meier Curve of Overall Survival by Treatment (CAP vs. 5FU/LV).

The multivariate Cox regression survival analysis revealed no significant differences in risk of death between CAP compared with 5-FU/LV (HR, 0.94; 95% CI, 0.89-1.23). This finding was confirmed in the propensity weighted Cox regression. Age, stage IV disease, greater number of positive lymph nodes, higher tumor grade, higher comorbidity score and lower income levels were identified as significant predictors of mortality in the adjusted model (Table 6). We conducted a sensitivity analysis keeping the 439 5-FU/LV and 197 CAP stage IV disease patients who were excluded due to having surgery prior to chemotherapy initiation and confirmed very similar findings in the multivariate Cox regression analysis (HR, 0.99; 95% CI, 0.91-1.20).

Covariates	N	Unadjusted Model		Adjusted Model[5]		Propensity Score-Weighted Model[6]	
		HR	95% CI	HR	95% CI	HR	95% CI
Treatment							
5-FU/LV (ref)	2213	1.00		1.00		1.00	
CAP	617	0.97	0.84 - 1.11	0.94	0.89 - 1.23	0.98	0.88-1.29
Age							
66-70 (ref)	599	1.00		1.00			
71-75	778	1.12	0.97 - 1.30	1.19	1.02 - 1.37		
76-80	751	1.27	1.10 - 1.47	1.39	1.20 - 1.61		
> 80	702	1.45	1.25 - 1.68	1.68	1.45 - 1.96		
Sex							
Male(ref)	1272	1.00					
Female	1558	0.94	0.85 - 1.04				
Race/ethnicity							
White(ref)	2349	1.00					
Non-White	481	0.98	0.86 - 1.12				
Stage							
Stage III(ref)	1408	1.00		1.00			
Stage IV	1422	4.44	3.93 – 5.01	4.56	3.97 - 5.24		
Positive lymph nodes							
0 (ref)	278	1.00		1.00			
1-3	1362	0.73	0.62 - 0.86	1.42	1.19 - 1.69		
≥ 4	1024	1.34	1.13 - 1.58	2.02	1.71 - 2.40		
Tumor grade							
1-3 (ref)	1877	1.00		1.00			
3-4	857	1.32	1.19 - 1.47	1.24	1.11 - 1.38		
NCI comorbidity score							
0 (ref)	1645	1.00		1.00			
1	735	1.06	0.94 - 1.19	1.08	0.95 - 1.21		
≥ 2	450	1.07	0.92 - 1.23	1.23	1.06 - 1.43		
Treatment Initiation							
2000-2004 (ref)	1672	1.00					
2005-2009	1158	0.46	0.41 – 0.53				
Geographic region							
Midwest (ref)	342	1.00					
Northeast	179	0.85	0.67 - 1.09				
South	1353	0.86	0.74 - 1.01				
West	956	0.97	0.82 - 1.14				
Median income quartiles							
1-Low (ref)	768	1.00		1.00			
2	720	0.94	0.81 - 1.07	0.95	0.83 - 1.10		
3	656	0.91	0.79 - 1.04	0.91	0.79 – 1.05		
4-High	673	0.96	0.83 - 1.10	0.85	0.74 – 0.98		

Table 6: Cox Regression Models of Overall Survival (CAP vs. 5-FU/LV).

---

[5] Reduced model by backward elimination; full model included treatment, age, sex, race, stage, positive lymph nodes, tumor grade, comorbidity score, treatment initiation year, geographic region, and income.

[6] Propensity score weighted for age, sex, race, stage, positive lymph nodes, tumor grade, comorbidity score, treatment initiation year, geographic region, and income.

While the median survival time was not reached, the three-year unadjusted survival rates for CAPOX and FOLFOX were 71.6% (95% CI, 54.1-83.3) and 68.5% (95% CI, 64.2-72.3), respectively (log rank $P = 0.6737$).

There were no significant differences in adjusted overall survival between CAPOX and FOLFOX (HR, 0.88; 95% CI, 0.56 – 1.37). The propensity weighted Cox regression analysis also confirmed these findings (Table 7). Age, stage, tumor grade and year of treatment initiation were independent predictors of mortality and after backwards elimination, these covariates maintained statistical significance in the model, adjusting for all other variables. After adjustment, NCI comorbidity score of 1 showed prognostic significance in survival with a 43% higher mortality risk compared to patients with an NCI comorbidity score of 0. We also conducted a sensitivity analysis keeping the 225 FOLFOX and 47 CAPOX stage IV disease patients who were excluded due to undergoing surgery prior to chemotherapy initiation and confirmed almost identical risk ratios in the multivariate Cox regression analysis (HR, 0.87; 95% CI, 0.62-1.22).

4   Discussion

This population-based retrospective cohort analysis of elderly patients in community settings revealed similar benefits in overall survival and complications requiring medical resource utilization as compared to younger patients in clinical trial settings (Cartwright, 2012; C. J. Twelves et al., 2005). Clinical trials confirm that therapy with agents including 5-FU, oxaliplatin, capecitabine, and oxaliplatin are associated with improved survival of patients with stage III and IV mCRC (Braun et al., 2004; J. Cassidy et al., 2006; J. Cassidy et al., 2011; J. Cassidy et al., 2004; Comella, Massidda, et al., 2005; Comella, Natale, et al., 2005; de Gramont et al., 2000; Diaz-Rubio et al., 2007; Douillard et al., 2008; Ducreux et al.; Giacchetti et al., 2000; Grothey, Sargent, Goldberg, & Schmoll, 2004; investigators, 1995; Koukourakis et al., 2008; Moertel et al., 1995; O'Connell et al., 1997; Porschen et al., 2007; Thirion et al., 2004; Van Cutsem et al., 2001; Welles L, 2004; Wolmark et al., 1993). Patient characteristics such as age, gender, race, and comorbidity burden, appear to be important factors in prescribing chemotherapy treatment, but after adjusting for these factors in the multivariate survival analyses, there were no significant differences in OS between the CAP-based and 5-FU/LV-based regimens. This is an encouraging finding for all patients diagnosed with advanced stage CRC, suggesting that currently available and recommended systemic therapies are equally effective for patients with diverse clinical and demographic characteristics.

In the present study, patients treated with CAP were the oldest, and had more comorbidities, compared to other treatment groups. Provided that treatment efficacy is not compromised, the elderly patient may prefer oral chemotherapy due to the convenience in administration, concerns over infusion-related problems, as well as limited mobility and access to transportation (Borner et al., 2002; Liu, Franssen, Fitch, & Warner, 1997). Even if patients receive their chemotherapy through an ambulatory pump, they still experience discomfort, potential complications (including deep-vein thrombosis), and the need to have a malfunctioning pump replaced (Chu et al., 2012). Physicians may also perceive the option of an oral chemotherapy to be of value to elderly patients and tend to weigh the short remaining natural life expectancy of these patients against the potential benefits of more aggressive treatment (Castiglione, Gelber, & Goldhirsch, 1990). Further, there is a belief among physicians that el-

Covariates	N	Unadjusted Model		Adjusted Model[7]		Propensity Score-Weighted Model[8]	
		HR	95% CI	HR	95% CI	HR	95% CI
Treatment							
FOLFOX (ref)	1298	1.00		1.00		1.00	
CAPOX	122	0.97	0.63 - 1.50	0.88	0.56 - 1.37	0.93	0.60 – 1.43
Age							
66-70 (ref)	538	1.00		1.00			
71-75	449	1.02	0.77 - 1.36	1.11	0.84 - 1.48		
76-80	334	1.16	0.86 - 1.56	1.14	0.84 - 1.55		
> 80	99	1.70	1.12 - 2.58	1.72	1.13 - 2.62		
Sex							
Male(ref)	688	1.00		1.00			
Female	732	1.12	0.89 - 1.40	1.28	1.02 – 1.62		
Race/ethnicity							
White(ref)	1234	1.00					
Non-White	186	0.76	0.53 - 1.09				
Stage							
Stage III(ref)	1041	1.00		1.00			
Stage IV	379	5.72	4.50 – 7.27	5.27	4.03 – 6.89		
Positive lymph nodes							
0 (ref)	70	1.00		1.00			
1-3	729	0.83	0.22 - 1.30	0.99	0.64 - 1.52		
≥ 4	575	0.96	0.44 - 1.38	1.55	1.03 – 2.35		
Tumor grade							
1-3 (ref)	940	1.00		1.00			
3-4	437	1.82	1.43 - 2.30	1.55	1.21 – 1.98		
NCI comorbidity score							
0 (ref)	884	1.00		1.00			
1	374	1.21	0.93 - 1.56	1.43	1.10 - 1.86		
≥ 2	162	1.04	0.71 - 1.53	1.04	0.88- 1.98		
Treatment Initiation							
2000-2004 (ref)	296	1.00		1.00			
2005-2009	1124	0.40	0.31 – 0.50	0.72	0.56 – 0.93		
Geographic region							
Midwest (ref)	177	1.00					
Northeast	95	1.13	0.65 - 1.99				
South	597	1.20	0.81 - 1.77				
West	551	0.97	0.65 - 1.45				
Median income quartiles							
1-Low (ref)	330	1.00					
2	358	0.83	0.60 - 1.16				
3	358	1.06	0.78 - 1.44				
4-High	372	0.79	0.57 - 1.09				

Table 7: Multivariate Cox Regression of Overall Survival (CAPOX vs. FOLFOX).

---

[7] Reduced model by backward elimination; full model included treatment, age, sex, race, stage, positive lymph nodes, tumor grade, comorbidity score, treatment initiation year, geographic region, and income.

[8] Propensity score weighted for age, sex, race, stage, positive lymph nodes, tumor grade, comorbidity score, treatment initiation year, geographic region, and income.

derly patients are frail and less able to tolerate aggressive or more toxic treatments. A recent review of the medical records of patients aged 65 or older diagnosed with stage III colon cancer between 2003 and 2006 revealed that 61% received a regimen containing oxaliplatin, 54% were treated with FOLFOX, 19% received 5-FU/LV, and 12% were administered CAP. Among those not treated with oxal iplatin, the primary reason cited for not administering oxaliplatin for 19% of patients was comorbid health conditions with age (O'Grady *et al.*, 2011).

Product-Limit Survival Estimates
With Number of Subjects at Risk and 95% Confidence Limits

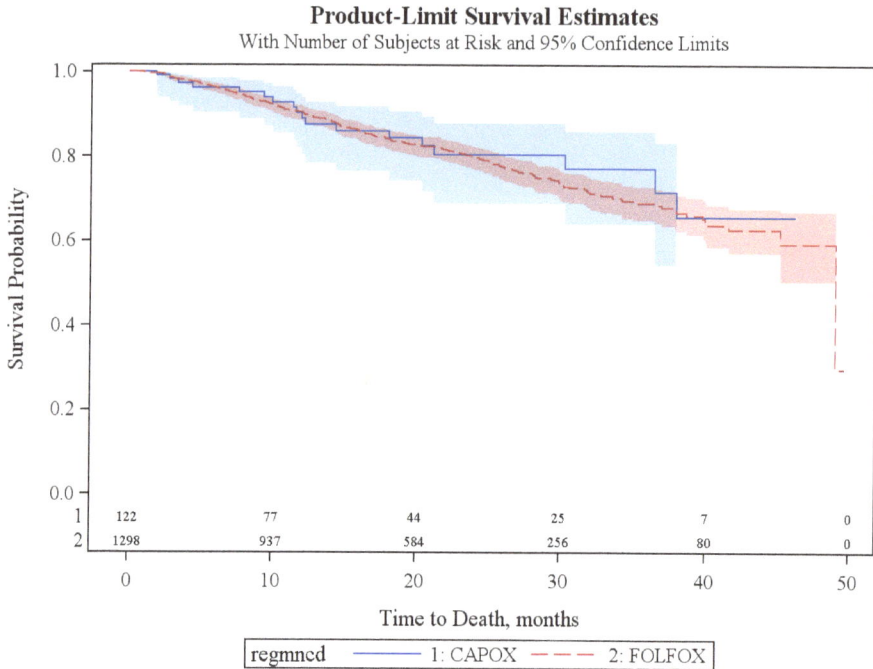

Figure 4: Kaplan Meier Curve of Overall Survival by Treatment (CAPOX vs. FOLFOX).

Complications requiring medical resource utilization were less frequent for CAP +/- oxaliplatin regimens but achieved equivalent survival benefits compared with 5-FU/LV +/- oxaliplatin regimens. This confirms similar observations from randomized clinical trials that CAP monotherapy is associated with a lower rate of adverse events and reduced medical resource utilization (Hoff *et al.*, 2001; Van Cutsem *et al.*, 2001). Randomized clinical trials report comparative safety profiles for CAP +/- oxaliplatin regimens vs. 5-FU/LV +/- oxaliplatin with more Grade 3 or 4 neutropenia and neutropenic fever associated with FOLFOX and more Grade 3 hand-foot syndrome and grade 3 or 4 diarrhea associated with CAPOX (J. Cassidy *et al.*, 2006; J. Cassidy *et al.*, 2008; J. Cassidy *et al.*, 2011). However, the incidence of medically significant diarrhea, i.e. requiring medical resources, was reduced in patients receiving CAPOX vs. FOLFOX in this study. Dose selection was at the discretion of the physician and dosing information could not be determined retrospectively from available data within the claims dataset. Regional differences in tolerance to both CAP and 5-FU/LV have been reported with US patients more likely to experience grade 3 or 4 fluoropyrimidine-related toxicities compared with patients from other parts of world, particularly Asia (Haller *et al.*, 2008; Hochster *et al.*, 2008; Rothenberg, 2008). Furthermore, physicians sometimes administer lower chemotherapy doses in elderly patients to increase the tolerability of treatment (Field *et al.*, 2008; C. Twelves *et al.*, 2005). RCT patients are also monitored closely for the occurrence of AEs; but in this analysis only more serious treatment complications are likely to have been reported given that patients were seen by a physician or received treatment that resulted in a medical claim for payment.

Initiation of chemotherapy for all four treatment regimens was longer (mean time: 74 to 81 days) than the typical 30 days that would be expected. Prior research show that not only do treatment rates decline dramatically with increasing age, (Schrag, Gelfand, *et al.*, 2001) but older age is associated with delayed chemotherapy initiation (Hershman *et al.*, 2006) and lower rates of chemotherapy completion (Dobie *et al.*, 2006). These age disparities in treatment patterns are associated with higher mortality (Dobie *et al.*, 2006; Hershman *et al.*, 2006) and the current results provide further support that demographic factors such as age should not deter the use of guideline-recommended therapies.

5 Strengths and Limitations

Unlike clinical trials, this observational study provides insight into the determinants and effectiveness of chemotherapy treatment in routine oncology practice. The study includes a large sample size and wide geographic representation of patients diagnosed with CRC in the United States. The SEER-Medicare database offers comprehensive information about inpatient and outpatient claims, covered services, all claims regardless of residence or service area, and longitudinal data with claims for services from the time a person is eligible for Medicare until their death.

However, use of the SEER-Medicare data for this type of analysis has some limitations, particularly for determining accurate utilization rates of oral chemotherapeutic agents such as capecitabine. A recent comparison of Medicare claims with the National Cancer Institute's Patterns of Care studies showed that among patients with various cancers receiving chemotherapy (including stage II/III CRC), Medicare claims data more accurately identified agents that were intravenously administered (Lund *et al.*, 2011).

This observational, retrospective, non-randomized analysis is limited in the ability to account for the biases inherent to treatment assignment in clinical practice. It is therefore possible that the observed associations are the result of unobserved differences among patients (confounding). To account for this, we utilized two approaches for adjustment and compared findings for both the propensity score-weighted and traditional covariate adjustment in survival analyses. The propensity scores are intended to account for underlying factors that affect treatment selection. It is the conditional probability of each patient receiving a specific treatment based on baseline characteristics. In essence, the effect of the propensity score weights was to balance the groups to reduce potential bias associated with treatment selection in order to compare patients with similar likelihood of receiving a treatment, similar to randomization in clinical trials. Our findings between both approaches yielded comparable results and underscores the importance of using multiple approaches to adjustment.

As evidenced by the wider confidence intervals, the relatively small number of patients receiving treatment with CAPOX may affect the power of the comparative analyses to detect differences in survival outcomes and estimates of complication rates may be unstable. In general, small samples may not provide a good representation of the general population receiving

CAPOX and may be affected by outliers which would highlight or conceal differences which in reality do not exist.

An examination of possible interactions between performance status and survival, as well as performance status and incidence of treatment-related complications were not possible as performance status was not available in the SEER-Medicare database. Lifestyle factors such as tobacco history were also not available, and these factors may have influenced clinicians' decisions regarding specific therapeutic regimens to administer.

This analysis also does not yield information about patient characteristics and treatment patterns of patients enrolled in health maintenance organizations (HMOs) since these data are not collected by Medicare. It is conceivable that treatment patterns, prognosis, and complications may differ between HMO and Medicare enrollees. Previous studies found that Medicare HMO enrollees with colon cancer had better OS compared with fee-for-service (FFS) plan members (Kirsner *et al.*, 2006; Merrill *et al.*, 1999). These mortality differences might have been due to higher use of screening and preventive services for HMO patients or the possibility that HMO enrollees tend to be healthier than FFS enrollees. An examination of treatment patterns, prognosis, and complications between alternative health care plans enrollees would be a productive area for additional evaluation.

6   Conclusions

Overall survival for elderly mCRC patients who were treated under conditions of routine medical oncology practice was comparable between CAP and 5-FU/LV and between CAPOX and FOLFOX. These results are consistent with those reported among younger patients in randomized clinical trials. The rate of treatment-related complications requiring medical resource use was lower for patients administered capecitabine monotherapy and in combination with oxaliplatin compared with 5-FU/LV and FOLFOX, respectively. These findings confirm that capecitabine-based regimens are an appropriate treatment choice for elderly patients with mCRC. These data also offer support for the use of treatments for elderly patients that are consistent to those administered to younger patients, and imply that age should not discourage the use of guideline-recommended therapies for mCRC.

Authors

Sacha Satram-Hoang
Department of Epidemiology, Q.D. Research Inc., USA

Carolina Reyes
Department of Health Economics & Outcomes Research, Genentech Inc., USA
Department of Clinical Pharmacy, University of California, San Francisco, USA

Edward McKenna
U.S. Medical Affairs, Genentech Inc., USA

Khang Q. Hoang
Medical Affairs, Q.D. Research Inc., USA

Acknowledgements

Funding for this study was provided by Genentech, Inc. Luen Lee, PhD and Shui Yu, PhD, are acknowledged for their contributions to the statistical analysis plan. The authors would also like to acknowledge Sridhar Guduru, MS and Ashok Gunuganti, MS for programming support. This study used the linked SEER–Medicare database. The efforts of the Applied Research Program, NCI (Bethesda, MD), the Office of Information Services and the Office of Strategic Planning, Health Care Financing Administration (Baltimore, MD), Information Management Services, Inc. (Silver Spring, MD), and the Surveillance, Epidemiology, and End Results (SEER) Program tumor registries are acknowledged in the creation of the SEER–Medicare database. The interpretation and reporting of these data are the sole responsibility of the authors.

References

Arkenau, H. T., Arnold, D., Cassidy, J., Diaz-Rubio, E., Douillard, J. Y., Hochster, H., . . . Porschen, R. (2008). *Efficacy of oxaliplatin plus capecitabine or infusional fluorouracil/leucovorin in patients with metastatic colorectal cancer: a pooled analysis of randomized trials.* J Clin Oncol, 26(36), 5910-5917.

Ayanian, J. Z., Zaslavsky, A. M., Fuchs, C. S., Guadagnoli, E., Creech, C. M., Cress, R. D., . . . Wright, W. E. (2003). *Use of adjuvant chemotherapy and radiation therapy for colorectal cancer in a population-based cohort.* J Clin Oncol, 21(7), 1293-1300.

Borner, M. M., Schoffski, P., de Wit, R., Caponigro, F., Comella, G., Sulkes, A., . . . Fumoleau, P. (2002). *Patient preference and pharmacokinetics of oral modulated UFT versus intravenous fluorouracil and leucovorin: a randomised crossover trial in advanced colorectal cancer. [Clinical Trial Comparative Study Randomized Controlled Trial].* Eur J Cancer, 38(3), 349-358.

Braun, A. H., Achterrath, W., Wilke, H., Vanhoefer, U., Harstrick, A., & Preusser, P. (2004). *New systemic frontline treatment for metastatic colorectal carcinoma.* Cancer, 100(8), 1558-1577.

Cartwright, T. H. (2012). *Treatment decisions after diagnosis of metastatic colorectal cancer.* Clin Colorectal Cancer, 11(3), 155-166.

Cassidy, J., Clarke, S., & Diaz-Rubio, E. (2006). *First efficacy and safety results from XELOX-I/NO16966, a randomized 2x2 factorial phase III trial of XELOX vs. FOLFOX4 + bevacizumab or placebo in first-line metastatic colorectal cancer (MCRC). Paper presented at the Annual Meeting of the European Society of Medical Oncology, Istanbul, Turkey.*

Cassidy, J., Clarke, S., Diaz-Rubio, E., Scheithauer, W., Figer, A., Wong, R., . . . Saltz, L. (2008). *Randomized phase III study of capecitabine plus oxaliplatin compared with fluorouracil/folinic acid plus oxaliplatin as first-line therapy for metastatic colorectal cancer.* J Clin Oncol, 26(12), 2006-2012.

Cassidy, J., Clarke, S., Diaz-Rubio, E., Scheithauer, W., Figer, A., Wong, R., . . . Saltz, L. (2011). *XELOX vs FOLFOX-4 as first-line therapy for metastatic colorectal cancer: NO16966 updated results.* Br J Cancer, 105(1), 58-64.

Cassidy, J., Tabernero, J., Twelves, C., Brunet, R., Butts, C., Conroy, T., . . . Diaz-Rubio, E. (2004). *XELOX (capecitabine plus oxaliplatin): active first-line therapy for patients with metastatic colorectal cancer.* J Clin Oncol, 22(11), 2084-2091.

Castiglione, M., Gelber, R. D., & Goldhirsch, A. (1990). *Adjuvant systemic therapy for breast cancer in the elderly: competing causes of mortality. International Breast Cancer Study Group. [Clinical Trial Randomized Controlled Trial Research Support, Non-U.S. Gov't].* J Clin Oncol, 8(3), 519-526.

Chagpar, R., Xing, Y., Chiang, Y. J., Feig, B. W., Chang, G. J., You, Y. N., & Cormier, J. N. (2012). *Adherence to stage-specific treatment guidelines for patients with colon cancer.* J Clin Oncol, 30(9), 972-979.

Charlson, M. E., Pompei, P., Ales, K. L., & MacKenzie, C. R. (1987). A new method of classifying prognostic comorbidity in longitudinal studies: development and validation. [Comparative Study Research Support, Non-U.S. Gov't]. J Chronic Dis, 40(5), 373-383.

Chu, E., Haller, D. G., Cartwright, T. H., Twelves, C., McKenna, E., Scotto, N., . . . Schmoll, H.-J. (2012). Epidemiology and natural history of central venous access device (CVAD) use and infusion pump performance among patients (pts) treated for metastatic colorectal cancer (mCRC): Analysis from the NO16966 trial. Paper presented at the 2012 Gastrointestinal Cancers Symposium, San Francisco, CA. http://www.asco.org/ASCOv2/Meetings/Abstracts? &vmview=abst_detail_view&confID=115&abstractID=88795

Comella, P., Massidda, B., Palmeri, S., Farris, A., Lucia, L. D., Natale, D., . . . Casaretti, R. (2005). Biweekly oxaliplatin combined with oral capecitabine (OXXEL regimen) as first-line treatment of metastatic colorectal cancer patients: a Southern Italy Cooperative Oncology Group phase II study. Cancer Chemother Pharmacol, 56(5), 481-486.

Comella, P., Natale, D., Farris, A., Gambardella, A., Maiorino, L., Massidda, B., . . . Cannone, M. (2005). Capecitabine plus oxaliplatin for the first-line treatment of elderly patients with metastatic colorectal carcinoma: final results of the Southern Italy Cooperative Oncology Group Trial 0108. Cancer, 104(2), 282-289.

de Gramont, A., Figer, A., Seymour, M., Homerin, M., Hmissi, A., Cassidy, J., . . . Bonetti, A. (2000). Leucovorin and fluorouracil with or without oxaliplatin as first-line treatment in advanced colorectal cancer. J Clin Oncol, 18(16), 2938-2947.

Diaz-Rubio, E., Tabernero, J., Gomez-Espana, A., Massuti, B., Sastre, J., Chaves, M., . . . Aranda, E. (2007). Phase III study of capecitabine plus oxaliplatin compared with continuous-infusion fluorouracil plus oxaliplatin as first-line therapy in metastatic colorectal cancer: final report of the Spanish Cooperative Group for the Treatment of Digestive Tumors Trial. J Clin Oncol, 25(27), 4224-4230.

Dobie, S. A., Baldwin, L. M., Dominitz, J. A., Matthews, B., Billingsley, K., & Barlow, W. (2006). Completion of therapy by Medicare patients with stage III colon cancer. [Research Support, N.I.H., Extramural]. J Natl Cancer Inst, 98(9), 610-619.

Douillard, J. Y., Bennouna, J., & Senellart, H. (2008). Is XELOX equivalent to FOLFOX or other continuous-infusion 5-fluorouracil chemotherapy in metastatic colorectal cancer? Clin Colorectal Cancer, 7(3), 206-211.

Ducreux, M., Bennouna, J., Hebbar, M., Ychou, M., Lledo, G., Conroy, T., . . . Douillard, J. Y. Capecitabine plus oxaliplatin (XELOX) versus 5-fluorouracil/leucovorin plus oxaliplatin (FOLFOX-6) as first-line treatment for metastatic colorectal cancer. Int J Cancer, 128(3), 682-690.

Field, K. M., Kosmider, S., Jefford, M., Michael, M., Jennens, R., Green, M., & Gibbs, P. (2008). Chemotherapy dosing strategies in the obese, elderly, and thin patient: results of a nationwide survey. J Oncol Pract, 4(3), 108-113.

Giacchetti, S., Perpoint, B., Zidani, R., Le Bail, N., Faggiuolo, R., Focan, C., . . . Levi, F. (2000). Phase III multicenter randomized trial of oxaliplatin added to chronomodulated fluorouracil-leucovorin as first-line treatment of metastatic colorectal cancer. J Clin Oncol, 18(1), 136-147.

Goldberg, R. M., Sargent, D. J., Morton, R. F., Fuchs, C. S., Ramanathan, R. K., Williamson, S. K., . . . Alberts, S. (2006). Randomized controlled trial of reduced-dose bolus fluorouracil plus leucovorin and irinotecan or infused fluorouracil plus leucovorin and oxaliplatin in patients with previously untreated metastatic colorectal cancer: a North American Intergroup Trial. J Clin Oncol, 24(21), 3347-3353.

Goldberg, R. M., Sargent, D. J., Morton, R. F., Fuchs, C. S., Ramanathan, R. K., Williamson, S. K., . . . Alberts, S. R. (2004). A randomized controlled trial of fluorouracil plus leucovorin, irinotecan, and oxaliplatin combinations in patients with previously untreated metastatic colorectal cancer. J Clin Oncol, 22(1), 23-30.

Greenland, S. (1998). Introduction to Stratified Analysis (2nd Edition ed.). Philadelphis: Lippincott-Raven Publishers

Grothey, A., Sargent, D., Goldberg, R. M., & Schmoll, H. J. (2004). Survival of patients with advanced colorectal cancer improves with the availability of fluorouracil-leucovorin, irinotecan, and oxaliplatin in the course of treatment. J Clin Oncol, 22(7), 1209-1214.

Haller, D. G., Cassidy, J., Clarke, S. J., Cunningham, D., Van Cutsem, E., Hoff, P. M., . . . Twelves, C. (2008). Potential regional differences for the tolerability profiles of fluoropyrimidines. J Clin Oncol, 26(13), 2118-2123.

Hershman, D., Hall, M. J., Wang, X., Jacobson, J. S., McBride, R., Grann, V. R., & Neugut, A. I. (2006). Timing of adjuvant chemotherapy initiation after surgery for stage III colon cancer. Cancer, 107(11), 2581-2588.

Hochster, H. S., Hart, L. L., Ramanathan, R. K., Childs, B. H., Hainsworth, J. D., Cohn, A. L., . . . Hedrick, E. (2008). Safety and efficacy of oxaliplatin and fluoropyrimidine regimens with or without bevacizumab as first-line treatment of metastatic colorectal cancer: results of the TREE Study. J Clin Oncol, 26(21), 3523-3529.

Hoff, P. M., Ansari, R., Batist, G., Cox, J., Kocha, W., Kuperminc, M., . . . Wong, R. (2001). Comparison of oral capecitabine versus intravenous fluorouracil plus leucovorin as first-line treatment in 605 patients with metastatic colorectal cancer: results of a randomized phase III study. J Clin Oncol, 19(8), 2282-2292.

Howlader, N., Noone, A. M., Krapcho, M., Neyman, N., Aminou, R., Waldron, W., . . . Edwards, B. K. (2011). SEER Cancer Statistics Review, 1975-2008. Retrieved from http://seer.cancer.gov/csr/1975_2008/

Hutchins, L. F., Unger, J. M., Crowley, J. J., Coltman, C. A., Jr., & Albain, K. S. (1999). Underrepresentation of patients 65 years of age or older in cancer-treatment trials. N Engl J Med, 341(27), 2061-2067.

investigators, I. M. P. A. o. C. C. T. I. (1995). Efficacy of adjuvant fluorouracil and folinic acid in colon cancer. International Multicentre Pooled Analysis of Colon Cancer Trials (IMPACT) investigators. Lancet, 345(8955), 939-944.

Kahn, K. L., Adams, J. L., Weeks, J. C., Chrischilles, E. A., Schrag, D., Ayanian, J. Z., . . . Fletcher, R. H. (2010). Adjuvant chemotherapy use and adverse events among older patients with stage III colon cancer. JAMA, 303(11), 1037-1045.

Kirsner, R. S., Ma, F., Fleming, L., Federman, D. G., Trapido, E., Duncan, R., & Wilkinson, J. D. (2006). The effect of medicare health care delivery systems on survival for patients with breast and colorectal cancer. Cancer Epidemiol Biomarkers Prev, 15(4), 769-773.

Klabunde, C. N., Legler, J. M., Warren, J. L., Baldwin, L. M., & Schrag, D. (2007). A refined comorbidity measurement algorithm for claims-based studies of breast, prostate, colorectal, and lung cancer patients. Ann Epidemiol, 17(8), 584-590.

Koukourakis, G. V., Kouloulias, V., Koukourakis, M. J., Zacharias, G. A., Zabatis, H., & Kouvaris, J. (2008). Efficacy of the oral fluorouracil pro-drug capecitabine in cancer treatment: a review. Molecules, 13(8), 1897-1922.

Kurth, T., Walker, A. M., Glynn, R. J., Chan, K. A., Gaziano, J. M., Berger, K., & Robins, J. M. (2006). Results of multivariable logistic regression, propensity matching, propensity adjustment, and propensity-based weighting under conditions of nonuniform effect. Am J Epidemiol, 163(3), 262-270.

Liu, G., Franssen, E., Fitch, M. I., & Warner, E. (1997). Patient preferences for oral versus intravenous palliative chemotherapy. J Clin Oncol, 15(1), 110-115.

Lund, J. L., Sturmer, T., Harlan, L. C., Sanoff, H. K., Sandler, R. S., Brookhart, M. A., & Warren, J. L. (2011). Identifying Specific Chemotherapeutic Agents in Medicare Data: A Validation Study. Med Care.

Merrill, R. M., Brown, M. L., Potosky, A. L., Riley, G., Taplin, S. H., Barlow, W., & Fireman, B. H. (1999). Survival and treatment for colorectal cancer Medicare patients in two group/staff health maintenance organizations and the fee-for-service setting. Med Care Res Rev, 56(2), 177-196.

Moertel, C. G., Fleming, T. R., Macdonald, J. S., Haller, D. G., Laurie, J. A., Tangen, C. M., . . . Mailliard, J. A. (1995). Fluorouracil plus levamisole as effective adjuvant therapy after resection of stage III colon carcinoma: a final report. Ann Intern Med, 122(5), 321-326.

Murthy, V. H., Krumholz, H. M., & Gross, C. P. (2004). Participation in cancer clinical trials: race-, sex-, and age-based disparities. JAMA, 291(22), 2720-2726.

NCCN, N. C. C. N. (2012). Clinical Practice Guidelines in Oncology. <http://www.nccn.org/professionals/physician_gls/pdf/colon.pdf>. , V. 3.2012.

O'Connell, M. J., Mailliard, J. A., Kahn, M. J., Macdonald, J. S., Haller, D. G., Mayer, R. J., & Wieand, H. S. (1997). Controlled trial of fluorouracil and low-dose leucovorin given for 6 months as postoperative adjuvant therapy for colon cancer. J Clin Oncol, 15(1), 246-250.

O'Grady, M. A., Slater, E., Sigurdson, E. R., Meropol, N. J., Weinstein, A., Lusch, C. J., . . . Cohen, S. J. (2011). Assessing compliance with national comprehensive cancer network guidelines for elderly patients with stage III colon cancer: the Fox Chase Cancer Center Partners' initiative. Clin Colorectal Cancer, 10(2), 113-116.

Porschen, R., Arkenau, H. T., Kubicka, S., Greil, R., Seufferlein, T., Freier, W., . . . Schmoll, H. J. (2007). Phase III study of capecitabine plus oxaliplatin compared with fluorouracil and leucovorin plus oxaliplatin in metastatic colorectal cancer: a final report of the AIO Colorectal Study Group. J Clin Oncol, 25(27), 4217-4223.

Potosky, A. L., Riley, G. F., Lubitz, J. D., Mentnech, R. M., & Kessler, L. G. (1993). Potential for cancer related health services research using a linked Medicare-tumor registry database. Med Care, 31(8), 732-748.

Rothenberg, M. L. (2008). Tolerability of fluoropyrimidines in combination with oxaliplatin appears to differ by region. Paper presented at the ASCO: 2008 Gastrointestinal Cancers Symposium.

Schrag, D., Cramer, L. D., Bach, P. B., & Begg, C. B. (2001). Age and adjuvant chemotherapy use after surgery for stage III colon cancer. J Natl Cancer Inst, 93(11), 850-857.

Schrag, D., Gelfand, S. E., Bach, P. B., Guillem, J., Minsky, B. D., & Begg, C. B. (2001). Who gets adjuvant treatment for stage II and III rectal cancer? Insight from surveillance, epidemiology, and end results--Medicare. J Clin Oncol, 19(17), 3712-3718.

Siegel, R., Naishadham, D., & Jemal, A. (2012). Cancer statistics, 2012. CA Cancer J Clin, 62(1), 10-29.

Suissa, S. (2008). Immortal time bias in pharmaco-epidemiology. Am J Epidemiol, 167(4), 492-499.

Thirion, P., Michiels, S., Pignon, J. P., Buyse, M., Braud, A. C., Carlson, R. W., . . . Piedbois, P. (2004). Modulation of fluorouracil by leucovorin in patients with advanced colorectal cancer: an updated meta-analysis. J Clin Oncol, 22(18), 3766-3775.

Townsley, C. A., Selby, R., & Siu, L. L. (2005). Systematic review of barriers to the recruitment of older patients with cancer onto clinical trials. J Clin Oncol, 23(13), 3112-3124.

Twelves, C., Wong, A., Nowacki, M. P., Abt, M., Burris, H., 3rd, Carrato, A., . . . Scheithauer, W. (2005). Capecitabine as adjuvant treatment for stage III colon cancer. [Clinical Trial Multicenter Study Randomized Controlled Trial Research Support, Non-U.S. Gov't]. N Engl J Med, 352(26), 2696-2704.

Twelves, C. J., Butts, C. A., Cassidy, J., Conroy, T., Braud, F., Diaz-Rubio, E., . . . Van Cutsem, E. J. (2005). Capecitabine/ oxaliplatin, a safe and active first-line regimen for older patients with metastatic colorectal cancer: post hoc analysis of a large phase II study. Clin Colorectal Cancer, 5(2), 101-107.

Van Cutsem, E., Hoff, P. M., Harper, P., Bukowski, R. M., Cunningham, D., Dufour, P., . . . Schilsky, R. L. (2004). Oral capecitabine vs intravenous 5-fluorouracil and leucovorin: integrated efficacy data and novel analyses from two large, randomised, phase III trials. Br J Cancer, 90(6), 1190-1197.

Van Cutsem, E., Twelves, C., Cassidy, J., Allman, D., Bajetta, E., Boyer, M., . . . Harper, P. (2001). Oral capecitabine compared with intravenous fluorouracil plus leucovorin in patients with metastatic colorectal cancer: results of a large phase III study. J Clin Oncol, 19(21), 4097-4106.

Warren, J. L., Harlan, L. C., Fahey, A., Virnig, B. A., Freeman, J. L., Klabunde, C. N., . . . Knopf, K. B. (2002). Utility of the SEER-Medicare data to identify chemotherapy use. Med Care, 40(8 Suppl), IV-55-61.

Warren, J. L., Klabunde, C. N., Schrag, D., Bach, P. B., & Riley, G. F. (2002). Overview of the SEER-Medicare data: content, research applications, and generalizability to the United States elderly population. Med Care, 40(8 Suppl), IV-3-18.

Welles L, H. H., Ramanathan R, et al. . (2004). Preliminary results of a randomized study of the safety and tolerability of three oxaliplatin-based regimens as first-line treatment for advanced colorectal cancer (CRC) ("TREE" study). Paper presented at the Am Soc Clin Oncol

Wolmark, N., Rockette, H., Fisher, B., Wickerham, D. L., Redmond, C., Fisher, E. R., . . . et al. (1993). The benefit of leucovorin-modulated fluorouracil as postoperative adjuvant therapy for primary colon cancer: results from National Surgical Adjuvant Breast and Bowel Project protocol C-03. J Clin Oncol, 11(10), 1879-1887.

The Implementation of a Standardized Approach to Laparoscopic Rectal Surgery: A Paradigm Shift

Katrine Kanstrup Aslak, Orhan Bulut

1 Background

Colorectal cancer is the fourth most common cancer in men and third most common in women worldwide, accounting for approximately 436,000 incident cases and 212,000 deaths in 2008. This cancer has an important economic impact, estimating that in the initial, continuing and last year of life phases of care a total of more than $7 billion were spent (American cancer Society Website Cancer Facts and Figures, 2004). Colorectal cancer accounts for 11% of cancers diagnosed. The worldwide incidence of colorectal cancer is increasing: in 1975 the worldwide incidence of colorectal cancer was only 500,000 (Boyle & Langman, 2000). In western countries, some of the increase is attributable to the aging of the population and perhaps better diagnostic abilities; however, in countries with a low baseline rate of colorectal cancer, an increase in incidence after adjustment of age has been found. There is substantial geographic variation in the incidence of colorectal cancer with relatively high rates in North America, Western Europe, and Australia and relatively low rates in Africa and Asia (Lagiou P, 2002). Interestingly, there is less variation in the incidence of rectal cancer between countries as compared with the incidence of colon cancer (Parkin DM *et al.*, 1999; Wingo PA *et al.*, 2003).

There have been great improvements of surgical and medical treatment over the last 20 years. This means that the patients that previously had metastatic disease and those patients that were not previously assessed for surgery can now be considered for surgical treatment. Hence, the increasing number of patients that need not only surgery but also radiological examinations and oncological treatment is a challenge for the workload in healthcare institutions worldwide.

2 Introduction

In recent years laparoscopic surgery has become increasingly popular in several fields of general surgery. In 1987 laparoscopic cholecystectomy was introduced by the French gynecologist Mouret and it quickly became the golden standard for treatment of symptomatic gall stone disease due to less postoperative pain and faster recovery. Similarly, laparoscopic appendectomy has become the standard choice of operation for treatment of acute appendicitis since the method was introduced by K Semm in 1983. Also in colorectal surgery several studies have analyzed benefits of laparoscopic surgery – especially during the last decade. However, the laparoscopic technique was not rapidly adapted by colorectal surgeons – partly due to the technically difficulty of the laparoscopic procedure but also due to uncertainty of the oncological safety. In 1995 Fodera (Fodera *et al.*, 1995) raised concern of risk of port site metastasis after laparoscopic assisted colectomy. It took several years and studies to conclude, that this risk was minimal and that the oncological outcomes (short- and long-term results) were equal to the outcomes after laparoscopic surgery. Not until 2005 two large scale randomized clinical trials (Guillou *et al.*, 2005; Van der Pas *et al.*, 2005) concluded that laparoscopic surgery for colon cancer is safe with satisfying oncological results. Further the authors concluded that laparoscopic surgery lead to smaller peroperative blood-loss, earlier recovery of bowel function, less postoperative pain and shorter hospital stay. Morbidity and mortality was equal to open surgery. However, the duration of laparoscopic surgery was significantly longer and furthermore, laparoscopic colorectal surgery is technically challenging with a steep learning curve for even experienced surgeons, and finally it is economically straining for any surgical department to invest in laparoscopic equipment. Hence, the implementation of laparoscopic colorectal surgery can be described as a challenging "bottle neck" when looked upon in a global as well as in a local perspective.

Recently a large American review (Kang CY *et al.*, 2012) of the Nationwide Inpatient Sample (NIS) data from 2007 and 2009, including data from more than 200,000 patients undergoing colorectal surgery, described how laparoscopic surgery has evolved. In 2007 13.8% of the registered patients underwent laparoscopic surgery for colorectal diseases (colon and rectal cancers and diverticulitis) but two years later a dramatic increase was registered with 42.6% of the patients now being laparoscopically operated. The in-hospital mortality was significantly lower for patients undergoing laparoscopic surgery (0.6 vs. 1.2 respectively) and the length of hospital stay was shorter (5 vs. 6 days). In 2007 the cost of laparoscopic surgery per patient was more expensive than open surgery, but in 2009 laparoscopic surgery had become the cheaper choice of surgical treatment. The study illustrates how a new method of surgery begins as a minor experimental, expensive treatment for few patients, but over time the method becomes more popular and established.

The evolution of laparoscopic surgery for rectal cancer is similar to that of colon cancer. Many studies have found good results with shorter hospital stay, less postoperative pain, morbidity and oncological results similar to results after open surgery (Miyajima N *et al.*, 2008; Lujan J *et al.*, 2009; Ströhlein *et al.*, 2008). However, most studies were not properly randomized and all were of too small sample sizes. In 2013 a large multicenter prospective randomized study (van der Pas MH *et al.*, 2013) including 1103 patients from eight different countries was finally published. The patients were randomized to either laparoscopic or open surgery for rectal cancer. The authors found more extensive use of epidural analgesia in the open group, shorter hospital stay in the laparoscopic group and equal results of mortality (30 days), morbidity and oncological short-term outcomes (histopathologic evaluation of specimen) between groups. The long-term oncological follow-up still remains to be published.

In Denmark 1200-1400 patients are diagnosed with rectal cancer every year. National guidelines (Danish Colorectalcancer Database, 2011) ensure that every patient-case is discussed on a multidisciplinary colorectal cancer team conference (MDT). Here individual plans for treatment are made for the patients after evaluation of computed tomography (CT) scan of the abdomen and thorax, magnetic resonance imaging (MR) of the rectum, histology after biopsy taken during colonoscopy or sigmoideoscopy, and if indicated ultrasound of the liver.

The patients are staged according to international guidelines (UICC – Union for International Cancer Control). Patients with ≥T3 tumors and with threatening of the circumferential resection margin are referred to preoperative neoadjuvant radiochemotherapy. Approximately 20% of the patients receive preoperative oncological treatment in order to down-stage tumor. In 2011 62.2% of the patients referred to surgery underwent laparoscopic surgery for rectal cancer.

The operative methods are chosen according to the location of the rectal tumor and after evaluation of the patient's general health status. Very brief, the low anterior resection (LAR) is chosen for patients with tumors in the upper two thirds of the rectum. After resection of the tumor-carrying part of the rectum (at least 2 cm free resection margin distal of the tumor (measured by the length of the free bowel wall) is recommended) a primary anastomosis is performed between the sigmoid colon and the low rectum. Depending on the height of the anastomosis and comorbidities of the patient it is often advisable to supply with a temporary loop-ileostomy in order to protect the patient from severe infection in case of anastomotic leak. The abdominoperineal resection (APR) is chosen for patients with low rectal cancers, where primary anastomosis is not possible. In these cases the rectum and anus is removed "en bloc" and the sigmoid colon is used to construct a stoma in the left fossa. The perineal defect can if chosen be reconstructed with a gluteus maximus flap – the so called "ad modum Holm" procedure (Holm T *et al.*, 2007). If the tumor is extended with severe invasion of neighboring organs or the patient is suffering from severe comorbidity it may be proper to offer a Hartmann's operation (HO) with resection of the rectal tumor and construction of a left colostomy. The anal part of the rectum that remains after resection is left in situ.

Our institution has been a pioneer of fast track surgery programs ever since it was introduced in 2000 (Basse L *et al.*, 2000). The program was originally designed for open surgery for colon cancer and included early mobilization, early oral feeding, optimal analgesia (epidural catheter) and early removal of urinary catheter. Hence, most patients can be discharged 2 days after open colon resection. Our rectal cancer surgery patients are likewise, after modification of the above mentioned fast track program, scheduled for discharge on the third postoperative day. When laparoscopic surgery for rectal cancer was implemented in our department the operative approach was standardized into a stepwise procedure in order to ensure equal and optimal treatment for all patients.

The purpose of this chapter is to audit the clinical and oncological results of an observational retrospective study in our institution during the implementation of laparoscopic surgery for rectal cancer within a fast track recovery setting as an alternative to traditional open surgery. Until 2009 all patients with colorectal cancer underwent open surgery. The decision to introduce laparoscopic surgery was primarily made for highly selected patients. Hence, at the beginning of our experience only benign rectal resections and highly selected rectal cancer patients went through laparoscopic surgery. As the surgeons gained more experience during the study-period the criteria for laparoscopic surgery got wider.

3   Materials and Methods

3.1   Patient Selection

From January 2009 to February 2011, 100 consecutive patients underwent laparoscopic surgery on an intention to treat basis for rectal cancer in our department. The clinical, operative and pathological data of these patients were retrospectively reviewed from a prospectively collected database. Every patient who was operated laparoscopically for rectal cancer in an elective setting in the period was included. There were no exclusion criteria. Hence, some patients had previously gone through abdominal surgery, mainly smaller operations like appendectomy, laparoscopic cholecystectomy and hysterectomy.

3.2   Preoperative Work-Up

The preoperative work-up included biopsy, endoscopy, CT, liver ultrasound, chest x-ray and MR. All patients were staged according to national guidelines. Each patient was reviewed at our MDT meetings before and after surgery. Tumors staged as ≥ T3, and those with a threatened circumferential resection margin (CRM) underwent neoadjuvant chemoradiotherapy. Surgery was carried out 6-8 weeks after completion of treatment. Patient characteristics, tumor size and location as well as perioperative data, pathological results, morbidity, length of hospital stay (LOS), readmission rate, 30 days mortality and follow-up were recorded prospectively. All procedures were performed by the same surgical team.

Tumors were considered rectal cancers if located below 15 cm from the anal verge measured with a rigid rectoscope. Rectal cancer suitable for surgery was defined as a biopsy-proven adenocarcinoma. Patients were considered suitable for laparoscopic surgery if they had no serious health conditions precluding a laparoscopic procedure. Patients with CT or MR evidence of tumor infiltration of adjacent organs and T4 cancers were considered as unsuitable for laparoscopic surgery in this implementation period. All patients were informed about possible risks and benefits of laparoscopic surgery and informed written consent was obtained. A phosphate enema was given as bowel preparation prior to surgery. Stoma sites were marked preoperatively. All patients received epidural anesthesia (bupivacaine/fentanyl) or intravenous morphine as postoperative pain relief. Perioperative care was previously described and primarily developed for open colonic surgery in fast track settings (Basse L *et al.*, 2000). The fast track settings included initiation of mobilization and full oral feeding (minimal oral intake of 1500 ml of fluid, but full diet was allowed) on the evening of surgery, removal of epidural catheter and urinary or suprapubic catheter on the third day of surgery and planning of discharge as soon as possible hereafter. During hospital stay all patients received thromboembolic prophylaxis. Nasogastric tubes and drains were not used routinely.

3.3   Surgical Method

Our surgical approach is based on the steps primarily described by Dr. J Leroy of France who is one of the pioneers in laparoscopic rectal surgery (http://www.websurg.com). We used 5 port sites. The standardized operative steps for laparoscopic rectal resection are: 1) open insertion of the umbilical port for establishment of pneumoperitoneum and peritoneal inspection. The patient was then placed in steep Trendelenburg's position and the operating table was rotated towards the right side. 2) Placement of three or four ports at variable sites. 3) Mesocolic dissection and inferior mesenteric pedicle isolation was achieved with medial approach and the inferior mesenteric artery was ligated close to its origin with clips or Endo-GIA. The superior rectal artery was divided just below the inferior mesenteric artery after application of 5 mm clips in the cases of APR and Hartmann's operation (HO). 4) The left ureter was recognized and subsequently, with the patient placed supine and rotated left side up medial-to-lateral dissection was continued cranially up until the left colon was mobilized. 5) The patient was returned to the Trendelenburg's position, and the small bowel was reflected cranially after the completion of mobilization of the left colon. A grasper was used to elevate the rectosigmoid colon out of pelvis and away from the retroperitoneum and sacral promontory, to enable entry into the presacral space. 6) The posterior aspect of the mesorectum was easily identified and the mesorectal plane dissected with harmonic scalpel, preserving the hypogastric nerves. Dissection was continued down to the presacral space in this avascular plane toward the pelvic floor. 7) Dissection proceeded laterally on both sides of rectum until circumferential mobilization of lower rectum was accomplished. 8) Digital examination was performed to verify the distance between the inferior margin of the tumor and the line of resection and the adequacy of distal margin was marked with a clip. 9) An EndoGIA roticulator stapler (Covidien Ltd., Norwalk, Conn. USA) 45-mm was fired twice to divide the lower rectum safely. The abdomen was then deflated and a suprapubic incision of 4-6 cm performed to extract the left colon and resect the specimen. A wound protector (Alexis OTM, Applied Medical Rancho Santo Margarita, CA) was placed at the incision. 10) Extracorporal preparation of the proximate colon was completed with placement of the anvil of a 29–mm circular stapler (Proximate ILS circular stapler, Ethicon, Endo-surgery, Cincinnati,OH, USA) in position to perform a side-to-end or end-to-end colorectal anastomosis in the cases of low anterior resection (LAR). Bowel anastomosis was performed intracorporally by double staple technique. The splenic flexure was not routinely mobilized. For tension-free anastomosis, full splenic flexure mobilization was performed in case of lack of redundancy of the sigmoid colon during surgery. The low pelvic dissection in APR was performed first posteriorly, then anteriorly, and finally with lateral dissection. The remainder of deep pelvic dissection was performed through perineal approach including removal of the tip of os coccyx together with the specimen ad modum T. Holm (Holm T et al., 2007). In cases of HO and APR a stoma was placed in the lower left quadrant according to the pre-operatively marked stoma-site. A standardized perioperative care protocol was used.

Conversion to an open procedure was defined as any abdominal incision larger than the above mentioned to extract the specimen. A protective loop ileostomy was performed for the patients needing anastomosis within 5 cm of the anal verge. Intestinal continuity was reestablished 3 months later or after completion of postoperative adjuvant therapy.

3.4 Follow-Up

Postoperative complications were defined as any morbidity, including wound-infection, in the postoperative period in hospital or in the outpatient clinic up to 30 days after the operation. Perioperative death was defined as death occurring within 30 days after surgery. Anastomotic leaks were defined as any dehiscence of the anastomosis observed by endoscopy, digital examination, CT scan or gastrograffin enema. All patients were referred to colonoscopy and CT-scan after the first and third year of surgery.

3.5 Pathologic Method

All specimens were examined by local pathologists with special attention to the number of harvested lymph nodes, CRM, distal resection margin (DRM) and completeness of the mesorectal fascia (MRF).

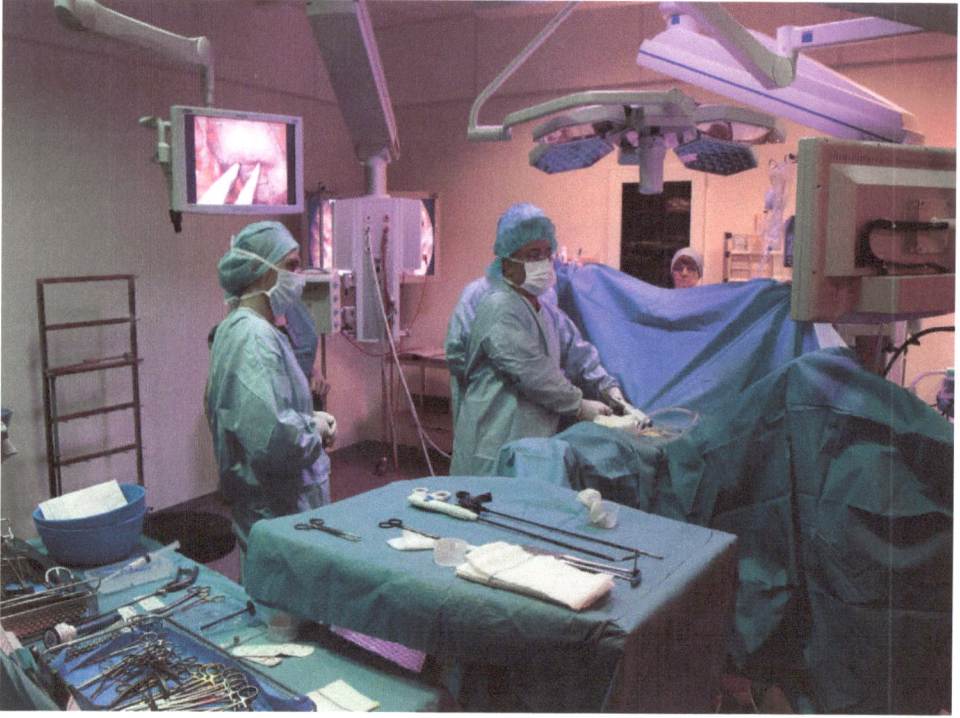

Figure 1: Operative set-up.

3.6 Statistical Analysis

Data was collected in a SPSS work-sheet (SPSS version 19; SPSS INC. Chicago, IL). All values are presented as median (range). When appropriate, Fisher's Exact Test (Chi-square test) was used for nonparametric data. P <.05 was considered statistically significant.

4 Results

Patients' characteristics are summarized in Table 1 and Perioperative data are shown in Table 2.

Gender, m/f (n)	61 / 39
Age, median (years)	66 (range 30-88)
Body mass index, median (kg/m^2)	24 (range 17-40)
ASA-score, median*	2 (range 1-3)
Tumor location, median (cm from anal verge)	10 (range 2-15)
Previous intraabdominal surgery (n)	31
Preoperative chemoradiotherapy:	
• None	76
• Chemo- and radiotherapy	24

Table 1: Patients demographics. * ASA = American Society of Anesthesiologists.

Surgical procedure (n)	
• Low anterior resection	26
• Low anterior resection with loop-ileostomy	39
• Hartmann's operation	14
• Abdominoperineal resection	21
Operative time, median (min)	250 (range 51-397)
• Low anterior resection	181 (range 51-353)
• Low anterior resection with loo-ileostomy	261 (range 100-376)
• Hartmann's operation	186 (range 114-345)
• Abdominoperineal resection	280 (range 131-397)
Loss of blood, median (ml)	100 (range 0-1145)
Hospital stay, median (days)	7 (range 3-80)
Re-admission (n)	9

Table 2: Perioperative data.

Nine patients (9%) were readmitted for a median of 3 days (range 1-13). There were 9 operations where conversion to open surgery were necessary. Indication for coversion included fixation of the tumor to the surrounding organs (n=6), dense adherences (n=1), tumor-growth into the bladder (n=1) and progressive respiratory insufficiency related to establishment of pneumoperitoneum (n=1).

Intraoperative complications occurred in 3 cases. One bladder injury and one superficial laceration of the rectum occurred during laparoscopic resections. These injuries were repaired laparoscopically without conversion. Finally one perforation of the anal canal occurred during perineal dissection in an APR-procedure.

In the postoperative period we registered 11 cases of anastomotic leaks in accordance to our previously mentioned criteria among the 65 patients who underwent low anterior resection. Amongst those, 6 patients (9%) required reoperation. The remaining 5 patients (8%) were treated conservatively or with endoscopic vacuum assisted closure. Table 3 outlines all postoperative complications encountered. Two patients developed compartment syndrome of one leg, probably as a result of improper positioning during the surgical procedure. We found a 30-days mortality-rate of 5% (5 patients). Mean follow-up was 9 months (range 1-27). The oncologic outcomes are shown in Table 4.

Twenty-four patients underwent neoadjuvant treatment prior to surgical procedure. Five of these (20.8%) had a complete pathological response with no residual tumor detectable in the resected specimen. The median length of the specimen was 17 cm (range 10-35), the median distal resection margin (DRM) was 30 mm (range 2.5-35), the median CRM was 10 mm (range 0-55) and CRM were positive in 6 patients. The overall median number of harvested lymph nodes was 15 (range 2-48). The median lymph node harvest in patients who underwent preoperative neoadjuvant treatments (n=24) were 12 (range 4-35) and in patients who underwent primary resection without neoadjuvant treatment (n=76) the median lymph node harvest was 16 (range 2-28). The mesorectal fascia (MRF) was complete or near-complete in 84 cases and not complete in 14 cases. The MRF was not described in the histopathological reports in two cases. One patient with disseminated cancer developed port-site metastasis.

Complication	No. of patients (n)	Treatment
Urine tract infection	5	Antibiotics
Gastrointestinal bleeding	1	Self-resolved
Superficial wound-infection	2	Drainage
Leakage of the rectal "stump"	3	Ultrasound-guided drainage
Compartment syndrome	2	Fasciotomy
Necrosis of stoma	2	Stoma refashioned
Ileus (adhesions)	1	Lysis of adhesions
Early port-site hernia	1	Repaired
Peritonitis	2	Laparotomy
Parastomal hernia	2	Repaired
Presacral abscess	3	Ultrasound-guided drainage
Anastomotic leak	5	Conservative treament/Endo-VAC*
Anastomotic leak	6	Reoperation
Total	35	

Table 3: Postoperative complications. *Endo-VAC = Endoscopic Vacuum-assisted closure.

Circumferential resection margin, median (mm)	10 (range 0-55)
Distal resection margin, median (mm)	30 (range 2,5-70)
Length of specimen, median (cm)	17 (range 10-35)
Harvested lymph-nodes, median (n)	15 (range 2-48)
Mesorectal fascia (n)	
• Complete	68
• Near-complete	16
• Incomplete	14
Radical resection	94

Table 4: Oncologic results.

5   Discussion

The results of this study reflect the circumstances that are present when an operating team adapts to a new surgical set-up. The surgeon and assisting surgeon is obviously challenged with the new laparoscopic technique, but also surgical nurses and the staff on the surgical ward must adapt to the new method and solve unforeseen problems as they occur. The results therefore may differ from other studies. For instance the operative time in this study was relatively long. Lindsetmo and Delaney (Lindsetmo RO & Delaney CP 2009) described a standard, stepwise laparoscopic procedure for rectal resections. As described earlier we have adapted this technique, which makes the operation predictable and reproducible for the whole surgical team. The process of adapting this standardized technique is however most likely one of the causes for the median operative time of 250 minutes, which is longer than comparable studies (Guillou PJ *et al.*, 2005; Ströhlein MA *et al.*, 2008). Other causes could be that two new surgeons in our team were trained to perform laparoscopic rectal surgery during the study-period. Furthermore there were a high number of patients with a history of previous abdominal surgeries in our series (31%). This may lead to intraabdominal adhesions which may prolong the phase of dissection during surgery.

There have been reports about increasing complication rates in patients converted from laparoscopic to open surgery (Lujan J *et al.*, 2009). Our rate of conversion was 9% which is lower than other studies (Guillou PJ *et al.*, 2005; Ströhlein MA *et al.*, 2008). This may reflect some degree of bias as our patients were selected candidates for laparoscopic surgery and not randomized to either open or laparoscopic surgery. Morbidity and length of hospital stay for converted patients were however similar to those who completed laparoscopic surgery. Our data therefore confirm that careful selection of patients for laparoscopic surgery makes the procedure practicable and the need to convert small. This study also confirms that our strategy to convert whenever there was failure to progress in the very difficult operative field was safe. At present, our approach is to initially plan laparoscopic method for almost all patients, only exclusions being T4 tumors or local growth into neighboring organs.

A median postoperative hospital stay of only 7 days in this series is short when compared to other studies with a median hospital stay of 8 to 15 days (Guillou PJ *et al.*, 2005; Lujan J *et al.*, 2009; Good DW *et al.*, 2011; Kang S-B et al., 2010; Sartori CA *et al.*, 2010). This great variety of results is probably due to cultural and economic differences in health care systems between countries. In Denmark all expenses for surgery and postoperative care lay with the state. The national welfare-system also include possibility for nursing assistance in the home, for instance in case of need for help with stoma- or wound care. These conditions perhaps facilitate early discharge. In our department there are very well established routines in our fast-track surgery program. As before mentioned it was originally evolved for postoperative care after colon surgery (Basse L *et al.*, 2000). It has over the years been adjusted for rectal surgery. Hence, all patients were prepared for stoma self-care already prior to surgery by one of the specialist nurses from our ward. Furthermore all patients, if possible, received epidural analgesia up to 3 days after surgery, all patients were encouraged to early oral feeding and mobilization as soon as possible after surgery - at latest the first day after surgery, and drains and catheters were withdrawn the third postoperative day. Our readmission rate of 9% with a median secondary hospital stay of 3 days is comparable to similar studies where up to 23% of the patients were readmitted after fast-track rectal cancer surgery (Schwenk *et al.*, 2006).

Table 3 shows that the majority of complications were surgical. There is no difference in complication-rates between the first and the last 50 patients in this series. Our overall complication rate of 35% matches results of other studies (Guillou PJ *et al.*, 2005; Lujan J *et al.*, 2009). There is a small tendency towards increased risk of complications, if the patient had received preoperative radio therapy as 40.9% of the radiated patients experienced complications versus 35.9% of the non-radiated patients. The tendency is however not statistically significant (p=0,803). Although a total of 15 reoperations seem to be a high figure, it is comparable to other reported series of laparoscopic rectal surgery (Bärlehner E *et al.*, 2005; Morino M *et al.*, 2003).

Much depends on the author's definition of anastomotic leakage when it comes to calculating leakage rates. We have used wide spanning criteria for our definition of anastomotic leaks. Our rate of leakages that required reoperation (9%) is acceptable in comparison of other series (Guillou PJ *et al.*, 2005; Lujan J *et al.*, 2009; Sartori CA *et al.*, 2010). Neither conversion nor neoadjuvant therapy resulted in higher risk of development of anastomotic leakage in this series. However Figure 2 shows that there is a decreasing tendency in the leakage rate in the latter part of the study period (study period B), where the standardized surgical approach had

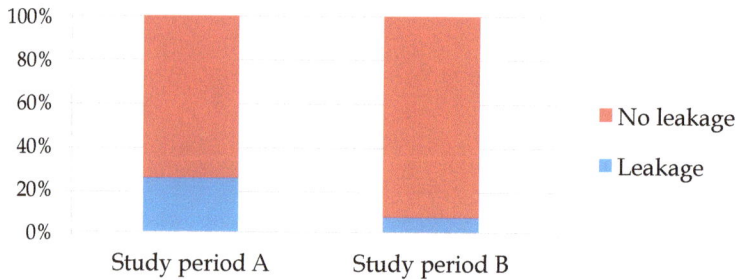

Figure 2: Anastomotic leakage rates. In study period A, patients no. 1-50 underwent surgery and 9 had anastomotic leakage (25%). In study period B, patients no. 51-100 underwent surgery, and 2 had anastomotic leakage (6,9%) (p=.094)

been fully implemented. The difference between these rates of leakages is however not significant (p=0,094).

Our 30-days mortality was 5% which is relatively high when compared to other studies (Ströhlein MA *et al.*, 2008; Kang S-B *et al.*, 2010). The postoperative morbidity and mortality in fast track settings remain challenging and controversial due to mainly a non-selected, high risk elderly population with co-existing illness (Stottmeier S *et al.*, 2012; Vlug MS *et al.*, 2011). In the present series the 5 patients who died were 78 to 88 years of age at the time of operation. They all preoperatively suffered from severe degrees of ischemic heart failure. Moreover one of the patients suffered from severe chronic obstructive lung-disease and non-insulin dependent diabetes mellitus, one patient suffered from renal failure and obesity (BMI=33) and one patient had recently been hospitalized due to lung embolia. After primary surgery all five patients experienced surgical complications and underwent re-operations. In two cases reoperation was needed because of fecal peritonitis (anastomotic leak and small bowel perforation), in two cases because of severe ischemia of the stoma and in one case because of non-fecal peritonitis of unknown origin. All five patients died due to sepsis and failure of multiple organs.

Large randomized trials comparing laparoscopic versus open resection for colorectal cancer have shown an equivalent oncological outcome (The COlon cancer Laparoscopic or Open Resection Study Group, 2005; The Clinical Outcomes of Surgical Therapy Study Group, 2004). Adequate surgical margin clearance remains crucial for local recurrence rates. The results of the CLASICC trial (Guillou PJ *et al*, 2005) with a trend towards increased rate of involved CRM (6% open vs. 12% laparoscopic) for anterior resection were initially alarming. However, a recent meta-analysis suggests that there are no differences between laparoscopic and open surgery for rectal cancer in terms of number of harvested lymph nodes, involvement of CRM and local recurrence (Huang M-J *et al.*, 2010). The rate of positive CRM was 6% in our study. All positive margins occurred in patients with T4 tumors or node positive (N2) disease. This rate is comparable with other reports (Guillou PJ *et al.*, 2005; Lujan J *et al.*, 2009). The number of lymph nodes harvested from the mesorectum during surgery is also an important predictor of prognosis (Nagtegaal ID *et al.*, 2002). In our study there was a median harvest of 15 lymph nodes and 80% of the specimens contained 12 lymph nodes or more which is equal to results of several studies (Ströhlein MA *et al.*, 2008; Lujan J *et al.*, 2009; Kang S-B *et al.*, 2010; Miyajima N *et al.*, 2008) and in accordance with international and national guidelines for lymph node harvest.

The mesorectal fascia was not complete in 16% of our patients. Macroscopic evaluation of the mesorectal fasciae is considered an important quality measure in rectal cancer surgery. Tears and shallow breaks in the mesorectum, however, are difficult to avoid, particularly when dealing with large bulky tumors in laparoscopic colorectal cancer surgery. Other factors such as a narrow pelvis and a fatty mesorectum increase the risk of damaging the mesorectal fascia with the laparoscopic instruments as well. For that reason, the grading of the mesorectal fasciae was characterized as only nearly complete in some cases, even though dissection was carried out in the correct surgical plane. Nagtegaal (Nagtegaal ID *et al.*, 2002) have shown that a complete or nearly complete mesorectal fascia is prognostic for good long-term oncological outcomes whereas an incomplete fascia is prognostic for unfortunate oncological long-term outcomes. Because of the short follow-up period it is not possible to conclude, if our oncologic result influences the long term oncologic outcome. Only one patient with disseminated cancer developed a port-site metastasis.

Amongst limitations of this study are furthermore that this retrospective series with prospectively registered data does not include a large number of patients. More data are needed from ongoing large randomized controlled trials regarding long-term oncological outcome.

6   Conclusions

Our results which included a small number of patients support the literature that finds advantages of lesser pain, faster recovery, lower postoperative morbidity and shorter length of hospital stay in comparison to open surgery. At present we need to confirm this evidence with the long term results of ongoing randomized studies (van der Pas MH *et al.*, 2013; Kang S-B *et al.*, 2010).

We believe that it is important to continuously evaluate the daily routines, such as choice of operative technique, and we found the given epidemiologic method, a prospective cohort study, efficient and conclusive. After finishing the study, laparoscopic surgery for rectal cancer continued to be "first choice" in our surgical treatment of patients with rectal cancer. In 2009 when this study took its beginning only few carefully selected patients underwent laparoscopic surgery for rectal cancer. At the beginning of our experience only benign rectal resections and highly selected rectal cancer patients were selected for laparoscopic surgery. Before 2009 all patients were operated by open approach

The fraction of laparoscopic surgery increased during the study-period to 87.8% in 2011 and today more than 90% of the patients with rectal cancer undergo laparoscopic surgery. It seems logical that minimizing the surgical trauma leads to less pain and discomfort for the patient and therefore we keep straining ourselves to refine the laparoscopic technique without compromising the oncological and surgical safety. In the near future we find it likely that new techniques, for instance single port surgery and use of the robotic platform, will gain access to the surgical everyday life.

Authors

Katrine Kanstrup Aslak, Orhan Bulut

Department of Surgical Gastroenterology, Hvidovre University Hospital, Copenhagen University, Copenhagen, Denmark

References

Adamsen S, Hansen OH, Fuch-Jensen P et al. Bile duct injury during laparoscopic cholecystectomy: a prospective nationwide series. J Am Coll Surg 1997; 184;571-78.

Akiyoshi T, Kuroyanagi H, Ueno M, et al. Learning curve for standardized laparoscopic surgery for colorectal cancer under supervision: a single center experience. Surg Endosc 2011;25:1409-14.

American cancer Society Website Cancer Facts and Figures. 2004. Available at: http://www.cancer.org/downloads/STT/CAFF2004PWSecured.pdf.

Bachmann MO, Alderson D, Peters TJ, et al. Influence of specialization on the management and outcome of patients with pancreatic cancer. Br J Surg 2003;90:171-7.

Barbas AS, Turley RS, Manynth CR et al. Effect of surgeon specialization on long-term survival following colon cancer resection at an NCI-designated cancer center. J Surg Oncol 2012;106:219-23

Basse L, Hjort Jakobsen D, Billesbolle P, Werner M, Kehlet H. A Clinical Pathway to Accelerate Recovery After Colonic Resection. Ann Surg. 2000;232(1):51–7.

Bärlehner E, Benhidjeb T, Anders S, Schicke B. Laparoscopic resection for rectal cancer: Outcomes in 194 patients and review of the literature. Surg Endosc 2005;19(6):757–66.

Boyle P, Langman JS. ABC of colorectal cancer: epidemiology BMJ 2000;321:805-808

Braga M, Frasson M, Zuliani W, et al. Randomized clinical trial of laparoscopic versus open left colonic resection. Br J Surg 2010;97:1180-6.

Chan ACY, Poon JTC, Fan JKM, et al. Impact of conversion on long-term outcome in laparoscopic resection of colorectal cancer. Surg Endosc 2008;22:2625-30

Danish Colorectalcancer Database. Annual report. Available at: http://www.dccg.dk/03_Publikation/02_arsraport_pdf/aarsrapport_2011.pdf

Danish National Board of Health. Guidelines concerning population screening of colorectal cancer. Available at: http://www.sst.dk/publ/Publ2010/PLAN/Tarmkraeft/AnbefalingerScreeningTarmkraeft2010.pdf

Delaney CP, Chang E, Senagore AJ, et al. Clinical outcomes and resource utilization associated with laparoscopic and open colectomy using a large national database. Ann Surg 2008;247:819-24.

Dowson HM, Huang A, Soon Y, et al. Systematic review of the costs of laparoscopic colorectal surgery. Dis Colon Rectum 2007;50:908-19.

Dowson HM, Gage H, Jackson D, et al. Laparoscopic and open colorectal surgery: a prospective cost analysis. Colorectal Dis 2012 [epub ahead of print].

Fodera M, Pello MJ, Atabek U, Spence RK, Alexander JB, Camishion RC. Trocar site tumor recurrence after laparoscopic-assisted colectomy. J Laparoendosc Surg. August 1995;5(4):259–62.

Good DW, O'Riordan JM, Moran D, Keane FB, Eguare E, O'Riordain DS, et al. Laparoscopic surgery for rectal cancer: a single-centre experience of 120 cases. Int J Colorectal Dis 2011;26(10):1309–15.

Guillou PJ, Quirke P, Thorpe H, Walker J, Jayne DG, Smith AMH, Heath RM, Brown JM. Short-term endpoints of conventional versus laparoscopic-assisted surgery in patients with colorectal cancer (MRC CLASICC trial): multicentre, randomized controlled trial. Lancet 2005;365:1718-1726

Holm T, Ljung A, Häggmark T, Jurell G, Lagergren J. Extended abdominoperineal resection with gluteus maximus flap reconstruction of the pelvic floor for rectal cancer. Br J Surg. 2007;94(2):232–8.

Huang M-J, Liang J-L, Wang H, Kang L, Deng Y-H, Wang J-P. *Laparoscopic-assisted versus open surgery for rectal cancer: a meta-analysis of randomized controlled trials on oncologic adequacy of resection and long-term oncologic outcomes.* Int J Colorectal Dis. 2010;26(4):415–21.

Janson M, Björholt I, Carlsson P, Haglind E, Henriksson M, Lindholm E, et al. *Randomized clinical trial of the costs of open and laparoscopic surgery for colonic cancer.* Br J Surg. 2004;91(4):409–17.

Kang CY, Halabi WJ, Luo R, Pigazzi A, Nguyen NT, Stamos MJ. *Laparoscopic colorectal surgery: A better look into the latest trends.* Arch Surg 2012;147(8):724–31.

Kang JC, Jao SW, Chung MH, et al. *The learning curve for hand-assisted laparoscopic colectomy: a single surgeon's experience.* Surg Endosc 2007;21:243-7.

Kang S-B, Park JW, Jeong S-Y, Nam BH, Choi HS, Kim D-W, et al. *Open versus laparoscopic surgery for mid or low rectal cancer after neoadjuvant chemoradiotherapy (COREAN trial): short-term outcomes of an open-label randomised controlled trial.* Lancet Oncol 2010;11(7):637–45.

Kim J, Edwards E, Bowne W, et al. *Medial-to-lateral laparoscopic colon resection: a view beyond the learning curve.* Surg Endosc 2007;2

Lapco Newsletter summer, 2010. http://www.lapco.nhs.uk/userfiles/file/lapco%20 newsletter%202010.pdf. Published 2010.1:1503-7.

Lagiou P. *Burden of cancer.* In: Adami HO, Hunter D, Tricholpoulos D, eds. Textbook of Cancer Epidemiology. Oxford: Oxford University Press; 2002:3-28

Leung KL, Kwok SPY, Lam SCW, et al. *Laparoscopic resection of rectosigmoid carcinoma; prospective randomised trial.* Lancet 2004;363:1187-92.

Law WL, Poon JTC, Fan JKM, et al. *Survival following laparoscopic versus open resection for colorectal cancer.* Int J Colorectal Dis 2012;27:1077-85.

Li JCM, Hon SSF,Ng SSM, et al. *The learning curve for laparoscopic colectomy: experience of a surgical fellow in an university colorectal unit.* Surg Endosc 2009;23:1603-8

Liang JT, Huang KC, Lai Hs, et al. *Oncologic results of laparoscopic versus conventional open surgery for stage II or III left-sided colon cancers: a randomized controlled trial.* Ann Surg Oncol 2007;14:109-17.

Lindsetmo R-O, Delaney CP. *A Standardized Technique for Laparoscopic Rectal Resection.* J Gastrointest Surg 2009;13(11):2059–63.

Lujan J, Valero G, Hernandez Q, Sanchez A, Frutos MD, Parrilla P. *Randomized clinical trial comparing laparoscopic and open surgery in patients with rectal cancer.* Br J Surg 2009;96(9):982–9.

Miskovic D, Ni M, Wyles SM, et al. *Is competency assessment at the specialist level achievable? A study for the national training programme in laparoscopic colorectal surgery in England.* Ann Surg 2013;257:476-82.

Morino M, Parini U, Giraudo G, Salval M, Brachet Contul R, Garrone C. *Laparoscopic total mesorectal excision: a consecutive series of 100 patients.* Ann Surg 2003;237(3):335–42.

Miyajima N, Fukunaga M, Hasegawa H, Tanaka J, Okuda J, Watanabe M, et al. *Results of a multicenter study of 1,057 cases of rectal cancer treated by laparoscopic surgery.* Surg Endosc 2008;23(1):113–8.

Nagtegaal ID, Velde CJH van de, Worp E van der, Kapiteijn E, Quirke P, Krieken JHJM van. *Macroscopic Evaluation of Rectal Cancer Resection Specimen: Clinical Significance of the Pathologist in Quality Control.* J Clin Oncol. 2002;20(7):1729–34.

Norwood MG, Stephens JH, Hewett PJ, et al. *The nursing and financial implications of laparoscopic colorectal surgery: data from a randomized controlled trial.* Colorectal Dis 2011;13:1303-7.

Park IJ, Choi GS, Lim KH, et al. *Multidimensional analysis of the learning curve for laparoscopic colorectal surgery: lessons from 1,000 cases of laparoscopic colorectal surgery.* Surg Endosc 2009;23:839-46.

Parkin DM, Pidani P, Ferlay J. *Global cancer statistics.* CA Cancer J Clin 1999;49:33-64

Rea JD, Cone MM, Diggs BS, et al. *Utilization of laparoscopic colectomy in the United States before and after the Clinical Outcomes of Surgical Therapy study group trial.* Ann Surg 2011;251:281-8.

Sartori CA, Dal Pozzo A, Franzato B, Balduino M, Sartori A, Baiocchi GL. *Laparoscopic total mesorectal excision for rectal cancer: experience of a single center with a series of 174 patients.* Surg Endosc 2010;25(2):508–14.

Schwenk W, Neudecker J, Raue W, Haase O, Müller JM. *"Fast-track" rehabilitation after rectal cancer resection.* Int J Colorectal Dis 2006;21(6):547–53.

Stottmeier S, Harling H, Wille-Jørgensen P, Balleby L, Kehlet H. *Postoperative morbidity after fast-track laparoscopic resection of rectal cancer. Colorectal Dis. 2012;14(6):769–75.*

Ströhlein MA, Grützner K-U, Jauch K-W, Heiss MM. *Comparison of Laparoscopic vs. Open Access Surgery in Patients with Rectal Cancer: A Prospective Analysis: Dis Colon Rectum 2008;51(4):385–91.*

Tekkis PP, Senagore AJ, Delaney CP et al. *Evaluation of the learning curve in laparoscopic colorectal surgery: comparison of right-sided and left-sided resections. Ann Surg 2005; 242:83-91.*

The Clinical Outcomes of Surgical Therapy Study Group. *A Comparison of Laparoscopically Assisted and Open Colectomy for Colon Cancer. N Engl J Med. 2004;350(20):2050–9.*

The Colon cancer Laparoscopic or Open Resection Study Group. *Laparoscopic surgery versus open surgery for colon cancer: short-term outcomes of a randomized trial. Lancet Oncol 2005;6:477-84*

Van der Pas MH, Haglind E, Cuesta MA, Fürst A, Lacy AM, Hop WC, et al. *Laparoscopic versus open surgery for rectal cancer (COLOR II): short-term outcomes of a randomised, phase 3 trial. Lancet Oncol 2013;14(3):210–8.*

Vlug MS, Wind J, Hollmann MW, Ubbink DT, Cense HA, Engel AF, et al. *Laparoscopy in Combination with Fast Track Multimodal Management is the Best Perioperative Strategy in Patients Undergoing Colonic Surgery: A Randomized Clinical Trial (LAFA-study). Ann Surg 2011;254(6):868–75.*

Wingo PA et al. *Long-term trends in cancer mortality in the United States, 1930-1998. Cancer 2003;97:3133-3275*

Researching the Social Determinants of Health using Social Quality Theory: A National Survey in Australia

Paul R. Ward, Loreen Mamerow, Samantha Meyer, Fiona Verity

1   Introduction

The World Health Organisation (WHO) has urged governments around the world to focus public health policy, practice and research on the SDH in order to improve the health of the most vulnerable and marginalised groups (Pittman 2006; Gilson, Doherty *et al.*, 2007; Commission on Social Determinants of Health 2008). The Commission on the Social Determinants of Health (CSDH) drew global attention to the multiple forms of oppression and disadvantage experienced by the most vulnerable members of society which lead to unacceptable inequities in health (Commission on Social Determinants of Health 2008). Indeed, Professor Sir Michael Marmot recently referred to these health inequities as a "stain on our society" which require concerted political will and moral imperative to change (Kondro 2012). In order for governments to reduce inequities in health within their countries, the CSDH called for a 'joined up', multi-sectoral approach which recognises the multidimensional nature of the problem. In this way, reducing health inequities requires additional action in spheres of government policy outside of healthcare, such as poverty reduction, welfare support, community development and other health promotion activities. The CSDH also builds on seminal multi-national agreements such as the Ottawa Charter, the Alma Ata Declaration and the Bangkok Declaration which also argue for 'joined up government' in order to improve the health of the most vulnerable groups in society.

Recognition of the SDH, from a policy perspective, is essential for health sector policy decision-making (Makinen, Waters *et al.*, 2000) since health policies shape health systems, and consequently, the broader SDH. Despite the differences in political and economic climate in the countries under analysis, our findings highlight patterns of social quality which require policy responses. We argue that our data should be used as a means of deciding the most appropriate policy response for each country which includes, rather than excludes, socially marginalised population groups (Freedman, Waldman *et al.*, 2005). These findings should be of interest to those involved in health policy, but also in policy more generally because as we have identified, health is influenced by determinants outside of the health system (Lee, Fustukian *et al.*, 2002).

For well over twenty years policy makers, health and social reformers in Australia have advocated the practical sense of an integrated approach in policy making and service delivery; to move from 'silos to a system', towards 'whole of government approaches', and 'health in all' (Menedue 2003; Wood 2008; Kickbusch 2008: 9). However, an unsettled question remains how this best is done. Our purpose in this chapter is to demonstrate the practical utility of the social quality approach as a means to guide the development of policies, practices and systems in accord with this objective.

Whilst we agree with the need to focus on multiple forms of disadvantage and thus complex and holistic policy responses, our previous paper argued that many conceptual frameworks currently used in public health research do not lend themselves easily to being useful for these purposes (Ward, Meyer et al., 2011). For example, there are large amounts of research which provide evidence that certain population groups are more socially excluded (Giddens 1994), have lower levels of social capital (Ahern and Hendryx 2003), have poorer access to financial resources, health promoting or curative services (Spicer 2009) and that some groups are disempowered (Ward and Coates 2006). All of these factors have been shown to be SDH, in that higher levels of social inclusion, social capital, access to finance and services and empowerment are all 'good for your health'; however, taken on their own, these studies are useful only in so far as they paint part of the picture as to both the problems and solutions for increasing the health of vulnerable groups. What they do not do is provide both a conceptual and methodological framework for linking these various concepts for the same population groups, which would then highlight the potentially multiple or cumulative 'problems' that certain population groups face, or the particular 'problems' that other groups face. This fragmented policy and research context has been described as '…a field of turbulent discourses; different problems, different analyses and different strategies sweeping across the policy field like storm clouds under time lapse photography (p. 22)" (Legge, Wilson et al., 1996). Research studies may highlight the need to implement policy to increase the social capital for particular groups, or to facilitate more socially inclusive policies or systems, but rarely can such studies (due to their conceptual limitations) provide evidence for policies and systems which attend to the multiplicity of needs highlighted by the CSDH. Therefore, research is required to unify theories and analyses that on their own, concentrate on one aspect of a dynamic and fragmented health and social policy context.

This chapter has two main aims. Firstly we introduce a theoretical and conceptual framework developed in social policy in Europe, known as social quality theory (van der Maesen and Walker 2005; Ward 2006; Ward, Redgrave et al., 2006; Walker 2009; Ward and Meyer 2009), which aims to overcome the 'silo' problem mentioned above and provides a holistic approach to understanding the SDH and potentials for policy initiatives. Secondly, we go on to describe a study of social quality in Australia, and in so doing, highlight the utility of such an approach for researchers and policy makers in public health interested in both understanding and responding to the SDH for the most vulnerable groups in society.

1.1   Policy Context in Australia

Australia in the early 21st century is varied in the cultures and socio-economic status of its inhabitants. Whilst in the main Australia escaped the severe hardships resulting from the Global Financial Crisis, unlike the European and North American experience, it is increasingly a society of contrasts. This is seen in socio-economic and health chasms opening up between population groups living in the same cities and between cities and regions (Gleeson 2004:3; Vinson 2007; ACOSS 2011). It is also evident in the different fortunes of sectors of the Australian economy. Australia's connections to Asian markets, especially to China and India, the strength of mining activity and exports relative to the retail sector, and the recent strong Australian dollar are contributors to what is called a two speed economy (OECD 2010). Nowhere is this gap more manifest than in the circumstances for Indigenous Australians relative to non-Indigenous Australians (Thomson, MacRae *et al.*, 2010).

To close these gaps and advance social quality, there has been a plethora of public policy programs developed at different levels of the federated system of government. These include initiatives to support economic objectives and social objectives. The latter include means tested social security payments, social service and health provision and programs under the rubrics of strengthening social capital and stronger families and communities. In more recent times social inclusion has taken on policy prominence and informed measures to lift community and economic participation and tackle disadvantage. The South Australian Labor government was first to develop a dedicated Social Inclusion Unit, followed by the establishment in 2007 of a national Labor Government's Social Inclusion Initiative (http://www.social inclusion.gov.au/aus_inclusion_board/inclusion_board.htm). These policies sit within a changing Australian welfare state, which for more than three decades has been increasingly dominated by values and practices supportive of self-responsibility, a resurgence of private market provision to meet social objectives and reduced direct government provision. Bryson and Verity call this a 'radical neo-liberal economic turn of social policy' (Bryson and Verity 2009: 67). The implementation of Welfare-to-Work reform is an example informed by this ideology as is privatisation and outsourcing policies.

It is against this backdrop of growing inequities and a neo-liberal welfare state that we focus in this Chapter on an assessment of individual and social well-being in Australia in late 2009. We do this using the tool known as theory of social quality as an innovative theoretical and methodological tool for researchers and policy makers wanting to understand and respond to the SDH (Beck, van der Maesen *et al.*, 1998; Beck, van der Maesen *et al.*, 2001; Walker and van der Maesen 2004; van der Maesen and Walker 2005; Ward 2006; Ward 2006; Ward, Redgrave *et al.*, 2006; Taylor-Gooby 2006c; Ward and Meyer 2009; Meyer, Luong *et al.*, 2010). One of the advantages is that it enables what we view as complex understandings of social problems and potentials for social change. In other words it links between personal domains and agency and the structural context which impact on SDH.

Measuring social quality of life in the Australian context is not in new. Australia has a tradition of social research about quality of life (Eckersley 1999) in the form of market research like the national 'Mind and Mood' Reports by Hugh MacKay now Ipsos MacKay and measures administered by the Australian Bureau of Statistics. The first national Australian Survey of Social Attitudes was in 2003 (Wilson, Meagher *et al.*, 2005) and in 2004 the Australian Bureau of Statistics released indicators on measuring social capital (Australian Bureau of Statistics 2004) with metrics for quality and the strength of social networks. There has, however, been limited application in public health research and social policy of the European approach known as the TSQ (van der Maesen and Walker 2005; Ward 2006; Ward, Redgrave *et al.*, 2006; Walker 2009; Ward and Meyer 2009). We have provided a detailed account of social quality theory elsewhere, in which we argued that social quality provides a comprehensive conceptual and methodological framework for measuring the SDH (Ward, Meyer *et al.*, 2011). However, we provide a brief summary here in order to provide necessary context for this chapter.

1.2   Social Quality Theory

Social quality theory is gaining international recognition as an innovative theoretical and methodological tool for researchers and policy makers in social policy and political science (Beck, van der Maesen *et al.*, 1998; Beck, van der Maesen *et al.*, 2001; Walker and van der Maesen 2004; van der Maesen and Walker 2005; Ward 2006; Ward 2006; Ward, Redgrave *et al.*, 2006; Taylor-Gooby 2006c; Ward and Meyer 2009; Meyer, Luong *et al.*, 2010), although little attention has been given within public health research and policy. Social quality has been defined as "the extent to which people are able to participate in the social, economic life and development of their communities under conditions which enhance their wellbeing and individual potential (p.3)" (Beck, van der Maesen *et al.*, 1998).

Social quality theory was initially developed by the European Network Indicators of Social Quality (ENISQ) (van der Maesen and Walker 2005). The ENISQ developed indicators (or metrics) of social quality so that governments and researchers could assess social quality within and between societies or Nation States, using only routinely available data sources. Whilst this has benefits in terms of not needing to design and implement primary research, it also relies on existing datasets, which are often collected for administrative purposes and are often relatively old. Therefore, we used the indicators to develop a new social quality questionnaire to measure social quality. In this way, we have advanced the methodological and practical aspects of social quality theory by providing researchers and policy makers with a readily available instrument to measure social quality, and thus the SDH.

Social quality theory has both ideological and methodological underpinnings. In terms of its underlying ideology, social quality theory argues that there four key normative factors that determine the quality of the social structures, policies and relationships within a society: social justice; solidarity; equal value of all humans; and human dignity (Beck, van der Maesen *et al.*, 2001). A society can be judged according to these normative factors, both in a global sense (i.e. how good is the social quality of a particular society) but also in terms of the specific normative factors (i.e. which factors require policy response in a particular society). However, on their own, these normative factors are not easily operationalised and do not have a methodological framework. Therefore, within social quality theory, there are a set of conditional factors which are aimed at rendering the normative factors 'researchable'. The four conditional factors are socio-economic security (linked to social justice), social cohesion (linked to solidarity), social inclusion (linked to equal value) and social empowerment (linked to human dignity). These four conditional factors were measured using the newly developed social quality survey.

Socio-economic security is concerned with the extent to which people or groups have access to, utilisation of and successful outcomes related to a variety of resources over time. These resources may be related to, among other things, finance, housing, healthcare, employment and education. Socio-economic security has great historical credence in public health policy and practice in terms of the importance of such factors in shaping inequalities in health and inequities in health care. Huge effort has been put into both public health policy (Commission on Social Determinants of Health 2005; Commission on Social Determinants of Health 2007; Commission on Social Determinants of Health 2008) and research around understanding the causes and mechanisms of socio-economic inequalities in health, with most authors regarding it as a key SDH (Marmot and Wilkinson 2006; Wilkinson and Pickett 2006; Wilkinson and Pickett 2007; Ostlin, Schrecker *et al.*, 2010).

Social cohesion relates to the extent to which people and groups share social relations. Such relations may refer to shared identities, values and norms. This domain relates closely to issues of solidarity and trust, which are again, particularly important in terms of public health (Ward and Coates 2006; Meyer, Ward et al., 2008; Meyer, Luong et al., 2012). In many ways, this domain relates to the concept of social capital, which is now commonplace in public health policy and research (Lochner, Kawachi et al., 2003; Subramanian, Lochner et al., 2003; Kim, Subramanian et al., 2006), although has its roots in sociological theory (Bourdieu 1984; Colclough and Sitaraman 2005; Carpiano 2006; Poortinga 2006; Poortinga 2006). Indeed, early sociologists such as Durkheim argued for the centrality of social cohesion for protecting health (Durkheim 1951) and contemporary sociologists such as Giddens and Luhmann argue that trust and social networks are the glue that hold society together, providing existential security, thereby protecting mental health (Luhmann 1979; Giddens 1990; Giddens 1994; Luhmann 2000).

Social inclusion, is in many ways, similar to social cohesion, although the difference is that social inclusion is related to the extent to which people and groups have access to and are integrated into the different institutions and social relations of 'everyday life'. This domain relates to the extent to which people and groups 'feel part of' or included in society, at an everyday level, and thus attempts to integrate dualistic processes at the level of systems (i.e. institutions and social systems) and individuals. In so doing, it extends Parsons' notions of social systems by seeing their interconnectedness with individual lifeworlds (Parsons 1951), which Giddens called the duality of structure (Giddens 1984). In this way, the domain of social inclusion fits neatly with system/lifeworld theories expounded by Habermas (Habermas 1997) and structure/agency argued by Giddens (Giddens 1984; Giddens 1990; Giddens 1991) and Archer (Archer 2003) in addition to public health research which provides empirical evidence on the links between social inclusion and health (Scambler 2001; Scambler and Britten 2001; Williams and Popay 2001).

Social empowerment relates to the extent to which the personal capabilities of individual people are enhanced by social relations, culminating in individuals feeling empowered within their country. In many ways, this builds on both social cohesion and social inclusion, revealing the integrated nature of social quality theory. In this way, this domain takes concepts of social inclusion and cohesion, and explores the enabling factors which empower people to act as social agents. This domain builds on, and empirically develops, notions of reflexivity outlined by Beck (Beck 1992; Beck, Giddens et al., 1994; Beck 2005) and Giddens (Giddens 1994) and extends the current evidence base on the positive effects of empowerment on both individual and public health (Laverack 2004; Laverack 2006; Wallerstein 2006).

As can be seen in this brief overview, the multi-dimensional and multi-level approach represents an advancement of public health policy and research, which is not solely aimed at either individuals or systems, but instead realises the intimate linkages between structure and agency and thus aims at understanding both within the same theoretical framework. The four conditional factors within social quality have all been shown individually to lead to better health, and as such are regarded as SDH, although have not been brought together into a single theoretical framework.The long-term aim of developing and implementing social quality theory is to enhance the social quality of peoples' lives (especially vulnerable groups), but as already stated, we firstly need to have empirical data on the domains of social quality (and the groups who have lower social quality) before we can inform changes in policy and/or practice. The aim of this chapter is to describe the patterns with regards to social quality (as measures of the SDH) and to identify both consistent and divergent patterns between countries. This chapter therefore represents baseline data from which the effectiveness of any future policy initiatives in Australia can be assessed.

2   Methods

There were three main research stages within this study: Pre-Pilot; Pilot Test; and, the Full Survey. Firstly, pre-pilot testing was undertaken to assess the validity of the measuring instrument used for the research - the questionnaire. Secondly, a pilot test was conducted to assess the reliability of the questionnaire. This was achieved by conducting a test-retest reliability test where analyses were carried out statistically. Lastly, the full survey was carried out once the pre-pilot and pilot test qualified the questionnaire to be sufficiently valid and reliable, respectively.

2.1   Pre-Pilot Test – Assessing the Validity of the Questionnaire

Face validity may be defined as having 'experts' review the contents of the instrument being used for measurement to ensure that is relevant and useful (Reber 1985). Therefore, in this case the participants' feedback may be taken to be the expert opinions that are used as face validity to verify the researchers' assessment. Thus, face validity was obtained by asking some of the participants for feedback. Feedback from both the research team and the pilot test participants was then taken into consideration to address the relevance of the questions and to make appropriate amendments to a few of the questions and/or question items prior to the statistical analysis of the pilot study.

Questions from pre-validated questionnaires, including the World Values Survey (World Values Survey Association 2005/2006) and the General Social Survey (National Opinion Research Center), were also employed in the SQ survey since they had previously been validated. Initially, the survey consisted of 58 questions that were predominantly constituted by nominal and ordinal levels of measurement. Although the SQ survey up until this point had been comprehensively developed and validated, in particular, for face, content, and construct validity (Bowling 2009), the need to ensure that the Australian research team had constructed a valid set of questions needed to be verified.

The questions used in the pilot test were developed by the Asia-Pacific Scientific Steering Group on Social Quality - Seoul National University led the process. The questionnaire itself was developed from the Social Quality Indicators developed by the ENISQ. All of the questions used in the questionnaire were either demographically relevant or related to any one of the four conditional factors of SQ (socio-economic security, social inclusion, social cohesion and social empowerment).

The initial stages of validity checking involved collaborative efforts across the Asia-Pacific research team, which included numerous and extensive face-to-face discussions. Revision and modification of the questionnaire lasted for approximately three months, including meticulous discussions of the cultural relevance of each question. The final questionnaire was agreed upon between all international teams in July 2009, which was subsequently tested for both validity and reliability (Meyer, Luong *et al.*, 2010), including collaboration and agreement with the originators of the social quality indicators (Ferriss 2004).

Further amendments were made after receiving the final revised questionnaire from the Korean research team. Extensive meetings were carried out to meticulously discuss the cultural relevance, question by question. To check the validity of the amended 'Australian version' of the questionnaire, 33 participants were asked to answer the survey and provide feedback about their experience of answering the questionnaire.

2.2   Pilot Test – Assessing the Test-Retest and Inter-Item Reliability of the Questionnaire

A total of 33 Australian respondents (18 males and 15 females aged 19 to 63), residing in metropolitan Adelaide (South Australia) were recruited as a sample of convenience.

The original survey (before testing for reliability and face validity within this study) consisted of 58 questions (mostly nominal and ordinal levels of measurement) relating to the four domains of social quality, as well as demographic items.

Face validity, prior to the data analysis, was obtained through asking some of the respondents to offer feedback about their experience of answering the questionnaire. Face validity is often defined as having 'experts' review the contents of the instrument for usefulness, relevance, etc. (Reber 1985). It can be argued that the respondents have expertise. In addition to respondent feedback, two academics who have had research experience and taught on the subject of designing questionnaires have also reviewed drafts of the social quality questionnaire. Following feedback from both types of experts, some difficulties were established and appropriate amendments were made to a few of the questions prior to statistical data analysis.

The analyses were focussed on reliability testing using SPSS. Both test-retest and inter-item reliability analyses were conducted. If the results from the test re-test analyses (Kappa, or Spearman Correlation tests) and the inter-item reliability test (Cronbach's α) were statistically non-significant ($p > 0.05$; N = 10-33) or the coefficients were < 0.70 for any of the questionnaire items, then the questions were amended or removed. Questionnaire items were also removed if response rates for these items were found to be very low (< 33%).

Test-retest reliability and obtaining face validity were conducted prior to inter-item reliability and as a result, some of the questions had already been changed prior to inter-item testing. Consequently, some of the questions were not subject to inter-item reliability. Any questions that scored poorly in inter-item reliability were subsequently altered. SPSS statistical analyses were used to identify items within questions that lowered the reliability scores. The questionnaire items that lowered the reliability of the questions were removed until Cronbach's α was $\geq .70$. For readers interested in more information, the results of the pilot study have been published (Meyer, Luong *et al.*, 2010), as has the final questionnaire (Ward, Meyer *et al.*, 2011).

2.3   Full Survey

Full details of the methods used in the full survey can be found in a previous publication (Ward, Meyer *et al.*, 2011), but enough detail is provided here to give the reader sufficient information. A national postal questionnaire survey of a random sample of households was undertaken across Australia. It was necessary to divide the national population by state (Alreck and Settle 2004) due to the difference in population size in each State. Therefore, more surveys were sent out to states with higher population numbers (New South Wales 1650, Northern Territory 45, Queensland 971, South Australia 389, Tasmania 120, Victoria 1253, Western Australia 490, Australian Capital Territory 82). The sampling frame was the electronic white pages, which contains postal addresses for all households with a telephone listed. Therefore, a small proportion of households who either do not have a telephone or have "silent" numbers were excluded. However, this possible limitation is outweighed by the fact that the electronic white pages is one of the only representative sources from which a national random sample of postal addresses can be generated.

A copy of the questionnaire, a letter of information, a letter of introduction, and a stamped return envelope was sent to each mail-out address September 2009. A postcard reminder was only sent out to those who had not returned the questionnaire after two weeks.

The hypothesised response rate was around 20% (based on the experience of the research team of conducting similar surveys in Australia), and in order to obtain a final sample size of 1000, it was estimated that an initial sample of 5000 addresses was required. Out of the 5000 surveys that were sent out, 638 were returned due to invalid addresses and 1044 were returned completed surveys. The actual response rate of 24% (1044/4362) was regarded as acceptable for this type of survey because of the decline in participation in survey research - see our previous paper for literature supporting this (Ward, Meyer *et al.,* 2011). As noted earlier, reminders postcards were sent to non-responders to ensure as high a response rate as possible (Low, King *et al.,* 1998). Nevertheless, the potential for survey non-response bias is acknowledged.

After data entry had been completed, an extra two variables were created from the postcode of the respondent. Both variables are derived from the national census. The first variable is called the Socio-Economic Indicator For Areas (or SEIFA) and provides a score for the level of socio-economic deprivation or affluence of the area. The second variable is called Accessibility and Remoteness Indicator for Areas (or ARIA) which provides a score for the distance of the postcode from major service centres. Both of these variables were thought to be potentially important when analysing differences in social quality.

Initially, descriptive analyses were undertaken in order to explore overall levels of social quality. We then performed bivariate logistic regression analyses in order to explore simple associations between a range of socio-demographic variables and the indicators of social quality. For the regression models, four questions identified by the ENISQ in 2004 (Ferriss 2004) as indicators of the four domains of social quality were used as dependent variables (i.e. one variable per domain of social quality). The complete questionnaire contained many indicators of social quality that have all been shown to be valid proxies for their relevant social quality domain [20]. All of these variables were found to have statistical significance with the listed demographic variables. For example, questions such as 'Please indicate whether you or your family have experienced any of the following negative life events in the last 12 months?', 'How much do you trust various groups of people?' were found to be associated with demographic variables; however, for the purpose of this chapter we have limited our results to one variable per domain. The independent variables chosen to investigate associations between social quality and demographic variables were age, sex, SEIFA IRSD (Socio-economic Index for Areas Index of Relative Socio-economic Disadvantage), ARIA (Accessibility/ Remoteness Index of Australia), employment status and income.

Bivariate analyses were conducted using Chi Squares (Cramer's V and Phi) as well as T-tests, one-way ANOVAs, Mann-Whitney U, and Kruskal-Wallis H. Each test produced a table which was subsequently analysed for statistically significant associations. Any bivariate odds ratios with $p<0.25$ were then included in multivariate logistic regression analyses (Hosmer and Lemeshow 2000). The tables presented in our result section include only the results of bivariate analyses found to have a p value of <0.25. All models were checked for collinearity and goodness of fit (Hosmer and Lemeshow 2000). During the bivariate analysis, some of the data was found to have expected cell counts less than five. As a result, many of the categories within the independent variables were collapsed in order to help the data meet the assumption. This was done by recoding the variables using SPSS. Data that could not be collapsed to help meet the assumption have not been included in the results section.

This study was given ethical clearance by the Social and Behavioural Research Ethics Committee at Flinders University.

3   Results

This section of the chapter provides statistical description and analysis of the data, focussing specifically on the four conditional factors within the social quality theory, namely socio-economic security, social cohesion, social inclusion and social empowerment. One multivariate regression model is presented for each of the four domains as a means of introducing the practical application of social quality theory. Each of the four models includes one social quality variable (social inclusion, social cohesion etc) as the dependent variable with the socio-demographic variables (sex, age, income etc) as independent variables.

3.1   Socio-economic Security

There were a number of variables that related to socio-economic security within the dataset, but for the purpose of this chapter, we have just used one variable. The question used to measure socio-economic security in the survey is outlined below:

- *Please indicate whether you or your family have experienced any of the following in the last 12 months?*
  1. *Costly medical expenses*
  2. *Job loss or business bankruptcy*
  3. *Job insecurity*
  4. *Work injury*
  5. *Becoming a victim of crime*
  6. *Investment loss*

Overall, 31% of respondents had experienced costly medical experiences, 10% had experienced job loss or bankruptcy, 14% had experienced job insecurity, 6.5% had experienced work injury, 6% had been a victim of crime, and 50% had experienced investment loss. Overall, there was a fairly low level of experiences of these negative life events, although costly medical expenses and investment loss were experienced by larger proportions of the population.

The variable was then recoded into two categories, those that had experienced at least one of these events (71.7%) and those who had not experienced any (28.3%). The multivariate odds ratios are in Table 1. The main points to take from this table are the higher levels of negative life events for people aged 55-64 (OR 2.41; 95% CI 1.34-4.32) and 65-74 (OR 3.55; 95% CI 1.72-7.34), and lower for retired people (OR 0.57; 95% CI 0.33-0.98) (the model was checked for collinearity given that these two variables could have been measuring the same factor – age).

	OR (95% CI)	p value
Age		
18-34 years	1.00	
35-44 years	1.06 (0.60-1.87)	0.844
45-54 years	1.67 (0.97-2.86)	0.064
55-64 years	2.41 (1.34-4.32)	0.003
65-74 years	3.55 (1.72-7.34)	0.001
75 years and over	1.55 (0.71-3.38)	0.273
Employment status		
Work full time or self employed	1.00	
Work part time	1.18 (0.74-1.89)	0.478
Work without pay, unemployed, student, disability, other	1.33 (0.74-2.39)	0.342
Retired	0.57 (0.33-0.98)	0.042
Household duties	0.88 (0.45-1.73)	0.710

Model stable, Hosmer and Lemeshow, Chi square 8.19, p = 0.415

Table 1: Multivariate odds ratios of demographic factors associated with those who experienced at least one negative life event.

Overall, our data suggest fairly low levels of socio-economic insecurity in Australia, although there are some particular financial issues such as loss of investments and rising medical costs. The regression model shows that older people experience higher socio-economic insecurity than younger people.

3.2   Social Cohesion

The variable chosen for analysis relating to social cohesion was:

- *How much do you trust various groups of people?*
    1. *Your family*
    2. *Your neighbours*
    3. *People you meet for the first time*
    4. *Your regular doctor*
    5. *Doctors in general*
    6. *A doctor you are seeing for the first time*
    7. *People of another religion*
    8. *People of another nationality*
    9. *National political leader*
    10. *Your local politician*
    11. *Police officers*

The response categories were 'completely distrust', 'distrust a little', 'trust a little', and 'completely trust'. Overall, 82% of respondents trust their family completely, 34% trust neighbours completely, 22% trust doctors completely, 18% trust people of another religion completely, 15% trust people of another nationality completely, 2% trust national political leaders completely and 25% trust police officers completely. From a social perspective, the relatively low numbers of people that trust neighbours and even lower numbers that trust people of another nationality or religion is worrying. In addition, only 22% trust doctors completely, 25% trust police officers completely although only 2% trust the national political leader completely, all of which have serious policy ramifications.

The variable was then recoded so that those who trusted completely were given a score of 1 and those who completely distrusted were given a score of 4. Scores could range from 11 (most trust) to 44 (least trust). Scores ranged from 11 to 37 with a mean of 21.53 and SD 4.09. A variable was then created with two levels, those who trusted all of the groups completely or somewhat (20.6%) and those who did not trust all groups completely or somewhat (79.4%). Univariate odds ratios then examined the relationship between those who trusted at least one of the groups completely or somewhat and demographic characteristics (age, sex, marital status, work status, income, SEIFA IRSD and ARIA). The multivariate odds ratios are in presented in Table 2.

	OR (95% CI)	p value
Sex		
Male	1.00	
Female	1.77 (1.18-2.66)	0.006
Age		
18-34 years	1.00	
35-44 years	2.02 (0.87-4.71)	0.104
45-54 years	1.29 (0.56-2.98)	0.548
55-64 years	2.67 (1.18-6.05)	0.019
65-74 years	2.49 (1.07-5.80)	0.035
75 years and over	5.44 (2.12-14.01)	<0.001
Marital status		
Never married	1.00	
Separated/divorced	1.98 (0.67-5.85)	0.217
Married/defacto	3.33 (1.28-8.66)	0.014
Widowed	1.80 (0.54-6.02)	0.340

Model stable, Hosmer and Lemeshow, Chi square 1.14, p = 0.992

Table 2: Multivariate odds ratios of demographic factors associated with those who trusted all groups completely or somewhat.

Table 2 shows that women are approximately 80% more likely to have high trust than men (OR 1.77; 95% CI 1.18-2.66), older people are more likely to have high trust than younger people, and that married people are more likely to have high trust than never married people. Indeed, people aged over 75 years are almost 5.5 times more likely to have high trust than people aged 18-34 years (OR 5.44; 95% CI 2.12-14.01) and people who are married are 3.3 times more likely to have high trust than people who have never been married (OR 3.3; 95% CI 1.28-8.66). Therefore, our data show that social cohesion is higher for women, older people and married people.

3.3   Social Inclusion

Social inclusion deals with an individual's accessibility to institutions and the degree of social integration that the individual attains to (Walker and Wigfield 2004). The variable chosen to examine social inclusion was:

- *During the past 12 months, have you ever experienced discrimination against you due to any of the following reasons?*
    1. *Physical/mental disability*
    2. *Age*
    3. *Sexual harassment*
    4. *Gender*
    5. *Nationality*
    6. *Physical appearance*
    7. *Ethnic background*
    8. *Criminal record*
    9. *Religion*
    10. *Other*

The proportion of respondents who had experienced discrimination varied: 4% experienced disability discrimination, 14% age discrimination, 2% sexual discrimination, 7% gender discrimination, 4% nationality discrimination, 6% physical appearance discrimination, 3% ethnic background discrimination, 1% criminal record discrimination, 2% religious discrimination, and 4% other discrimination. The variable was then recoded into two categories, those who had experienced discrimination (23.9%) (excluding the 'other' responses due to the large number of missing) and those who had not experienced any discrimination (76.1%). Univariate odds ratios then examined the relationship between those who experienced discrimination and demographic characteristics (age, sex, marital status, work status, income, SEIFA IRSD and ARIA), and the multivariate analysis is presented in Table 3.

Table 3 shows that women are more likely to experience discrimination in addition to people on lower incomes (measured by the individual income and also the area based SEIFA score). However, older people are less likely to experience discrimination. Women are over 50% more likely to have experienced discrimination than men (OR 1.53; 95% CI 1.06-2.12), people in the lowest income group ($0-$44,999) are over 70% more likely to have experienced discrimination than the highest income group (OR 1.71; 95% CI 1.04-2.81) and people aged over 75 years are over 50% less likely to have experienced discrimination than the youngest group (OR 0.43; 95% CI 0.19-0.98). Overall, social inclusion is high in Australia as measured by generally low levels of perceived discrimination. Nevertheless, some groups are more likely to perceive discrimination, such as women, people on lower incomes and younger people.

3.4   Social Empowerment

The variable chosen for analysis relating to social empowerment was:

- *Please rate how strongly you agree/disagree with each of the following statements below:*
    1. *I am optimistic about the future*
    2. *In order to get ahead nowadays you are forced to do things that are not appropriate*
    3. *I feel left out of society*
    4. *Life has become so complicated today that I almost can't find my way*
    5. *I don't feel the value of what I do is recognised by others*

Descriptive analysis of the data from this question revealed that 75% of respondents were optimistic about the future, 20% were forced to do something that was not appropriate, 9% felt left out of society, 18% felt that life was too complicated, and 24% felt that the value of what

	OR	p value
Sex		
Male	1.00	
Female	1.53 (1.06-2.12)	**0.022**
Age		
18-34 years	1.00	
35-44 years	1.16 (0.62-2.17)	**0.651**
45-54 years	0.64 (0.35-2.17)	**0.141**
55-64 years	0.54 (0.29-1.03)	**0.060**
65-74 years	0.54 (0.28-1.08)	**0.080**
75 years and over	0.43 (0.19-0.98)	**0.044**
Income (financial year)		
$105,000-$150,000+	1.00	
$45,000-$104,999	1.09 (0.69-1.71)	**0.716**
$0-$44,999	1.71 (1.04-2.81)	**0.034**
SEIFA IRSD		
Lowest quintile	1.00	
Low quintile	0.93 (0.54-1.59)	**0.782**
Middle quintile	0.81 (0.47-1.41)	**0.453**
High quintile	0.45 (0.25-0.81)	**0.008**
Highest quintile	**0.86 (0.49-1.48)**	**0.575**

Model stable, Hosmer and Lemeshow, Chi square 2.22, p = 0.974

Table 3: Multivariate odds ratios of demographic factors associated with those who experienced discrimination.

they do is not recognised. Whilst three-quarters of respondents felt optimistic about the future, it is worrying that a fifth were forced to do something they did not want to do, and a quarter felt that they are not valued for what they do.

Each variable was then recoded into five variables, with the first variable comprising those who "agreed" and "strongly agreed" with the statement (compared to the remainder) and the remaining four variables those that "disagreed" or "strongly disagreed" with the statement (compared to the remainder). Finally a combined variable was created of those who were positive about at least one factor (94.9%) compared those who were not positive about any of the statements (5.1%). Univariate odds ratios then examined the relationship between those who experienced discrimination and demographic characteristics (age, sex, marital status, work status, income, SEIFA IRSD and ARIA) and the multivariate analysis is presented in Table 4.

	OR	p value
Income (financial year)		
$105,000-$150,000+	1.00	
$45,000-$104,999	0.52 (0.20-1.37)	**0.186**
$0-$44,999	**0.33 (0.13-0.82)**	**0.017**

Model stable, Hosmer and Lemeshow, Chi square 1.66, p = 0.976

Table 4: Multivariate odds ratios of demographic factors associated with those who had at least one positive feeling.

In Table 4, only one variable was left in the model, which is income. This model shows that people on lower incomes are almost 70% less likely to have positive feelings about being socially empowered, compared with people on higher incomes (OR 0.33; 95% CI 0.13-0.82).

4   Conclusions

The main aim of this chapter was to provide an analysis of the SDH in order to compare and contrast the predictors and vulnerable populations. We fulfilled this aim by using data from a population survey in Australia which used social quality as its conceptual framework. In terms of both conceptual and policy-related strengths, this paper presents the first attempt to conduct an analysis of social quality data with the specific purpose of identifying vulnerable population groups in terms of low socio-economic security, low social inclusion, low social cohesion and/or low social empowerment. Our analysis allows policy makers and researchers to identify population groups in need of policy and practice attention, both within and across countries. In particular, we have identified some population groups that have low levels of social quality across all four factors, identifying multiple and potentially cumulative disadvantage for these groups.

Social quality theory aims to move beyond partial understandings of social problems informed by single disciplinary knowledge, and partial explanations afforded by theories that examine only one area of social life. On the basis of the data reported upon in this chapter we contend social quality is useful because of this emphasis on a more complete and integrated picture. The picture developed in this chapter, using the four conditional factors of social quality, is that the social quality of life in Australia is relatively high across the four domains. Socio-economic security is high (except for approximately 30% of people who had costly medical expenses), social cohesion is fairly high (relatively high levels of trust in family, lower levels of trust in neighbours, and worryingly low levels of trust in people of another religion or nationality), social inclusion is high (low levels of perceived discrimination) and social empowerment is fairly high (three-quarters of respondents were optimistic about the future, but a fifth were forced to do something they did not want to do, and a quarter felt that they are not valued for what they do).

However social quality theory, in drawing together individual measures, does more than provide a holistic picture. It develops a picture of systematic differences in social quality between population groups at a point in time. As seen in this chapter, notwithstanding the relatively positive picture of social quality in Australia, there were systematic differences in social quality between population groups. People with the lowest annual income and/or in the most disadvantaged social group (measured by SEIFA) experienced higher levels of discrimination (lower social inclusion) and had more negative views about their place in society and their future (lower social empowerment). Therefore, on the basis of social inclusion and social empowerment, people with lower incomes have lower social quality than people on higher incomes.

Our findings showed a rather mixed picture on the basis of age, whereby older people experienced more negative financial experiences (lower socio-economic security) than younger people, although they also had higher levels of trust (higher social cohesion) and experienced lower levels of discrimination (high social inclusion). The lower socio-economic security may be indicative of the fact that older individuals are likely to be living off of pensions and/or retirement plans and more likely to require medical care. However, this finding remains an important consideration in view of the estimations of population numbers who will be over 65 years by the year 2040 and that life expectancy is lengthening. However, the fact that younger people experience more discrimination and have lower levels of trust will require policy initiatives in order to increase trust and reduce discrimination in the future.

In terms of gender, women experience more discrimination (lower social inclusion) but have higher levels of trust (higher social cohesion) than men. Anti-discrimination and gender-mainstreaming policy is required to redress the difference in social inclusion and more research is required to understand and suggest policy options for increasing trust in men.

It is recognised globally that public health policy, practice and research needs to focus on addressing the SDH in order to increase the health of the most vulnerable and disadvantaged groups (WHO 2005; WHO Task Force on Research Priorities for Equity in Health 2005; Wilkinson and Pickett 2006; Commission on Social Determinants of Health 2008; Ostlin, Schrecker *et al.*, 2010). Given the multiple and complex nature of the SDH, this chapter used a new conceptual framework called social quality, which we argue allows researchers and policy makers to measure and respond to the SDH. In a previous paper, we argued for the utility of social quality for researching the SDH (Ward, Meyer *et al.*, 2011), and in this paper, we provided new empirical evidence. Our analyses focused on the four domains of social quality: socio-economic security, social cohesion, social inclusion and social empowerment, which we argue are key SDH. As such, our paper represents a key social epidemiological analysis of the SDH, and in particular, an important contribution to identifying vulnerable populations groups in need of policy and practice responses in Australia. Our results also provide baseline measures for identifying where and how policy should be altered to improve social quality and therefore, the SDH. Furthermore, these data can be used for future policy evaluation to identify whether changes in policy have indeed improved social quality and the SDH, particularly for marginalised and vulnerable populations with low levels of social quality.

Authors

Paul R. Ward, Loreen Mamerow
Discipline of Public Health, Faculty of Medicine, Nursing and Health Sciences, Flinders University, Australia

Samantha B Meyer
School of Public Health and Health Systems, University of Waterloo, Canada

Fiona Verity
School of Social Work and Social Policy, Flinders University, Australia

Acknowledgements

We would like to thank members of the Asian Social Quality Network for assisting in developing the questionnaire on which this chapter is based. In particular, we would like to thank Prof

Jaeyeol Yee and Prof Dukjin Chang from Seoul National University, Korea for driving the development of the questionnaire. We would like to thank Dr. George Tsourtos and Dr Tiffany Gill for their early contributions to the study and Tini Luong for her contribution towards data collection. Additionally we would like to acknowledge Flinders University for funding this research via a faculty seeding grant.

References

ACOSS (2011). Australian Community Services Sector Survey Volume 1. Australian Council of Social Services. Sydney.

Ahern, M. M. and M. S. Hendryx (2003). "Social capital and trust in providers." Social Science and Medicine 57: 1195-1203.

Alreck, P. L. and R. B. Settle (2004). The Survey Research Handbook. New York, McGraw-Hill.

Archer, M. (2003). Structure, Agency and the Internal Conversation. Cambridge, Cambridge University Press.

Australian Bureau of Statistics (2004). 8159.3 - Household Telephone Connections, Queensland.

Beck, U. (1992). Risk Society. Towards a new modernity. London, Sage.

Beck, U. (2005). World Risk Society. Cambridge, Polity Press.

Beck, U., A. Giddens, et al., (1994). Reflexive Modernization. Politics, Tradition and Aesthetics in the Modern Social Order. Cambridge, Polity Press.

Beck, W., L. van der Maesen, et al., Eds. (1998). The Social Quality of Europe. Bristol, Policy Press.

Beck, W., L. van der Maesen, et al., (2001). Introduction: Who and What is the European Union For? Social Quality: A Vision for Europe. W. Beck. The Hague, Kluwer Law International.

Beck, W., L. van der Maesen, et al., Eds. (2001). Social Quality: A Vision for Europe. The Hague, Netherlands, Law International.

Bourdieu, P. (1984). Distinction: A Social Critique of the Judgement of Taste. London, Routledge.

Bowling, A., Ed. (2009). Research Methods in Health. New York, Open University Press.

Bryson, L. and F. Verity (2009: 67). Australia: From Wage Earners to Neo-Liberal Welfare State. International Social Policy: Welfare regimes in the developed world. G. Craig and P. Alcock. UK, Palgrave.

Carpiano, R. M. (2006). "Toward a neighborhood resource-based theory of social capital for health: Can Bourdieu and sociology help?" Social Science and Medicine 62(1): 165-175.

Colclough, G. and B. Sitaraman (2005). "Community and Social Capital: What is the Difference?" Sociological Inquiry 75: 474-496.

Commission on Social Determinants of Health (2005). Action on the Social Determinants of Health: Learning from Previous Experiences. Geneva, World Health Organisation.

Commission on Social Determinants of Health (2007). Achieving health equity: from root causes to fair outcomes. Geneva, World Health Organisation.

Commission on Social Determinants of Health (2008). Closing the gap in a generation: Health equity through action on the social determinants of health. Final report of the CSDH. Geneva, World Health Organisation.

Durkheim, E. (1951). Suicide: A Study in Sociology. Glencoe, Free Press.

Eckersley, R. (1999). Quality of Life in Australia - An analysis of public perceptions, Disucssion paper Number 23 September. National Centre for Epidemiology and Population Health. Australian National University.

Ferriss, A. L. (2004). "The quality of life concept in sociology." The American Sociologist 35(3): 37-51.

Freedman, L. P., R. J. Waldman, et al., (2005) "Who's got the power? Transforming health systems for women and chilren." UN Millennium Project Task Force on Child Health and Maternal Health.

Giddens, A. (1984). The Constitution of Society. Cambridge, Polity Press.

Giddens, A. (1990). *The Consequences of Modernity. Cambridge, Polity Press.*

Giddens, A. (1991). *Modernity and Self Identity. Cambridge, Polity Press.*

Giddens, A. (1994). *Beyond Left and Right. Cambridge, Polity Press.*

Giddens, A. (1994). *Risk, Trust, Reflexivity. Reflexive Modernization. U. Beck, A. Giddens and S. Lash. Cambridge, Polity Press.*

Gilson, L., J. Doherty, et al., (2007). *Challenging Inequity Through Health Systems. Final Report: Knowledge Network on Health Systems, WHO Commission on Social Determinants of Health.*

Gleeson, B. (2004:3). *The Future of Australia's Cities: Making Space for Hope. Professional Lecture, School of Environmental Planning.*

Habermas, J. (1997). *The Theory of Communicative Action. Volume 1. Reason and Rationalization of Society. Cambridge, Polity Press.*

Hosmer, D. W. and S. Lemeshow (2000). *Applied Logistic Regression. New Jersey, John Wiley & Sons.*

Kickbusch, I. (2008: 9). *Health Societies: Addressing 21st Century Health Challenges. Thinkers in Residence, Adelaide, Australia, Department of the Premier and Cabinate.*

Kim, D., S. V. Subramanian, et al., (2006). "Bonding versus bridging social capital and their associations with self rated health: a multilevel analysis of 40 US communities." *Journal of Epidemiology & Community Health* 60(2): 116-122.

Kondro, W. (2012). "The fiendish puzzle of health inequities." *Canadian Medical Association Journal* 184(13): 1456-1457.

Laverack, G. (2004). *Health Promotion Practice. Power & Empowerment. London, Sage.*

Laverack, G. (2006). "Improving health outcomes through community empowerment: a review of the literature." *Journal of Health, Population and Nutrition* 24(1): 113-120.

Lee, K., S. Fustukian, et al., (2002). *An introduction to global health policy. Health Policy in a Globalising World. K. Lee, K. Buse and S. Fustukian. Cambridge, Cambridge University Press.*

Legge, D., G. Wilson, et al., (1996). *Best Practice in Primary Health Care. Centre for Development and Innovation in Health and Commonwealth Department of Health and Family Services. Victoria, Australia.*

Lochner, K. A., I. Kawachi, et al., (2003). "Social capital and neighborhood mortality rates in Chicago." *Social Science and Medicine* 56(8): 1797-1805.

Low, L., S. King, et al., (1998). "Genetic discrimination in life insurance: empirical evidence from a cross sectional survey of genetic support groups in the United Kingdom." *BMJ* 17: 1632-1635.

Luhmann, N. (1979). *Trust and Power. New York, Wiley.*

Luhmann, N. (2000). *Familiarity, Confidence, Trust: Problems and Alternatives. Trust: Making and Breaking Cooperative Relations. D. Gambetta. Oxford, Blackwell.*

Makinen, M., H. Waters, et al., (2000). "Inequalities in health care use and expenditures: empirical data from eight developing countries and countries in transition." *Bulletin of the World Health Organization* 78(1): 55-65.

Marmot, M. and R. Wilkinson (2006). *Social determinants of health. Oxford, Oxford University Press.*

Menedue, J. (2003). *The Health of Our State, Briefing Paper. SA Government. Adelaide, SA, Generational Health Review.*

Meyer, S., T. Luong, et al., (2012). "Investigating Australians' trust: Findings from a national survey." *International Journal of Social Quality* 2(2): 3-23.

Meyer, S., P. R. Ward, et al., (2008). "Trust in the health system: an analysis and extension of the social theories of Giddens and Luhmann. ." *Health Sociology Review* 17: 177-186.

Meyer, S. B., C. N. Luong, et al., (2010). "Operationalising the theory of social quality: analysis of the reliability of an instrument to measure social quality." *Development and Society* 39(2): 327-356.

National Opinion Research Center General Social Survey. Chicago, NORC. www3.norc.org/gss+website/.

OECD (2010). "Economic Survey of Australia."

Ostlin, P., T. Schrecker, et al., (2010). *Priorities for research on equity and health: implications for global and national priority setting and the role of WHO to take the health equity research agenda forward. Geneva, World Health Organisation.*

Parsons, T. (1951). *The social system. Glencoe, Ill., Free Press.*

Pittman, P. M. (2006). "Beyond the sound of one hand clapping: experiences in six countries using health equity research in policy." *Journal of Health Politics, Policy & Law* 31(1): 33-49.

Poortinga, W. (2006). "Social capital: An individual or collective resource for health?" *Social Science and Medicine* 62(2): 292-302.

Poortinga, W. (2006). "Social relations or social capital? Individual and community health effects of bonding social capital." *Social Science and Medicine*.

Reber, A. S. (1985). *The Penguin Dictionary of Psychology*. Harmondsworth England, Penguin Books Ltd.

Scambler, G. (2001). *Habermas, Critical Theory and Health*. London, Routledge.

Scambler, G. and N. Britten (2001). *System, lifeworld and doctor-patient interaction: issues of trust in a changing world. Habermas, Critical Theory and Health*. G. Scambler. London, Routledge.

Spicer, N. (2009). "Places of Exclusion and Inclusion: Asylum-Seeker and Refugee Experiences of Neighbourhoods in the UK." *Journal of Ethnic and Migration Studies* 34(3): 491-510.

Subramanian, S. V., K. A. Lochner, et al., (2003). "Neighborhood differences in social capital: a compositional artifact or a contextual construct?" *Health & Place* 9(1): 33-44.

Taylor-Gooby, P. (2006c). "The rational actor reform paradigm: delivering the goods but destroying public trust?" *European Journal of Social Quality* 6(2): 121-141.

Thomson, N., A. MacRae, et al., (2010). "Overview of Australian Indigenous health status." Retrieved April 2010, from http://www.healthinfonet.ecu.edu.au/health-facts/overviews.

van der Maesen, L. and A. Walker (2005). *European Network Indicators of Social Quality. Social Quality: The Final Report*. Amsterdam, European Foundation on Social Quality.

van der Maesen, L. J. G. and A. Walker (2005). "Indicators of Social Quality: Outcomes of the European Scientific Network." *European Journal of Social Quality* 5(1/2): 8-24.

Vinson, T. (2007). *Dropping off the edge: the distribution of disadvantage in Australia*. Australia, Jesuit Social Services and Catholic Social Services.

Walker, A. (2009). "The social quality approach: bridging Asia and Europe." *Development and Society* 38: 209-235.

Walker, A. and L. van der Maesen (2004). *Social Quality and Quality of Life. Challenges for Quality of Life in the Contemporary World: Advances in Quality-of-Life Studies, theory and Research*. W. Glatzer, S. Von Below and M. Stoffregen. Dordrecht, The Netherlands, Kluwer Academic Publishers.

Walker, A. and A. Wigfield (2004). *The Social Inclusion Component of Social Quality*. Amsterdam, European Foundation on Social Quality.

Wallerstein, N. (2006). *What is the evidence on effectiveness of empowerment to improve health?* Copenhagen, WHO Regional Office for Europe (Health Evidence Network Report).

Ward, P. and A. Coates (2006). ""We shed tears but there is no one there to wipe them up for us": narratives of (mis)trust in a materially deprived community." *Health: An interdisciplinary journal for the social study of health, illness and medicine* 10: 283-302.

Ward, P., S. Meyer, et al., (2011). "Complex problems require complex solutions: the utility of social quality theory for addressing the Social Determinants of Health." *BMC Public Health* 11(1): 630.

Ward, P. R. (2006). "Social Quality and Modern Public Health: Developing a Framework for the Twenty-First Century." *European Journal of Social Quality* 6(2): 1-7.

Ward, P. R. (2006). "Trust, reflexivity and dependence: a 'social systems theory' analysis in/of medicine." *European Journal of Social Quality* 6(2): 121-133.

Ward, P. R. and S. B. Meyer (2009). "Trust, social quality and wellbeing: a sociological exegesis." *Development and Society* 38(2): 339-363.

Ward, P. R., S. M. Meyer, et al., (2011) "Complex problems require complex solutions: the utility of social quality theory for addressing the Social Determinants of Health." *BMC Public Health* 11, 630 DOI: 10.1186/1471-2458-11-630.

Ward, P. R., P. Redgrave, et al., (2006). "Operationalizing the Theory of Social Quality: Theoretical and Experiential Reflections from the Development and Implementation of a Public Health and Programme in the UK." European Journal of Social Quality 6(2): 9-18.

WHO (2005). The Bangkok Charter for Health Promotion in a Globalized World. Geneva, WHO.

WHO Task Force on Research Priorities for Equity in Health (2005). "Priorities for research to take forward the health equity policy agenda." Bulletin of the World Health Orgainsation 83: 948-953.

Wilkinson, R. G. and K. E. Pickett (2006). "Income inequality and population health: a review and explanation of the evidence." Social Science & Medicine 62(7): 1768-1784.

Wilkinson, R. G. and K. E. Pickett (2007). "The problems of relative deprivation: why some societies do better than others." Social Science & Medicine 65(9): 1965-1978.

Williams, G. and J. Popay (2001). Lay health knowledge and the concept of the lifeworld. Habermas, Critical Theory and Health. G. Scambler. London, Routledge.

Wilson, S., G. Meagher, et al., Eds. (2005). Australian Social Attitudes: The First Report. Sydney, UNSW Press.

Wood, C. (2008). "Time, Cycles and Tempos in Social-ecological Research and Environmental Policy." Time and Society 17: 261-282.

World Values Survey Association (2005/2006). World Values Survey. http://www.worldvaluessurvey.org/.

Assessment of Osmotic Characteristics of Influenza Viruses

Hyo-Jick Choi, Carlo D. Montemagno

1 Introduction

In natural enveloped organisms, intercellular/intracellular communication depends on the functionality of membrane proteins to maintain physiological life processes. For example, ion channels, ion pumps, and other transport proteins conduct ions and other materials across cellular membranes in a selective manner (Gouaux & Mackinnon, 2005). All enveloped organisms will inevitably be subjected to osmotic stress at some point, but many living cells may survive osmotic shocks due to the presence of water channel proteins, called aquaporins (Borgnia et al., 1999b). Aquaporins are exclusively permeable to water and function to dissipate osmotic gradient across the membrane in osmotic environments. However, to date no such osmoregulation mechanism has been reported for enveloped viruses.

In the case of enveloped viruses (i.e., influenza, human immunodeficiency virus, human herpes virus, hepatitis, etc.), viral infection (virus entry, replication, and budding) and general immune response can be ascribed to the stability and characteristics of both antigenic proteins and viral envelopes (Chan et al., 2010). According to previous reports, the stability of membrane proteins is strongly associated with membrane dynamics (Duwe et al., 1989). One of the most important parameters determining the stability of membrane proteins is the difference in hydrophobic thickness between proteins (l) and membranes (d_0) (Killian, 1998). Hydrophobic mismatch induces membrane and/or protein deformation (Figure 1). Membrane deformation energy is expressed as a quadratic function of the spring constant associated with the extent of membrane deformation ($u = (d_0 - d)/2$), where d_0 and d represent the hydrophobic thickness of the unperturbed and local membrane, respectively (Andersen & Koeppe, 2007):

$$\Delta G_{def} \propto (d_0 - l)^2$$

Thus, strong local stress ($F \propto (d_0 - l)$) to the integral proteins may result in a nonfunctional deformation, decreasing the protein lifetime (Elliott et al., 1983; Andersen & Koeppe, 2007). It is important to emphasize that such a membrane deformation can also be induced upon exposure to osmotic stress. Accordingly, it is thought that a loss of functional activity and/or structural integrity associated with osmotic pressure-induced membrane deformation could play an important role in the stability and infectivity of enveloped viruses and that a better understanding of this effect could assist in developing vaccines. While acknowledging the structural diversity of viruses and antigenic proteins, physicochemical and mechanical properties of the membrane are expected to be important in assessing the stability of viral envelope and antigenic proteins embedded in the membrane.

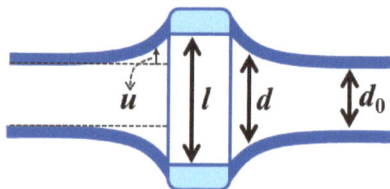

Figure 1: Schematic illustration of hydrophobic mismatch between protein (l) and membrane (d_0). u and d represent the extent of membrane deformation and the local hydrophobic thickness of the membrane, respectively.

Despite the important role of environmental factor-induced morphological change of the antigen-incorporated viral wall in stability, most research efforts have been directed to the structure and function of virus components. In the pat, there were limitations in the study of these damaging factors because there was no method for monitoring morphological changes of the virus over time. As a result, there was strong motivation to find a non-destructive method to quantitatively characterize morphological change of enveloped viruses. This led us to use a stopped-flow light scattering (SFLS) analysis method. SFLS was originally adopted to examine reaction kinetics after the rapid mixing of particle suspension with reagents. The change in size and shape of the particles is reflected in the variation of scattered light intensity. A major advantage of SFLS is the rapid data acquisition, enabling us to investigate morphological change of enveloped viruses on a millisecond time scale. Furthermore, the time scale can be adjusted to measure the reaction over various time periods by simply changing data acquisition rate. Therefore, SFLS shows potential application in probing the rapid osmotic behavior of enveloped viruses and vaccines with a millisecond resolution and the long-term stability under controlled environmental conditions.

To demonstrate the potential applications of SFLS in evaluating the stability of influenza virus, we seek to report our current understanding of the unique scattering behavior of A/PR/8/34 (H1N1) influenza virus and its relation to morphological and structural integrity of the virus (antigenic proteins and lipid envelope). For this purpose, a correlation between osmotic swelling/shrinking behavior and scattered light intensity change was established for liposomes as a model system for influenza virus. The relationship was then used to quantitatively analyze morphological variation in terms of influenza virus size change at different osmotic conditions in real time as well as membrane permeability characteristics. This was combined with other environmental stressors (temperature, pH, and incubation time), to obtain a cumulative understanding of the structural integrity of the virus and to determine the most detrimental factors.

2   Difference in SFLS Behavior between Liposomes and Influenza Virus

2.1   Osmotic Swelling/Shrinking Behavior of Liposomes

Osmotic stress-induced swelling/shrinking behavior of liposome was investigated by using a stopped-flow apparatus. Scattered light was recorded from liposomes made of phosphatidylcholine (PC), i.e. one of the major phospholipid components of egg-grown influenza viruses (Figure 2A) (Kates *et al.*, 1961; Blough, 1971). To investigate how liposomes respond to different types of osmotic gradients, SFLS analysis was performed for PC-liposomes in solutions at three representative osmotic stresses, corresponding to Δ = –0.3, 0, and 0.3 osM. As shown in Figure 2B, exposure to iso-osmotic (Δ = 0 osM) stress resulted in no significant level of time-dependent change in scattered light intensity (I), indicating no size change. In contrast, light scattering intensity increased due to shrinkage or decreased due to swelling upon exposure to hyper-osmotic (Δ > 0 osM) and hypo-osmotic (Δ < 0 osM) stresses, respectively. The rapid saturation of scattered light intensity in the hypo-osmotic stress compared to hyper-osmotic stress can be explained by a lower resistance of membrane to swelling than to shrinkage.

To evaluate the size change rate, the rate constant (k) was measured from a curve-fit of SFLS curves and is plotted in Figure 2C as a function of osmotic stress. As predicted from Figure 2B, k values of liposomes were significantly higher in the case of hypo-osmotic stress (k = 18.4 ± 2.0 s^{-1}, Δ = –0.3 osM) as compared with hyper-osmotic stress (k = 4.8 ± 0.4 s^{-1}, Δ = 0.3 osM) (*t*-test, P < 0.005), which is consistent with the membrane resistance discussed above. Thus, it is clear that PC-liposomes exhibit the typical osmotic behavior of envelope-membrane system in response to osmotic stimulus.

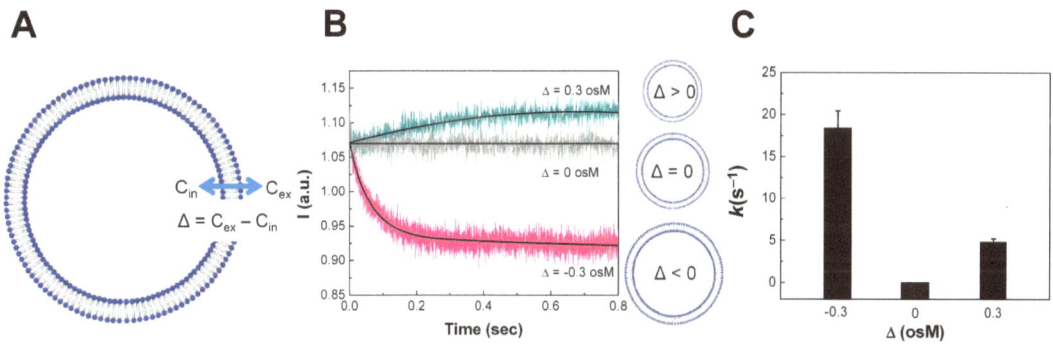

Figure 2: Osmotic response of liposomes. (A) Schematic of the liposome system. Osmotic gradient (Δ = C_{ex} – C_{in}) is defined as the difference in concentration (osmolarity (osM)) between internal (C_{in} = 0.3 osM) and external (C_{ex}) media. (B) Representative SFLS curves in response to hypo-, iso-, and hyper-osmotic stress (Δ = –0.3, 0, and 0.3 osM). Adapted from (Choi *et al.*, 2013b). The solid curve is a fit to the light scattering data using the equation I = a + b·e^{-kt} where a and b (> 0 and < 0 at hypo- and hyper-osmotic stress, respectively) at are constants and k [s^{-1}] is a rate constant (Choi *et al.*, 2013a), and (C) corresponding rate constants were presented as the mean ± standard deviation (SD) (n = 54). Hyper-osmotic (Δ > 0 osM) shrinkage and hypo-osmotic (Δ < 0 osM) swelling of liposomes result in an increase and a decrease of the scattered light intensity with time, respectively.

2.2   Osmotic Swelling/Shrinking Behavior of Influenza A Virus

2.2.1   Influenza Epidemics/Pandemics

Influenza viruses are enveloped, single-stranded RNA viruses, belonging to the family Orthomyxoviridae. Influenza has been responsible for a major epidemic- and pandemic-respiratory disease with substantial morbidity and mortality. Influenza epidemics account for

250,000 to 500,000 deaths per year worldwide, resulting in an enormous healthcare cost burden (Fauci, 2006). Influenza pandemics occur when new strain of influenza A virus emerges as a result of antigenic shift (World Health Organization, 2005; Kamps, 2006). There have been three particularly deadly influenza pandemics in the 20th century: an H1N1 subtype in 1918 (Johnson & Mueller, 2002), an H2N2 subtype in 1957, and an H3N2 subtype in 1968. All had high transmissibility and caused a combined total of more than 50 million deaths (Kamps, 2006). In 2003, an outbreak of highly pathogenic H5N1 avian influenza virus in Southeast Asia resulted in the death of more than 150 million birds. Since 2003, 306 deaths out of 519 human infections (59%) have been reported from 15 countries (World Health Organization, 2011; Centers for Disease Control and Prevention, 2012). Human infection was associated with direct contact with an infected poultry and person-to-person transmission (Ungchusak et al., 2005; Wang et al., 2008). The most recent pandemic occurred in 2009 due to the emergence of a new swine-origin influenza virus (H1N1). This H1N1 influenza strain was predicted to come from the reassortment of triple reassortant swine virus (human H3N2, North American avian, and swine virus) with a Eurasian avian-like swine virus (Novel Swine-Origin Influenza A (H1N1) Investigation Team, 2009). The rapid and worldwide spread of the new H1N1 pandemic influenza virus caused > 17,000 human cases (Malik Peiris et al., 2009). The zoonotic transmission of the strain showed age-specific infection rate: pre-school age (16%–28%), school age (34%–43%), young adults (12%–15%), and old adults (2%–3%) (Kelly et al., 2011). It has been predicted that next pandemic is inevitable and that for moderate pandemics, like the ones in 1957 and 1968, the health costs alone have been estimated to approach $181 billion (U.S. Department of Health and Human Services, 2006). Despite uncertainty about timing, it is clear that there will be another major pandemic influenza outbreak, that it will be major threat to public health and that it will have a tremendous impact on the economy and society.

2.2.2   Structure of Influenza A Virus

As shown in the schematic in Figure 3A, influenza envelope contains three transmembrane proteins; hemagglutinin (HA), neuraminidase (NA), and an ion channel (M2). HA is a trimeric glycoprotein and well known as a major influenza antigen. It is important to note that both receptor binding and antigenic sites are located at the globular head domain (H1) of the protein, mediating viral attachment to cells and acting as a target for neutralizing antibodies (Wiley & Skehel, 1987; Skehel & Wiley, 2000). Thus, the conformational stability of HA proteins plays a critical role in infectivity and immunogenicity. As a result, structural changes in trimer interface may affect the receptor binding activity of HA as well as the interaction with immune cells such as B lymphocytes and antigen-presenting cells, thus affecting broad immune response (Wiley & Skehel, 1987; Wilson & Cox, 1990; Cox et al., 2004; Staneková & Vareckova, 2010). NA is a tetrameric antigenic glycoprotein, responsible for cleavage of the sialic acid groups from glycoproteins, and promotes virus release. As can be seen from the transmission electron microscope (TEM) image of Figure 3B, the spikes on the surface of the influenza virus correspond to HA and NA. M2 is a proton channel that lowers the pH of virus core, leading to the disconnection of matrix protein (M1)-proteins, which facilitates membrane fusion and release of RNPs (Schnell & Chou, 2008). Matrix protein (M1) is the most abundant component of virions (Compans et al., 1970). It lines inside of lipid envelope, assisting viral assembly (Gregoriades & Frangione, 1981; Ruigrok et al., 2000). M1 is also known to play a critical role in the assembly and budding of virus during infection process (Lohmeyer et al., 1979; Nayak et al., 2004). Influenza A viruses have eight segments of RNA genes. The RNP

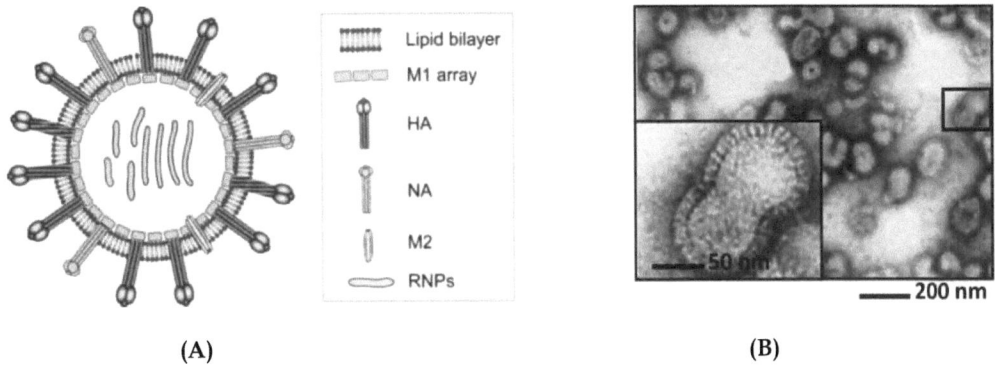

(A)   **(B)**

Figure 3: Influenza A virus. (A) Schematic representation of the influenza A virus: hemagglutinin glycoprotein (HA), neuraminidase (NA), matrix protein (M1), ion channel (M2), and ribonucleoprotein (RNP) complex. (B) Negative-stain TEM micrograph of formaldehyde-inactivated A/PR/8/34 influenza virus (2% phosphotungstic acid (pH 7.0)) (Choi *et al.*, 2013b).

complex consists of RNA transcriptase components (polymerase B1 protein (PB1), polymerase B2 protein (PB2), polymerase A protein (PA)) and NP (nucleocapsid protein). Non-structural protein 1 (NS 1) is an RNA-binding protein, inhibiting both the nuclear export of mRNAs and splicing of pre-mRNA (Fortes *et al.*, 1994; Qiu *et al.*, 1995; Wang *et al.*, 1999). Non-structural protein 2 (NS 2) is a minor component of virions and facilitates the transport of newly synthesized RNPs from the nucleus to the cytoplasm to accelerate virus production (O'Neill *et al.*, 1998).

2.2.3   Osmotic Response of Influenza A Virus

As compared in Figure 4A, the major structural difference between influenza viral wall and liposomal membranes lies in the presence of an additional protein layer (M1) below the lipid membrane. Since proteins are likely to be more rigid than fluidic lipids, the wall of influenza viruses can be viewed as a double-shelled composite structure, consisting of the flexible lipid bilayers supported by the rigid M1 protein shell. Such a difference in the wall structure is assumed to cause different mechanical properties and thus to directly influence the osmotic swell-shrink behavior between single-walled liposomes and double-walled influenza viruses.

SFLS analysis was performed for inactivated influenza virus to observe time-dependent evolution of the morphology. As shown in Figure 4B, the intensity of SFLS spectra of influenza virus (i) increased in a step-wise manner over time upon exposure to hyper-osmotic stress (Δ = 0.3 osM) unlike that of liposomes (ii). Considering that an increase in scattered light intensity is related to a size decrease, the intensity increase at the primary phase at 0 s can be attributed to an initial shrinkage of the virus. The intensity increase at the secondary phase at 45 s can be explained by the secondary shrinkage of the virus and/or morphological change of the viral envelope. During the primary shrinkage process, k and osmotic water permeability constant (P_f, (Borgnia *et al.*, 1999a)) were measured to be ~ 0.58 s^{-1} and ~ 1.5 × 10^{-4} cm s^{-1}, respectively, both of which are lower than those of liposomes. This implies that viral envelope develops a higher resistance to osmotic shrinkage and has more dense membrane than liposomes, based on the significantly lower levels of k and P_f, respectively. Although more research is needed, it can be estimated that the relatively fast, first shrinkage is induced mainly by the shrinkage of

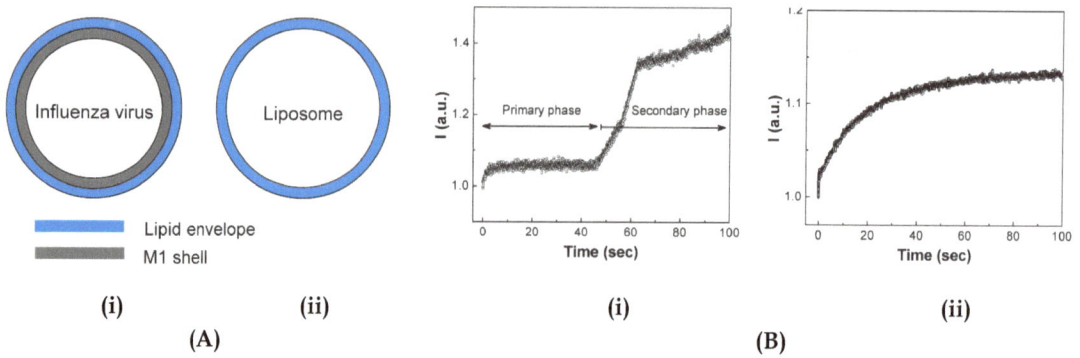

Figure 4: Composite wall structure of influenza virus leading to a different pattern in response to osmotic stress. (A) Schematic diagram showing the wall structure of (i) influenza virus and (ii) liposome. (B) SFLS spectra of (i) inactivated A/PR/8/34 influenza virus, adapted from (Choi *et al.*, 2013b), and (ii) liposome in response to hyper-osmotic gradient of 0.3 osM at 4 °C.

outer lipid membrane of the virus and the relatively slow, secondary shrinkage/morphological change is due to the resistance of the M1 layer to further change against the applied osmotic stress. Considering that the M1 layer plays the role of backbone in maintaining structural integrity of viral envelope, it is further predicted that light scattering pattern in the secondary phase, i.e. onset time for the secondary shrinkage/morphological change (t_{2nd}) and degree of undulation in scattered light intensity, is of great importance for the stability of the influenza virus.

It should be noted that the PC-liposomes used in this work may not represent an optimal model for estimating the osmotic response of influenza viruses or whole inactivated influenza virus vaccines. First, SFLS spectra of PC-liposomes may not reflect osmotic swelling/shrinkage of the virus due to the difference in lipid composition and the presence of antigenic proteins comprising the viral wall. The lipid composition of virus depends on the strain and host cells (Kates *et al.*, 1961; Blough, 1971), thus it is essential to determine the effects of lipid species and composition ratios on the osmotic behavior of the influenza virus (Gerl *et al.*, 2012). Moreover, our interpretation of the step-wise morphological change of the virus was mainly focused on the lipid membrane and M1 layer, as shown in Figure 4A(i). However, it is noteworthy that each influenza virus contains about 600 glycoproteins (HA and NA) in its envelope (Lamb & Choppin, 1983). Therefore, mechanical properties of viral membrane can be better predicted through the precise contribution of the integral proteins on the lipid membrane of the influenza virus, since the presence of globular proteins can possibly affect the mechanical property of the lipid membrane. Second, in this work we used whole inactivated influenza virus, which forms the basis of influenza vaccines, to estimate the osmotic stability of both influenza virus and influenza vaccine. This is based on the assumption that the inactivation of virus, in this case accomplished using formaldehyde, does not affect osmotic response of the virus. However, formaldehyde inactivation would increase stiffness/elastic modulus of proteins as a result of crosslinking (Fraenkel-Conrat & Olcott, 1948; Solomon & Varshavsky, 1985), while minimizing the structural change of antigens. As a result, there is a possibility that formaldehyde inactivation may contribute to the step-wise swelling/shrinkage process of the virus and/or may give rise to difference in the osmotic behavior between live influenza virus and whole activated influenza virus. Further research would be focused on the development of improved reference liposomes which exhibit similar mechanical characteristics to influenza virus/vaccine, and the systematic understanding on the origin and effects of step-wise morphological changes.

3   Applicability of SFLS in the Prediction of Influenza Virus Stability

The potential of SFLS in assessing the stability of influenza virus was first introduced while developing transdermal influenza vaccine delivery using microneedles. Current microneedle coating formulations are composed of a disaccharide sugar (e.g., trehalose or sucrose), a viscosity enhancer (e.g., carboxymethyl cellulose (abbreviated as CMC)), and a surfactant (e.g., poloxamer (abbreviated as Lutrol)) (Gill & Prausnitz, 2007). Disaccharides are a major component in the coating formulation. Although sugar has been commonly used to stabilize biomolecules during drying or freezing conditions (Crowe *et al.*, 1992), it is a well-known osmolyte, generating osmotic stress to the enveloped biological systems during the dehydration processes. Thus, it is important to include an excipient which can negate any drying-induced osmotic stress increase to minimize the destabilization of whole inactivated influenza virus. As shown in Figure 5A(i), the viscosity of the medium exhibited a significant increase with the addition of CMC,   compared with Lutrol. Viscosity is known not only to suppress phase transformation, but also to reduce osmotic stress (Loeb, 1921; Kunitz, 1926). This stabilizing effect of CMC was assessed by measuring HA activity for both inactivated and live influenza virus. As shown in Figure 5A(ii), the addition of CMC to the sugar formulation significantly increased vaccine stability with increasing CMC concentration (one-way ANOVA, $P < 0.0005$), consistent with the prediction.

   The effects of viscosity on the osmotic stability of inactivated influenza virus were evaluated by analyzing SFLS curves with various influenza vaccine coating formulations in terms of k during the primary shrinkage and t_{2nd}. Figure 5B(i) shows SFLS spectra performed on the inactivated influenza virus in response to increasing CMC concentration at constant trehalose and Lutrol concentration. The influenza virus showed step-wise morphological change. Importantly, the k of the primary shrinkage and t_{2nd} of the secondary shrinkage/morphological change were found to decrease or increase, respectively, with increasing CMC concentration (Figure 5B(ii)). Therefore, the CMC-induced stabilizing effect of the influenza virus may be accounted for, in part, by osmotic stress dampening due to an increase in viscosity. Further, mice immunized with CMC-containing formulations generated stronger antibody responses than groups immunized without CMC (Figure 5C(i)). As shown in Figure 5C(ii), formulations with CMC conferred complete protection against lethal challenge (T15C1, T15L2C1), in contrast to the 0% survival rate (T15L2) or 80% survival rate with severe body weight loss (T15). This *in vivo* study confirms that viscosity increase suppresses the destabilization of the influenza virus. Additionally, SFLS analysis was useful in estimating the effective osmotic stress applied to the influenza virus by comparing t_{2nd} values, and thus predicting the stability of the virus in osmotic environment.

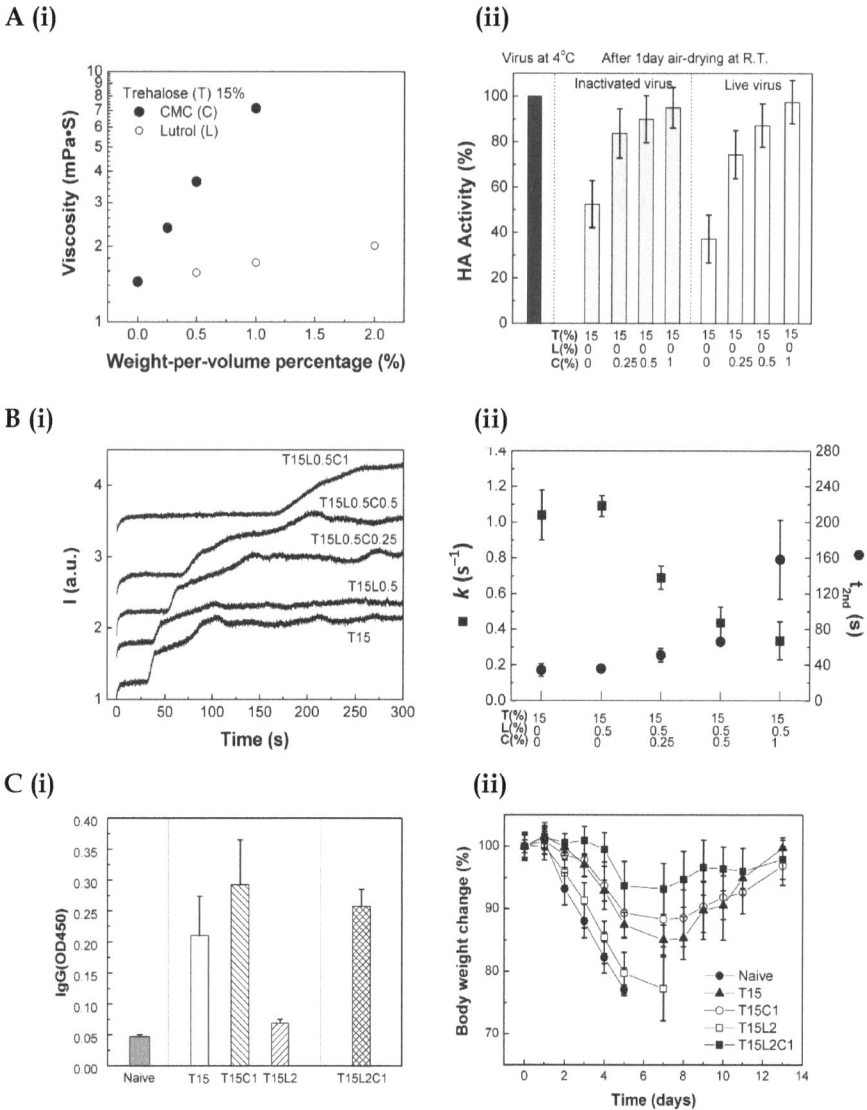

Figure 5: Application of SFLS analysis to predict the stability of inactivated A/PR/8/34 influenza virus. (A) (i) Viscosity of coating formulations at different concentrations of CMC and Lutrol. Unless otherwise stated, trehalose, Lutrol, and CMC have been abbreviated as T, L, and C, respectively. (Mean ± SD, n = 3.) (ii) Stabilizing effect of viscosity enhancer on the functional HA activity of dried influenza virus coatings on Ti plates. CMC concentration was varied at fixed trehalose concentration. (Mean ± SD; n = 8 – 23.) (B) (i) SFLS spectra in different coating formulations: trehalose-only and various CMC concentrations at fixed trehalose/Lutrol concentration in w/v % and (ii) the resulting rate constants and onset time for secondary shrinkage (t_{2nd}). SFLS curves are offset. (C) (i) Comparison of antibody responses after immunization using vaccine-coated microneedles. Total serum anti-A/PR/8/34 IgG levels were determined by reading optical densities using ELISA. IgG was measured from mice bled on the 2nd week following immunization (0.12 μg of viral protein). (Mean ± SD, n = 6 mice per group.) (ii) Protection of immunized mice against lethal challenge. (a) Body weight changes as a measure of protection of immunized mice against lethal challenge. At week 4 after vaccination, groups of mice were intranasally challenged with 10×LD_{50} of mouse-adapted A/PR/8/34 virus. (Mean ± SD, n = 6.) Adapted with permission from Elsevier (Choi *et al.*, 2013a).

4   Relationship between Scattered Light Intensity and Liposome size

Following the demonstration of the potential applicability of SFLS method in estimating osmotic stability of the influenza virus, research efforts have focused on the quantitative interpretation of scattered light intensity change of the influenza virus. For this purpose, the size of liposomes was measured using dynamic light scattering and the corresponding osmotic stress-induced SFLS spectra from the same liposome samples were recorded, which allowed for an empirical relationship between relative intensity and relative volume for liposomes. Thus, liposomes served as a reference for SFLS data interpretation of influenza virus under the hypothesis of a similar response to osmotic stress.

As a first step, SFLS analysis was performed at various osmotic conditions (Figure 6A) to obtain the relative scattering intensity ($I_{rel} = I_{sat}/I_0$, I_0: intensity at t = 0 s, I_{sat}: intensity at t $\rightarrow$ ∞) at each osmotic stress. As shown in Figure 6B and its caption, I_{rel} plots corresponding to hyper-osmotic and hypo-osmotic stresses were fitted to a double exponential equation, $I_{rel} = 1 + c \cdot e^{x/\Delta} + d \cdot e^{y/\Delta}$, where c, d, x, and y are constants. The next step was to find a relationship between the relative volume ($V_{rel} = V_\Delta/V_{iso}$, V_{iso}: volume at Δ = 0 osM, V_Δ: volume in hypo- or hyper-osmotic stress) and the magnitude of osmotic stress. The size of the liposomes at each osmotic stress was measured using the dynamic light scattering method and their relative volumes are plotted in Figures 6C and 6D for hypo-osmotic and hyper-osmotic stresses, respectively. For convenience of analysis, the V_{rel} values of hypo- and hyper-osmotic stresses were represented as a function of Δ ($C_{ex} - C_{in}$) and C_{in}/C_{ex}, respectively, and were subsequently analyzed by linear regression. As a consequence, both I_{rel} and V_{rel} could be described by a common variable, Δ. Therefore, from the time-dependent SFLS spectra of the influenza virus, the following procedures could be employed to convert scattered light intensity to volume as a function of time: (1) $I_{rel}(t)$ is obtained by dividing the scattering data with I_0; (2) effective osmotic stress (Δ_{eff}) corresponding to I_{rel} can be derived at each time point using the relationship between I_{rel} and Δ in Figure 6B; (3) V_{rel} at each time point can be calculated using the relationship between V_{rel} and Δ in Figures 6C and 6D. However, it should be noted that $V_{rel}(t)$ calculated in the way described here is based on three assumptions: (1) the liposomes behaves similarly to a perfect osmometer (Ponder, 1944), (2) influenza viruses have the same mechanical properties as liposomes, and (3) $I_{rel}(t)$ variation due to both size and morphological changes is interpreted only in terms of size variation ($V_{rel}(t)$). Although further optimizations are needed to find better reference system with similar mechanical properties to influenza virus and to differentiate the morphological change from the size change, this approach could offer a quantitative method in predicting time-dependent stability changes of enveloped viruses such as influenza virus in response to environmental stressors.

5   Effects of Environmental Factors on the Stability of Influenza Virus

5.1   Effects of pH and Temperature on the Hyper-osmotic Behavior of Influenza Virus

SFLS analysis was performed to investigate the influence of pH and temperature on inactivated A/PR/8/34 influenza virus at a hyper-osmotic gradient of 0.3 osM with different pHs (2.0

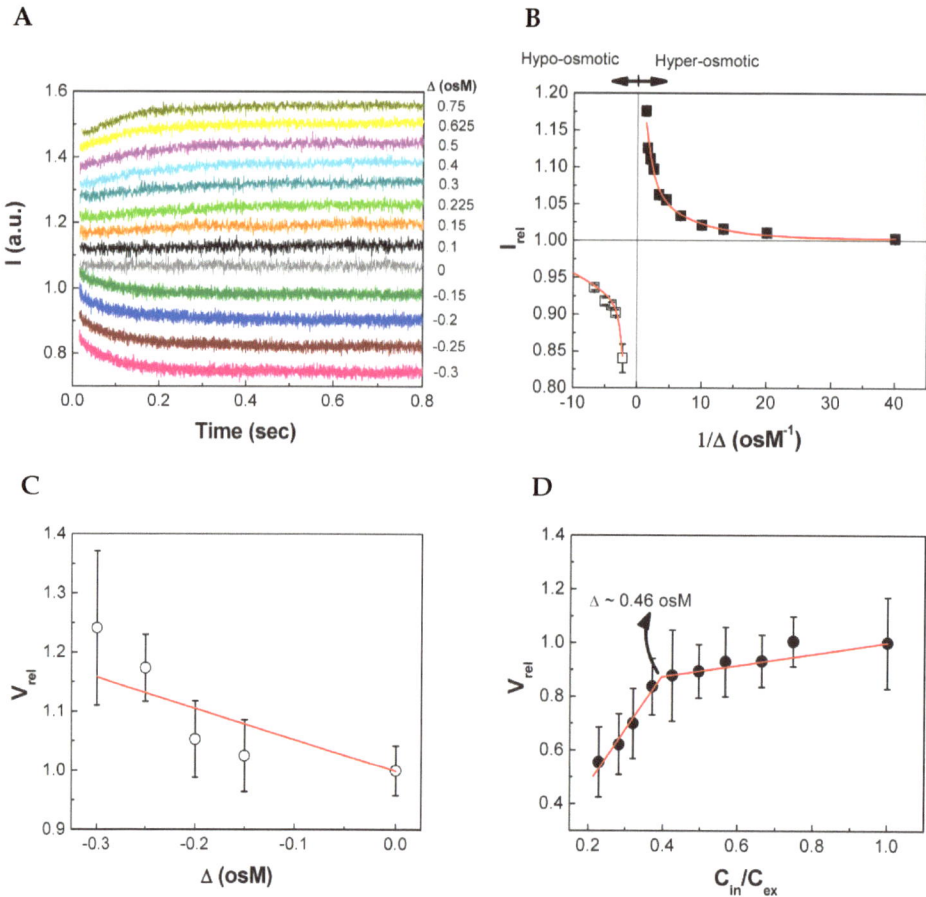

Figure 6: Relative scattering intensity-volume relationship of liposomes. (A) Time course of SFLS analysis of PC-liposomes. (B) Osmotic stress dependence of the relative light scattering intensity (I_{rel}) of PC-liposomes. (Mean ± SD; $n = 54$.) The plot was fitted to a double-exponential curve: $I_{rel} = 1 - 0.11653\,e^{0.09645/\Delta} - 2.28333\,e^{1.61951/\Delta}$ and $I_{rel} = 1 + 0.14824\,e^{-0.21065/\Delta} + 5.14043\,e^{-3.30994/\Delta}$ for hypo-osmotic stress and hyper-osmotic stress, respectively. The relative volume ($V_{rel} = V/V_{\Delta=0}$) of liposomes at (C) hypo-osmotic and (D) hyper-osmotic conditions $V_{rel} = 1 - 0.52879\,\Delta$ for $\Delta \leq 0$, $V_{rel} = 0.79 + 0.21\,(C_{in}/C_{ex})$ for $0 < \Delta \leq 0.46$, and $V_{rel} = 0.07 + 2.03\,(C_{in}/C_{ex})$ for $\Delta \geq 0.46$. (Mean ± SD; $n = 36 - 60$.) (Choi *et al.*, 2013b)

and 7.0). The change in scattered light intensity was recorded using two different scan ranges: 8 s for primary shrinkage process and 160 s for secondary shrinkage/morphological change.

To study the effect of temperature on the characteristics of I_{rel} and V_{rel} at pH 7.0, SFLS analysis was performed on the influenza virus after exposure to hyper-osmotic stress of 0.3 osM at five different temperatures. The I_{rel} spectra corresponding to 8 s and 160 s are shown in Figures 7A (i) and (ii), respectively. I_{rel} in Figure 7A(ii) was converted to V_{rel} (Figure 7A(iii)) following the procedure described in section 4. As shown in Figures 7A (i) and (ii), I_{rel} saturated earlier and t_{2nd} decreased with the increase of temperature due to faster shrinkage during the primary shrinkage process and lowered resistance of viral envelope to further shrinkage due to increased thermal energy. In terms of volume change, influenza virus shrank to ~ 90% and ~ 45% of the original volume upon exposure to $\Delta = 0.3$ osM as a consequence of step-wise morphological change (Figure 7A(iii)).

Time-dependent morphological change of influenza virus at pH 2.0 was investigated under the same test conditions as pH 7.0. Figure 7B shows the time-course of I_{rel} ((i) 8 s and (ii) 160 s) and V_{rel} (iii) at various temperatures. As shown in Figure 7B(i), influenza virus exhibited a typical hyper-osmotic shrinkage behavior as evidenced by increased I_{rel} at 4 °C and 15 °C due to the decrease of V_{rel}. Interestingly, I_{rel} at 25 °C exhibited an initial increase followed by a decrease at ~ 0.6 s. Such a reversal in the direction of virus size change can probably be attributed to virus aggregation in the acidic environment (Kim *et al.*, 1998), which became more dominant with increasing temperature. This explains why no evidence of hyper-osmotic shrinkage was observed at pH 2.0 and 37 °C in Figure 7B(i). Long-term analysis revealed a step-wise morphological change as shown in Figures 7B (ii) and (iii). Similarly to pH 7.0, t_{2nd} at pH 2.0 decreased with the increase of temperature and also, consistent with the short-term SFLS spectra in Figure 7B(i), a decrease in I_{rel} was observed at the first phase in SFLS curves measured at 25, 31, and 37 °C.

While the average virus size increased by aggregation in response to acidic hyper-osmotic solution at high temperatures (25, 31, and 37 °C), a longer incubation resulted in typical hyper-osmotic volume changes. As shown in Figure 7B(iii), at 4 °C, the primary and secondary phase resulted in 92% and 42% of the original size, respectively. At 37 °C, V_{rel} of influenza virus increased to 108% during the first phase followed by a decrease. It is important to note that at ≥ 25 °C, the secondary phase initiated after similar time lags to pH 7.0, but proceeded more slowly than at pH 7.0. This can be explained by the aggregation-induced physical hindrance effect resisting osmotic shrinkage, and/or by the decreased osmotic gradient across the membrane due to the low pH-induced membrane leakage, as evidenced by lower levels of shrinkage compared to that at pH 7.0. Furthermore, noticeably more fluctuation in V_{rel} at ≥ 25 °C showed that high temperature are more detrimental to the physical stability of the enveloped influenza virus under hyper-osmotic stress at pH 2.0, consistent with previous reports (Brown *et al.*, 2009).

Analyses of k during the primary stage, and t_{2nd} can provide valuable information about the shrinkage kinetics. As shown in Figures 7C and 7D, k and t_{2nd} values varied significantly depending on temperature (two-way ANOVA, $P < 0.005$). The k values for both pH 7.0 and 2.0 increased with temperature (Figure 7C), but varied with a significant statistical difference (two-way ANOVA, $P < 0.001$). However, compared to a significant decrease of t_{2nd} with increasing temperature (Figure 7D), the effect of pH on t_{2nd} was insignificant (two-way ANOVA, $P = 0.143$). If the virus size increase was caused by fusion, the osmolyte leakage through membrane defects during the fusion process might result in a decrease of the osmotic gradient, causing increased t_{2nd} (compare following Figure 8A(ii) with 8B(ii)). In addition, virus fusion would lead to smaller k values due to increased size. Therefore, based on the observations of (1) the statistically higher k values during the first shrinkage step at pH 2.0 than those at pH 7.0 with increasing temperature up to 25 °C and (2) the same t_{2nd} at both pH 7.0 and 2.0, the temporary increase in V_{rel} at pH 2.0 is estimated to come from aggregation, rather than fusion. These SFLS analyses indicate that exposure of virus to acidic environments reduced the resistance to the primary shrinkage, without any significant membrane integrity loss.

A (i)   **(ii)**

(ii)

B (i)   **(ii)**

(ii)

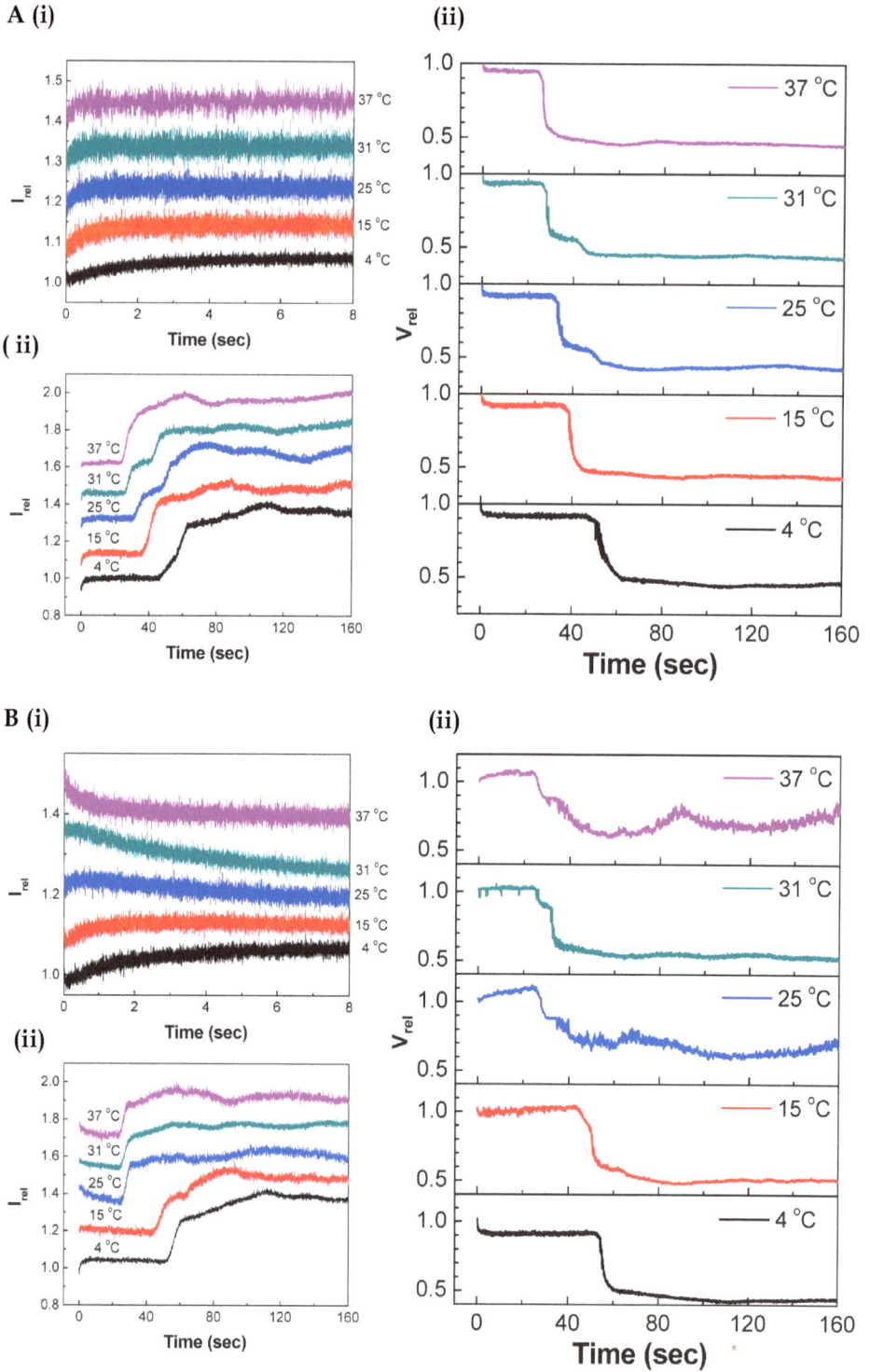

(continued on next page)

C

D

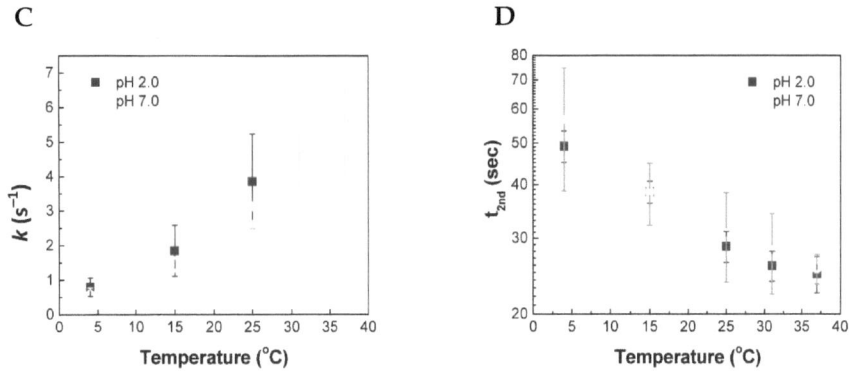

Figure 7: The effects of temperature and pH on the time-dependent osmotic response of inactivated A/PR/8/34 influenza virus. The osmotic shrinkage behavior of the virus was investigated at five different temperatures (4, 15, 25, 31, and 37 °C) by applying a hyper-osmotic gradient of 0.3 osM with different pH sucrose solutions (pH 2.0 and 7.0). 8-s (i) and 160-s (ii) scan of SFLS of influenza vaccine in response to sucrose solution at pH 7.0 (A) and 2.0 (B). I_{rel} of SFLS spectra in (i) and (ii) are offset to highlight the differences, but the relative intensity scale is identical for all spectra. (iii) V_{rel} of influenza virus corresponding to SFLS spectra in part (ii). Effective osmotic stress (Δ_{eff}) corresponding to I_{rel} at each time point was calculated from equations in Figure 6, and used to calculate V_{rel} from equations shown in Figures 6C and 6D. The V_{rel} misfit at $I_{rel} = 1$ was corrected by adding 0.02 (V_{rel}) for $I_{rel} > 1$ and subtracting 0.015 (V_{rel}) for $I_{rel} < 1$. (C) k at the primary phase as a function of temperature (Mean ± SD; $n = 96$). (D) t_{2nd} as a function of temperature (Mean ± SD; $n = 42$). Adapted from (Choi *et al.*, 2013b).

5.2   Effects of Osmotic Stress and pH on the Stability of Influenza Virus at 37 °C

To test the effects of osmotic stress and pH at physiological temperature, SFLS analysis was performed on the inactivated influenza virus at four different osmotic stresses ($\Delta = -0.15$, 0, 0.15, and 0.3 osM) at

pH 2.0/7.0 and 37 °C. At pH 7.0, SFLS spectra displayed a typical swell-shrink behavior depending on the direction and magnitude of osmotic stress (Figure 8A(i)). In the presence of the hyper- and hypo-osmotic stresses, the shrinkage and swelling of the influenza virus proceeded in a step-wise manner as indicated by the step-wise intensity change (Figure 8A(ii)). At equal magnitudes, hypo-osmotic stress resulted in lower t_{2nd} than hyper-osmotic stress and, in general, a higher magnitude of osmotic stress resulted in lower t_{2nd} values. When incubated in an iso-osmotic medium for 2 h, a gradual decrease of I_{rel} was observed from the influenza virus, which can probably be attributed to dilution-induced virus destabilization (Figure 8A(iii)). This resulted in a gradual size increase (113% after 2 h incubation, data not shown).

Unlike pH 7.0, SFLS spectra at pH 2.0 exhibited a decrease in I_{rel} for all tested osmotic stresses (Figure 8B(i)). Based on the observation in Figure 7, acid-induced virus aggregation is assumed to be a general phenomenon occurring at pH 2.0 and 37 °C. In spite of the I_{rel} decrease at the primary phase, influenza virus exhibited the step-wise size/morphological change similar to pH 7.0 (Figure 8B(ii)). When incubated for 2 h, dilution-induced I_{rel} decrease was more dominantly observed at pH 2.0 compared to pH 7.0 (compare I_{rel} at iso-osmotic condition in Figure 8A(iii) with 8B(iii)). In terms of volumetric change, this corresponds to 136% of the original size and, considering the dilution effect described in Figure 7A, the additional

23% increase in V_{rel} can be explained by low pH-induced aggregation. Most significant is the finding that 2 h incubation at hyper-osmotic, acidic medium generated very unstable light scattering behaviors (Δ = 0.15 and 0.3 osM in Figure 8B(iii)). The irregular light scattering could be explained by membrane deformation. Therefore, these SFLS data indicate that the presence of hyper-osmotic stress in acidic medium at physiological temperature can be more detrimental to the stability of influenza virus than hypo- or iso-osmotic stresses, because perturbation of lipid membrane and interfacial tension may induce conformational change of membrane proteins, as described briefly in the introduction.

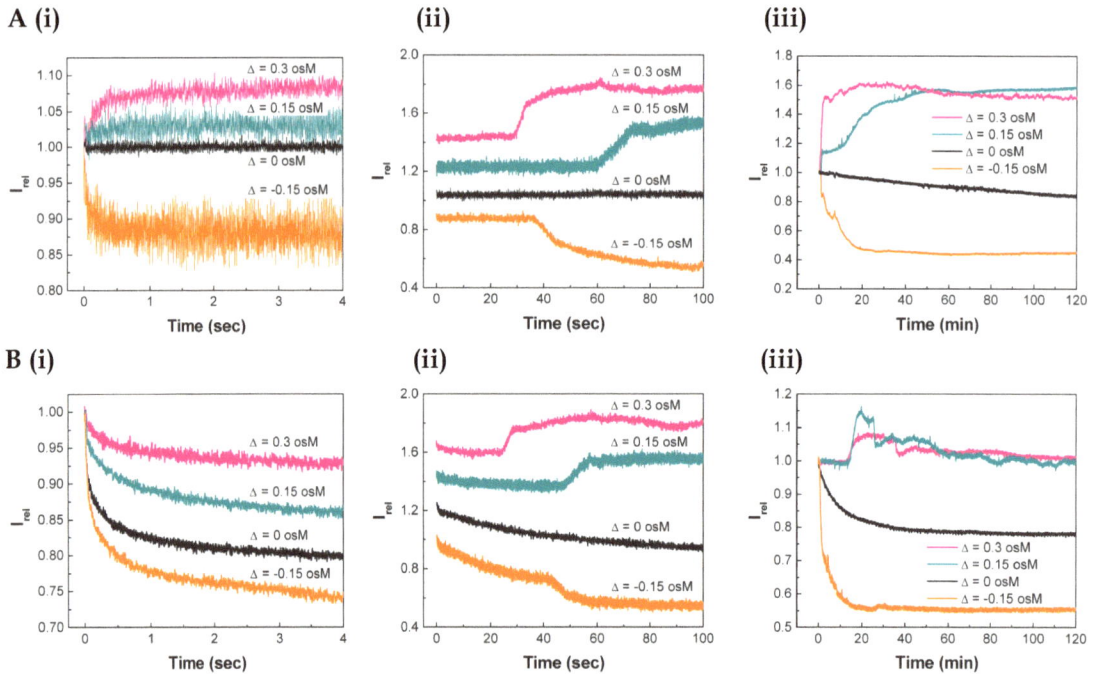

Figure 8: A comparison of pH-dependent osmotic swelling/shrinking behavior of inactivated influenza virus. SFLS analysis of the virus subjected to osmotic gradient of –0.15, 0, 0.15, and 0.3 osM using sucrose at (A) pH 7.0 and (B) pH 2.0 at 37 °C. Scan time of (i) 4 s, (ii) 100 s, and (iii) 120 min. 100-s scan spectra are offset for clarity. (Mean ± SD; n = 24 – 36 for (i)/(ii) and n = 9 for (iii).) Adapted from (Choi *et al.*, 2013b).

To evaluate destabilization mechanisms predicted by SFLS, TEM and intrinsic fluorescence analyses were performed for inactivated influenza virus exposed to Δ = 0 and 0.3 osM at pH 7.0/2.0 and 37 °C for 2 h. That is, conformational stability of antigenic proteins and morphological change of the influenza virus were measured using intrinsic fluorescence and TEM, respectively, in the presence of iso- and hyper-osmotic stress at pH 2.0 and 37 °C, which were then compared with those at pH 7.0. As shown in Figure 9A, a significant decrease in intensity and an increase in maximum emission wavelength were observed upon exposure to iso-osmotic stress at pH 2.0 within ~ 1 min, followed by additional changes due to further incubation. The initial rapid change of emission spectra can be explained by an acid-induced conformational change in the tertiary structure of antigenic proteins and the slow gradual change by membrane destabilization mentioned in Figure 8B (Choi *et al.*, 2013c). TEM micrograph in Figure 9A(iii) shows that the influenza viruses maintained an intact spherical membrane structure but displayed ill-defined spike-like morphology, implying the loss of protein structure (compare Figure 9A(iii) with 9C(i)). This observation correlates well with our interpretation of SFLS (Figures 8, 9A(i), 9C(ii)) and intrinsic fluorescence (Figure 9A(ii)) data.

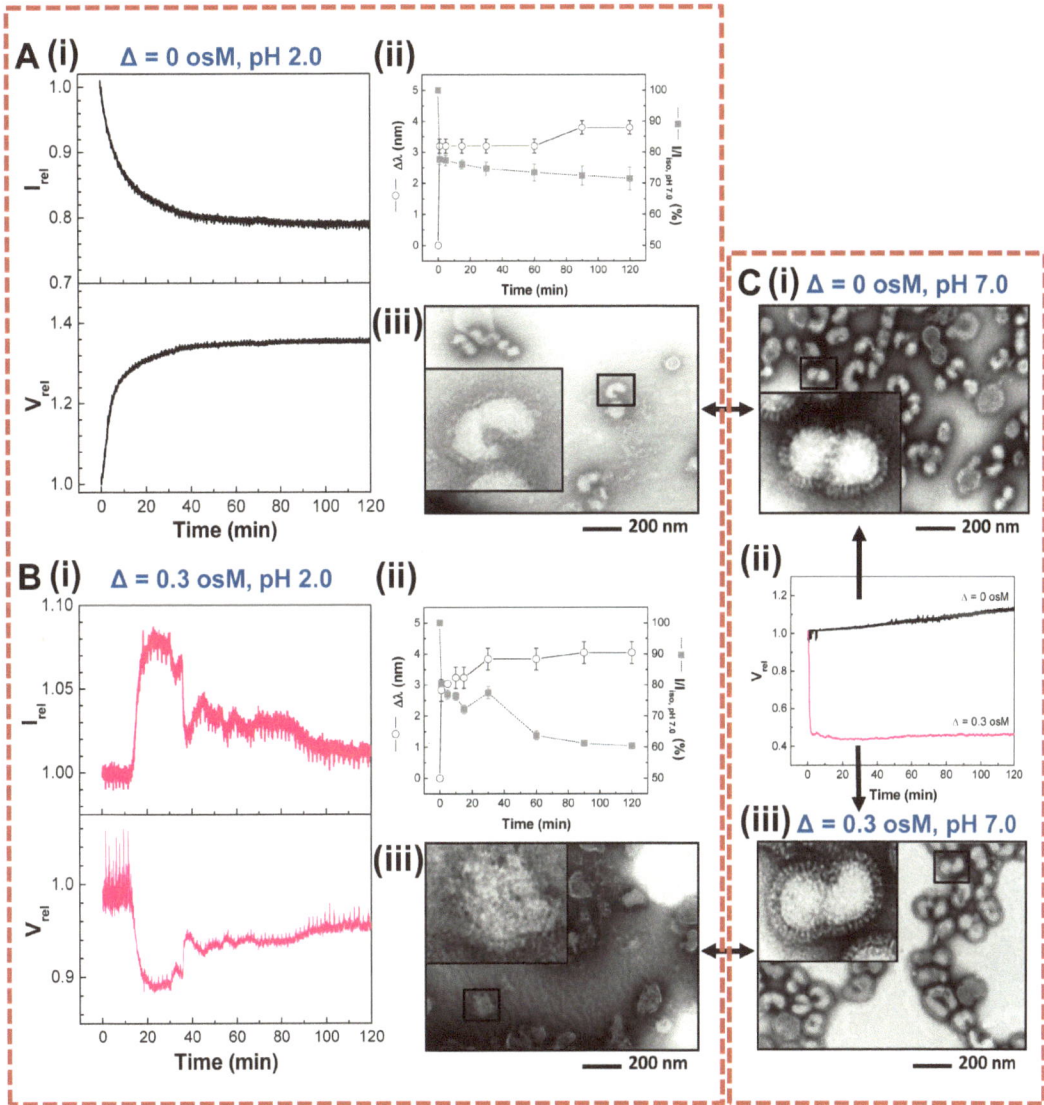

Figure 9: Effects of pH and osmotic stress on the morphological change of inactivated influenza virus. SFLS analysis (i), intrinsic fluorescence spectra (ii), and negative-stain TEM micrographs (iii) subjected to (A) $\Delta = 0$ osM and (B) $\Delta = 0.3$ osM at pH 2.0 (37 °C for 2 h) are compared with those at pH 7.0 (C). The maximum emission position and intensity of fluorescence spectra relative to control (pH 7.0) were measured at the excitation wavelength of 295 nm and plotted as a function of time. No significant fluorescence difference was observed between 4 °C and 37 °C. (Mean ± SD; $n = 9$ and 3 for SFLS and intrinsic fluorescence measurements, respectively.) Adapted from (Choi *et al.*, 2013b).

In the presence of hyper-osmotic stress, intrinsic fluorescence showed a red shift in wavelength and a large decrease in intensity at the initial stage, similarly to iso-osmotic stress. However, such a peak change was more noticeable than in iso-osmotic condition (compare Figure 9B(ii) with Figure 9A(ii)). As predicted in Figure 9B(iii), considering the substantial amount of irregular light scattering (compare Figure 9B(i) and Figure 9A(i)), the enhanced red shift and intensity decrease can be mainly due to the membrane perturbation and integrity loss under hyper-osmotic stress in addition to the pH-induced conformational change. TEM image in Figure 9B(iii) supports the conclusion (compare Figure 9B(iii) with Figure 9A(iii) and 9C(iii) to see the effects of osmotic-stress and pH, respectively). That is, upon exposure to hyper-osmotic acidic medium, the spherical shape of the influenza virus was partially lost and some of them had ruptured (Figure 9B(iii)). As can be seen in the TEM images in Figure 9, the observed destructive effects of pH and osmotic stress on the morphology of the virus are believed to be irreversible. Therefore, the TEM data support our SFLS analysis that virus destabilization in acidic, hyper-osmotic environments is mainly associated with the osmotic stress-induced morphological change as well as the low pH-induced denaturation.

The effect of osmotic stress on the destabilization of the inactivated influenza virus was examined by measuring HA activity through hemagglutination tests in the presence of various osmotic stresses (Δ = –0.15, 0, 0.15, 0.3, and 0.5 osM) at pH 2.0 and 37 °C. As shown in Figure 10, iso- and hypo-osmotic stresses exhibited a similar HA activity decrease over time. This indicates that hypo-osmotic swelling does not induce further destabilization of the influenza virus. In contrast, hyper-osmotic stresses generated significant level of HA activity decrease in a concentration dependent manner, which was associated with the membrane integrity loss and disruption as demonstrated by SFLS, intrinsic fluorescence, and TEM. Considering the fact that H1 subunit serves as a receptor by binding to sialic acid of host cells, the decrease of HA activity indicates that low pH treatment and osmotic stress induced conformational changes in H1 and/or the receptor binding sites, supporting our hypothesis that osmotic stress-induced structural destabilization as well as pH-induced conformational change of antigenic proteins of the influenza virus contributed to the decrease in HA activity under acidic environments.

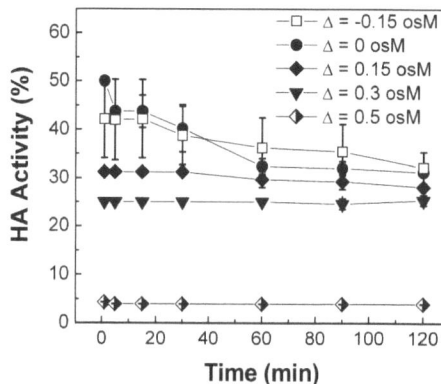

Figure 10: Effects of pH on functional HA activity of influenza virus. Hemagglutinating activity of vaccine in osmolyte solution (Δ = –0.15, 0, 0.15, 0.3, and 0.5 osM) was measured after 1, 5, 15, 30, 60, 90, and 120 min of incubation at pH 2.0 and 37 °C, and the remaining HA activity relative to control (pH 7.0 and 4 °C) is plotted as a function of time. (Mean ± SD; n = 8 – 16.) (Choi *et al.*, 2013b)

6 Conclusions

While the stability of influenza viruses in various environmental conditions has long been an important question, there is still very little understanding, mainly due to the lack of characterization method tracking changes in morphology. Quantitative and qualitative assessments of the virus stability can advance our ability to investigate pathogenicity of the influenza virus (e.g., such as the binding, fusion, replication, etc.) as well as immune reactions of the whole inactivated influenza vaccine. Physical and chemical parameters including temperature, pH, osmotic stress, and time would have a profound impact on the structural and functional stability of the influenza virus. The goal of this report was to overview current research activities in studying destabilization mechanisms of the influenza virus in environmental conditions by the use of SFLS method. For this reason, we showed the applicability of the SFLS technique to predict osmotic stability of inactivated influenza virus. The time-dependent changes in the magnitude and direction of I_{rel}, k, t_{2nd}, and fluctuation in scattered light as a whole allowed for the quantitative estimation of the stability of the influenza virus in terms of the osmotic swell-shrink kinetics, effective osmotic stress, degree of membrane deformation/membrane integrity, and structural change of antigenic proteins. Although initial research efforts were limited to the formaldehyde-inactivated influenza virus, SFLS analysis under different crosslinking conditions would provide valuable information about the effects of inactivation process on the stability of influenza envelope. A comparative study on the osmotic behavior of live influenza viruses among different strains, mutants, and genetically engineered strains may be of great interest in characterizing species-dependent physicochemical differences. This can probably contribute to better understanding basic questions about the stability of the influenza viruses, especially in regards to the influence of environment on the transmission and survival of influenza virus, which can be helpful in prevention and control of the virus. The enormous potential of the SFLS method lies in the fact that it can be used as a complementary technique to identify stability characteristics of a wide range of enveloped pathogens in the presence of osmotic stress.

Authors

Hyo-Jick Choi, Carlo D. Montemagno
Department of Chemical and Materials Engineering, University of Alberta, Canada

Acknowledgments

This project was funded by a grant from the Bill & Melinda Gates Foundation through the Grand Challenges Exploration Initiative (C.D.M. and H.J.C.).

References

Andersen, Olaf S & Koeppe, Roger E. (2007). *Bilayer thickness and membrane protein function: an energetic perspective. Annu Rev Biophys Biomol Struct, 36, 107-130.*

Blough, H. A. (1971). Fatty acid composition of individual phospholipids of influenza virus. J Gen Virol, 12(3), 317-320.

Borgnia, M. J., Kozono, D., Calamita, G., Maloney, P. C. & Agre, P. (1999a). Functional reconstitution and characterization of AqpZ, the E. coli water channel protein. J Mol Biol, 291(5), 1169-1179.

Borgnia, M., Nielsen, S., Engel, A. & Agre, P. (1999b). Cellular and molecular biology of the aquaporin water channels. Annu Rev Biochem, 68(1), 425-458.

Brown, J. D., Goekjian, G., Poulson, R., Valeika, S. & Stallknecht, D. E. (2009). Avian influenza virus in water: Infectivity is dependent on pH, salinity and temperature. Vet Microbiol, 136(1-2), 20-26.

Centers for Disease Control and Prevention. (2012). Highly pathogenic avian influenza A (H5N1) in people, from http://www.cdc.gov/flu/avianflu/h5n1-people.htm

Chan, R. B., Tanner, L. & Wenk, M. R. (2010). Implications for lipids during replication of enveloped viruses. Chem Phys Lipids, 163(6), 449-459.

Choi, H. J., Bondy, B. J., Yoo, D. G., Compans, R. W., Kang, S. M. & Prausnitz, M. R. (2013a). Stability of whole inactivated influenza virus vaccine during coating onto metal microneedles. J Control Release, 166(2), 159-171.

Choi, H. J., Ebersbacher, C. F., Kim, M. C., Kang, S. M. & Montemagno, C. D. (2013b). A mechanistic study on the destabilization of whole inactivated influenza virus vaccine in gastric environment. PLoS One, 8(6), e66316.

Choi, H. J., Ebersbacher, C. F., Quan, F. S. & Montemagno, C. D. (2013c). pH stability and comparative evaluation of ranaspumin-2 foam for application in biochemical reactors. Nanotechnology, 24(5), 055603.

Compans, R. W., Klenk, H. D., Caliguiri, L. A. & Choppin, P. W. (1970). Influenza virus proteins. I. Analysis of polypeptides of the virion and identification of spike glycoproteins. Virology, 42(4), 880-889.

Cox, R. J., Brokstad, K. A. & Ogra, P. (2004). Influenza virus: immunity and vaccination strategies. Comparison of the immune response to inactivated and live, attenuated influenza vaccines. Scand J Immunol, 59(1), 1-15.

Crowe, J. H., Hoekstra, F. A. & Crowe, L. M. (1992). Anhydrobiosis. Annu Rev Physiol, 54, 579-599.

Duwe, H. P., Eggl, P. & Sackmann, E. (1989). The cell-plasma membranes as composite system of two-dimensional liquid crystal and macromolecular network and how to mimick its physical properties. Angew Makromol Chem, 166(1), 1-19.

Elliott, J. R., Needham, D., Dilger, J. P. & Haydon, D. A. (1983). The effects of bilayer thickness and tension on gramicidin single-channel lifetime. Biochim Biophys Acta, 735(1), 95-103.

Fauci, A. S. (2006). Emerging and re-emerging infectious diseases: Influenza as a prototype of the host-pathogen balancing act. Cell, 124(4), 665-670.

Fortes, P., Beloso, A. & Ortin, J. (1994). Influenza virus NS1 protein inhibits pre-mRNA splicing and blocks mRNA nucleocytoplasmic transport. EMBO J, 13(3), 704-712.

Fraenkel-Conrat, Heinz & Olcott, Harold S. (1948). The reaction of formaldehyde with proteins. V. Cross-linking between amino and primary amide or guanidyl groups. J Am Chem Soc, 70(8), 2673-2684.

Gerl, Mathias J, Sampaio, Julio L, Urban, Severino, Kalvodova, Lucie, Verbavatz, Jean-Marc, Binnington, Beth, Lindemann, Dirk, Lingwood, Clifford A, Shevchenko, Andrej & Schroeder, Cornelia. (2012). Quantitative analysis of the lipidomes of the influenza virus envelope and MDCK cell apical membrane. J Cell Biol, 196(2), 213-221.

Gill, H. S. & Prausnitz, M. R. (2007). Coating formulations for microneedles. Pharm Res, 24(7), 1369-1380.

Gouaux, E. & Mackinnon, R. (2005). Principles of selective ion transport in channels and pumps. Science, 310(5753), 1461-1465.

Gregoriades, A & Frangione, B. (1981). Insertion of influenza M protein into the viral lipid bilayer and localization of site of insertion. J Virol, 40(1), 323-328.

Johnson, N. P. & Mueller, J. (2002). Updating the accounts: global mortality of the 1918-1920 "Spanish" influenza pandemic. Bull Hist Med, 76(1), 105-115.

Kamps, B. S.; Reyes-Teran, G. (2006). Influenza 2006. Paris: Flying Publisher.

Kates, M., Allison, AC, Tyrrell, DAJ & James, AT. (1961). Lipids of influenza virus and their relation to those of the host cell. Biochim Biophys Acta, 52(3), 455-466.

Kelly, Heath, Peck, Heidi A, Laurie, Karen L, Wu, Peng, Nishiura, Hiroshi & Cowling, Benjamin J. (2011). The age-specific cumulative incidence of infection with pandemic influenza H1N1 2009 was similar in various countries prior to vaccination. PLoS One, 6(8), e21828.

Killian, J Antoinette. (1998). Hydrophobic mismatch between proteins and lipids in membranes. Biochim Biophys Acta, 1376(3), 401-416.

Kim, C. H., Macosko, J. C. & Shin, Y. K. (1998). The mechanism for low-pH-induced clustering of phospholipid vesicles carrying the HA2 ectodomain of influenza hemagglutinin. Biochemistry, 37(1), 137-144.

Kunitz, M. (1926). An empirical formula for the relation between viscosity of solution and volume of solute. J Gen Physiol, 9(6), 715-725.

Lamb, Robert A & Choppin, Purnell W. (1983). The gene structure and replication of influenza virus. Annu Rev Biochem, 52(1), 467-506.

Loeb, J. (1921). The reciprocal relation between the osmotic pressure and the viscosity of gelatin solutions. J Gen Physiol, 4(1), 97-112.

Lohmeyer, J., Talens, L. T. & Klenk, H. D. (1979). Biosynthesis of the influenza virus envelope in abortive infection. J Gen Virol, 42(1), 73-88.

Malik Peiris, JS, Poon, Leo LM & Guan, Yi. (2009). Emergence of a novel swine-origin influenza A virus (S-OIV) H1N1 virus in humans. J Clin Virol, 45(3), 169-173.

Nayak, D. P., Hui, E. K. W. & Barman, S. (2004). Assembly and budding of influenza virus. Virus Res, 106(2), 147-165.

Novel Swine-Origin Influenza A (H1N1) Investigation Team. (2009). Emergence of a novel swine origin influenza A (H1N1) virus in humans. N Engl J Med, 360, 2605-2615.

O'Neill, R. E., Talon, J. & Palese, P. (1998). The influenza virus NEP (NS2 protein) mediates the nuclear export of viral ribonucleoproteins. EMBO J, 17(1), 288-296.

Ponder, E. (1944). The osmotic behavior of crenated red cells. J Gen Physiol, 27(4), 273-285.

Qiu, Y., Nemeroff, M. & Krug, R. M. (1995). The influenza virus NS1 protein binds to a specific region in human U6 snRNA and inhibits U6-U2 and U6-U4 snRNA interactions during splicing. Rna, 1(3), 304-316.

Ruigrok, R. W., Barge, A., Durrer, P., Brunner, J., Ma, K. & Whittaker, G. R. (2000). Membrane interaction of influenza virus M1 protein. Virology, 267(2), 289-298.

Schnell, J. R. & Chou, J. J. (2008). Structure and mechanism of the M2 proton channel of influenza A virus. Nature, 451(7178), 591-595.

Skehel, J. J. & Wiley, D. C. (2000). Receptor binding and membrane fusion in virus entry: the influenza hemagglutinin. Annu Rev Biochem, 69(1), 531-569.

Solomon, Mark J & Varshavsky, Alexander. (1985). Formaldehyde-mediated DNA-protein crosslinking: a probe for in vivo chromatin structures. Proc Natl Acad Sci U S A, 82(19), 6470-6474.

Staneková, Z. & Vareckova, E. (2010). Conserved epitopes of influenza A virus inducing protective immunity and their prospects for universal vaccine development. Virology Journal, 7, 351.

U.S. Department of Health and Human Services. (2006). HHS pandemic influenza plan 2005. Avai lable at: http://www. hhs. gov/pandemicflu/plan/pdf/hhspandemicinfluenzaplan. pdf. Accessed November, 8.

Ungchusak, Kumnuan, Auewarakul, Prasert, Dowell, Scott F, Kitphati, Rungrueng, Auwanit, Wattana, Puthavathana, Pilaipan, Uiprasertkul, Mongkol, Boonnak, Kobporn, Pittayawonganon, Chakrarat & Cox, Nancy J. (2005). Probable person-to-person transmission of avian influenza A (H5N1). N Engl J Med, 352(4), 333-340.

Wang, Hua, Feng, Zijian, Shu, Yuelong, Yu, Hongjie, Zhou, Lei, Zu, Rongqiang, Huai, Yang, Dong, Jie, Bao, Changjun & Wen, Leying. (2008). Probable limited person-to-person transmission of highly pathogenic avian influenza A (H5N1) virus in China. Lancet, 371(9622), 1427-1434.

Wang, W., Riedel, K., Lynch, P., Chien, C. Y., Montelione, G. T. & Krug, R. M. (1999). RNA binding by the novel helical domain of the influenza virus NS1 protein requires its dimer structure and a small number of specific basic amino acids. Rna, 5(2), 195-205.

Wiley, D. C. & Skehel, J. J. (1987). The structure and function of the hemagglutinin membrane glycoprotein of influenza virus. Annu Rev Biochem, 56(1), 365-394.

Wilson, I. A. & Cox, N. J. (1990). Structural basis of immune recognition of influenza virus hemagglutinin. Annu Rev Immunol, 8(1), 737-771.

World Health Organization. (2005). Avian influenza: assessing the pandemic threat. Acceso Nov, 2.

World Health Organization. (2011). Cumulative number of confirmed human cases of avian influenza A/(H5N1) reported to WHO.

Horizontal Transfer during the Evolution of Pathogens and their Hosts

Elena de la Casa-Esperón

1 Introduction

The genetic information is usually passed from progenitors to descendants, but vertical inheritance is not the only way of genetic transmission. Horizontal or lateral transfer of genes (HT) has also been observed between many organisms. The acquired sequences can be modified and adapted (*i.e.*, domesticated, co-opted) and play an important role in the evolution of the recipient species.

HT was first observed in prokaryotes, when bacteria were found to be able to incorporate drug resistance genes from other organisms. These findings revealed the importance of the acquired sequences in the survival and adaptation of the recipients to the environment (Filee *et al.*, 2007; Hughes & Friedman, 2005; Keeling, 2009). Since then, there have been countless reports of horizontally transferred (HTd) genes in bacteria and archaea (Boto, 2010; Gogarten & Townsend, 2005; Koonin *et al.*, 2001), mostly at the level of extrachromosomal elements, but also as an integral and significant proportion of their genomes. Consequently, HT blurs the boundaries between prokaryotic species.

HTd sequences can be originated from related or unrelated species. Prokaryotes can incorporate sequences from other prokaryotes, as well as viruses and, less often, from eukaryotes. In fact, viruses are also common receptors of foreign genes (Filee *et al.*, 2008; Filee *et al.*, 2007; Hughes & Friedman, 2005). However, both prokaryotes and viruses are not capable of processing introns, which is a major limitation for the domestication of many eukaryotic genes (Keeling & Palmer, 2008; Lefkowitz *et al.*, 2006; Moran *et al.*, 2012). Because of their abundance and close contact with other species, prokaryotes and viruses are also major donors of sequences to other organisms. In addition, prokaryotes have adapted to very diverse environments and, hence, may provide a large spectrum of genes that could be co-opted by other species (Keeling & Palmer, 2008).

It is important to distinguish between the process of transfer and the fixation of the foreign sequences. Close proximity or direct interaction between organisms facilitates the exchange of genetic material between them. But integration in the individual genome and fixation in populations depends on many factors, such as population dynamics and evolutionary forces operating on the acquired gene. In fact, most of the foreign sequences are eliminated in the recipient species within a few generations (Gogarten & Townsend, 2005). In addition, accumulation of substitutions over time can mask ancient HTd sequences; therefore, most HT reports are restricted to recent acquisitions or to conserved genes. Hence, the extent of HT has been largely underestimated (Huang, 2013). In particular, the reports about HT in eukaryotes have been very scarce for a long time. However, recent studies have revealed that HT in eu-karyotes is more common than previously thought (Andersson, 2005; Boto, 2014; Dunning Hotopp, 2011; Keeling, 2009; Keeling & Palmer, 2008; Syvanen, 2012). In this process, patho-gens appear to have played an important role, as donors, recipients and vectors of HTd genes (de la Casa-Esperon, 2012) (Figure 1). I will discuss how HT has contributed to the evolution of pathogens and their hosts.

2   Who can Receive a Foreign Sequence?

The importance and extent of HT has been recognized in prokaryotes and viruses for a long time (Boto, 2010; Haig, 2001; Koonin *et al.,* 2001; Lalani & McFadden, 1999; McClure *et al.,* 1987). However, HT is also relatively frequent in unicellular eukaryotes; the sequence donors are mostly bacteria they live in close contact with, as well as other unicellular organisms and viruses. This close interaction is more than a physical proximity: bacteria can infect, live in en-dosymbiosis or be phagocytized by protists and, hence, protists contain a relative large num-ber of HTd genes of bacterial origin (Andersson, 2005; Dunning Hotopp, 2011; Richards *et al.,* 2003). In addition, many bacteria can transfer large DNA molecules to eukaryotes through the type IV secretion system; but studies of yeast mutants have shown that not all recipients are equally susceptible to gene transfer by this secretion system (Moriguchi *et al.,* 2013).

Bacteria are very diverse and, hence, excellent donors of genes that might allow eukary-otes to colonize new niches or exploit novel resources (Andersson, 2005; Keeling & Palmer, 2008). An example is found in a thermo-acidophilic unicellular red alga, which contains several genes of bacterial and archaea origin that presumably facilitated the adaptation to an extreme environment (Schonknecht *et al.,* 2014). Examples of a   daptive HT of bacterial genes are also found in multicellular eukaryotes (Acuna *et al.,* 2012). Interestingly, HT is not restrict-ed to individual sequences: in several pathways, HT has been reported to be the source of multiple genes involved in them (Craig *et al.,* 2008; Monier *et al.,* 2009; Moran & Jarvik, 2010; Striepen *et al.,* 2004; Sun & Huang, 2011).

Hence, HTd sequences have the potential of supplying novel or improved functions that may benefit to the recipient species, whether they provide coding or regulatory sequences (Bernstein *et al.,* 2012; Boschetti *et al.,* 2012; Graham *et al.,* 2008). These sequences can be co-opted and successfully retained in the genome of the recipient species, not only for their own benefit, but also to modulate the relationship with the donor species. For instance, HT from endosymbionts to their hosts can facilitate their mutual relationship; an example is found be-tween aphids and an obligate mutualistic bacterium (Nikoh & Nakabachi, 2009). Endosymbi-onts are, in fact, a major source of HTd genes, exemplified by the relocation of mitochondrial and plastid genes to the eukaryotic nucleus, or by the massive transfer of *Wolbachia* genes to insects and nematodes (Andersson, 2005; Dunning Hotopp *et al.,* 2007; Keeling, 2009; Qiu *et al.,* 2013; Sloan *et al.,* 2014). In contrast, HT of genes originated in pathogens can provide a particu-lar advantage to their hosts: the ability to resist or tolerate the infection. While resistance strategies limit the pathogen growth, tolerance is achieved by lowering the effects of infection without eliminating the pathogen (Miller *et al.,* 2005; Roy & Kirchner, 2000). Fixation of genes that contribute to resistance or tolerance follows different dynamics, although both types of genes may be acquired by domestication of pathogen-derived sequences (Miller *et al.,* 2005; Roy & Kirchner, 2000). Several examples will be discussed in detail in the following sections, as well as the contribution of the reciprocal process (HT from host to pathogen) in the evolution and interactions between both organisms.

Although close proximity and selective advantages have facilitated the incorporation of foreign genes in eukaryotes, HT is not as frequent in multicellular organisms as it is in unicellular ones (Andersson, 2005; Huang, 2013). Besides their abundance and lifestyle differences, multicellular eukaryotes can only transmit HTd genes as long as they have been incorporated to their germline. This is particularly difficult in sexually reproducing organisms with a confined and sheltered reproductive system (Huang, 2013; Keeling, 2009; Schaack *et al.*, 2010). Therefore, successful HT is predicted to occur in germ cells/gametes or early developmental stages (*e.g.*, zygotes, embryos, spores, gametophytes), especially when they are more exposed to the environment or to interactions with other organisms (Huang, 2013; Yue *et al.*, 2012).

In spite of these difficulties, there are many examples of HTd genes in multicellular eukaryotes. In plants, exchange of mitochondrial and plastid genes is the most common form of HT (Andersson, 2005; Bock, 2010; Gao *et al.*, 2013; Keeling, 2009; Xi *et al.*, 2013); in addition, genes of viruses, bacteria, fungi, algal endosymbionts and other plants have contributed to the genome and evolution of plants (Gao *et al.*, 2013; Qiu *et al.*, 2013; Richardson & Palmer, 2007; Xi *et al.*, 2013; Yue *et al.*, 2012). In animals and fungi, HT has been observed in very diverse species, but is considered a rare event (Andersson, 2005; Denker *et al.*, 2008; Graham *et al.*, 2008; Haugen *et al.*, 2005; Mehrabi *et al.*, 2011; Richards *et al.*, 2009). Nevertheless, HTd genes represent a substantial part of the genome of bdelloid rotifers (at least 8-9%) and nematodes (about 3% of the protein-coding genes) (Boschetti *et al.*, 2012; Paganini *et al.*, 2012).

Not surprisingly, many of the HT sequences involve transposable elements. They represent a substantial part of the eukaryotic genome because of their intrinsic ability of propagating within the genome. Therefore, transposon expansion can have a significant impact in the structure of the genome (and, hence, in its function) and some of the copies can eventually acquire novel roles (as regulatory elements, protein-coding genes, etc.) (Bernstein *et al.*, 2012). Studies of these mobile elements in large animals have revealed a surprising number of HT events, even between distantly related species (Danchin, 2011; Daniels *et al.*, 1990; Graham *et al.*, 2008; Haring *et al.*, 2000; Jordan *et al.*, 1999; Moran & Jarvik, 2010; Schaack *et al.*, 2010; Yohn *et al.*, 2005). Moreover, some of the transposable elements present in tetrapods have been HTd several times, found in species separated by large geographical distances and even in insects (de Boer *et al.*, 2007; Gilbert *et al.*, 2012; Gilbert *et al.*, 2010; Kordis & Gubensek, 1998; Novick *et al.*, 2010; Pace *et al.*, 2008; Walsh *et al.*, 2013); the later include several animal parasites, which have been proposed as vectors for HT (de Boer *et al.*, 2007; Gilbert *et al.*, 2010; Pace *et al.*, 2008; Walsh *et al.*, 2013).

3   Pathogens as Sources of Horizontally Transferred Genes to their Hosts

Eukaryotes have incorporated several genes that were likely originated from their pathogens. These include prokaryotes and viruses, as well as parasitic eukaryotes (de Boer *et al.*, 2007; Gilbert *et al.*, 2010; Pace *et al.*, 2008). An example of the later is found in the *Trypanosome*-derived sequences found in infected patients, and transmitted to their children (Hecht *et al.*, 2010). Plants have also been found to contain sequences derived from parasitic plants (mitochondrial genes) and bacterial pathogens (Intrieri & Buiatti, 2001; Mower *et al.*, 2004). Among the prokaryotic donors, perhaps the best-known is *Wolbachia*, one of the most widespread intracellular bacteria found in the majority of insects, as well as in some crustaceans, mites, and nematodes. The effect of the *Wolbachia* infection is variable, depending on the host. This bacteria can be vertically transmitted thanks to its ability of colonizing (and even manipulating to its advantage) the germ cells of some hosts (Kondo *et al.*, 2002). These features made *Wolbachia* a perfect source of HT genes, as it has been observed in several insect and nematode sequences (Dunning Hotopp *et al.*, 2007; Nikoh *et al.*, 2008).

But the pathogens that have often made the largest contribution to their host genomes are viruses. Prophages constitute up to 20% of the bacterial genomes (Wang *et al.*, 2010); their sequences can be trapped by rearrangements and substitutions in the host genome and, occasionally, domesticated by the recipients. In fact, cryptic prophages have provided beneficial genes to bacterial hosts against very diverse adverse conditions (Wang *et al.*, 2010). Viral-derived sequences also constitute a large part of the eukaryote genome. Retroviruses can integrate into the genome of their hosts as proviruses, occasionally reaching the germline; therefore, they are a major source of exogenous sequences in vertebrates, constituting up to 8% of the human genome (Lander *et al.*, 2001). Other viruses, such as double-stranded RNA viruses, can also donate sequences to very diverse eukaryotic organisms, in which they can be adopted for novel functions -for instance, the defense against exogenous infections (Koonin, 2010; H. Liu *et al.*, 2010; Taylor & Bruenn, 2009).

Certainly, some pathogen-derived HTd genes have been co-opted by their hosts to protect themselves from infections. In some cases, the domestication of pathogen sequences leads to protection against related agents; in others, against competing infections. It has been long known that some viruses protect their prokaryote or eukaryote hosts against secondary infections and, hence, they could be donors of defense mechanisms (Barton *et al.*, 2007; Villarreal, 2011). In fact, two different, but widespread and fundamental antiviral defense mechanisms present in prokaryotes, appear to be derived from viruses. The first one comprises the restriction-modification systems, which have been suggested to have viral origin because related genes have been found in prophages (Stern & Sorek, 2011; Villarreal, 2011). The second is constituted by the clustered, regularly interspaced short palindromic repeat (CRISPR) loci and their associated proteins (Cas). The CRISPR loci contain sequences derived from viruses (and plasmids) that are used to generate RNA-mediated defenses against viral (and plasmidic) infections (Horvath & Barrangou, 2010; Sorek *et al.*, 2008; Villarreal, 2011). Interestingly, recent studies have suggested that the CRISPR immunity is inactivated in a small fraction of cells, allowing for the incorporation of potentially beneficial foreign sequences to the population (Jiang *et al.*, 2013).

Similarly, in eukaryotes, retroviral-derived sequences and other endogenous viral elements have been co-opted by the hosts in multiple instances, sometimes for defensive purposes. For instance, the mouse Friend-virus-susceptibility-1 gene (*Fv1*), which contributes to retrovirus resistance, is a domesticated version of the gag MuERV-L retroviral gene (Kozak, 2010; Patel *et al.*, 2011; Buckler-White *et al.*, 2009). This and other retrovirus-derived genes interfere with viral entry and the activity of viral receptors (Kozak, 2010; Patel *et al.*, 2011; Yan *et al.*, 2009). In addition, regulatory sequences of viral origin can also be adopted by hosts for antiviral purposes (Kozak, 2010; Sanville *et al.*, 2010).

Small RNAs participating in defense mechanisms that interfere or silence viral gene expression might also originate from pathogens: studies in *Caenorhabditis elegans* have suggested that the genes coding small RNAs may be derived from transposable elements and/or endogenous retroviral sequences (Villarreal, 2011). Moreover, several genes and mechanisms involved in the vertebrate immune response appear to be related to some viral sequences and processes (Du Pasquier, 2004; Villarreal, 2009, 2011). Therefore, it has been proposed that HT and domestication of multiple viral sequences could have originated the basal components of the adaptive immune system in vertebrates (Du Pasquier, 2004; Villarreal, 2009, 2011).

In these cases, the pathogen-derived sequences have provided a benefit to the hosts and, hence, have been maintained in their genomes. In addition, HTd between hosts that share common selective pressures may also be fixated. For instance, genes involved in defense mechanisms can be acquired from other hosts of the same plague. Such is the case of the drosomycin-type antifungal peptides present in moulting animals (arthropods, nematodes and tardigrades), as well as in plants (the likely donors) (Zhu & Gao, 2014). Several mechanisms have been proposed for the transfer of genetic material between hosts, such as the contribution of parasitic vectors that will be discussed in a later section (Gilbert et al., 2010; Houck et al., 1991; Pace et al., 2008; Walsh et al., 2013).

4 Pathogens as Recipients of Horizontally Transferred Genes from Their Hosts

Like host-to-host HT, pathogens can receive from other pathogens genetic material that facilitates their survival, infectivity, the adaptation to new hosts or the parasitic lifestyle. As previously discussed, unicellular organisms, especially prokaryotes and viruses, are prone to exchange genetic material. But pathogens can also receive beneficial genes from their hosts.

There are several examples of genes exchanged between pathogens (or even acquired from non-pathogenic organisms) that, once co-opted, have improved their pathogenic capability; moreover, HTd sequences have also contributed to the transformation of certain organisms into pathogens. The transfer of certain fungal genes, or of entire extranumerary chromosomes, allowed the transition from non-pathogenic fungi into pathogenic organisms (Ma et al., 2010; Mehrabi et al., 2011). Acquisition of foreign genes also seems to have played a role in the evolution of certain nematodes into plant parasites. These genes are related to bacterial sequences, including plant pathogens (Craig et al., 2008; Danchin, 2011; Haegeman et al., 2011; Paganini et al., 2012). Other plant pest, the coffee berry borer beetle, contains a gene of bacterial origin involved in coffee bean processing. The sequences appear absent in related species that do not infect coffee beans, suggesting that HT likely facilitated the adaptation to new niches (Acuna et al., 2012).

The close relationship between host and pathogen has resulted in many examples of homologous sequences present in both organisms that have shaped their individual evolution and co-evolution. Although it is not always clear the origin of the shared sequences (Monier et al., 2009), phylogenetic analyses have revealed that, in most instances, the receptor is clearly not the host, but the pathogen. Examples of host-to-pathogen HT are found in very diverse species, such as the reports of sequences of eukaryotic origin present in bacteria (Anderson & Seifert, 2011; Davis & Wurdack, 2004; de Felipe et al., 2005; Nembaware et al., 2004). For instance, the bacteria *Neisseria gonorrhoeae*, a strictly human pathogen, carries a sequence closely related to a human transposable element that is absent in other *Neisseria* species; hence, it was likely recently transferred (Anderson & Seifert, 2011). Within eukaryotes, several parasitic animals also carry transposable elements that appear derived from their animal hosts (Hecht *et al.*, 2010; Laha *et al.*, 2007). In plants, HT from host to parasite (and vice versa) of mitochondrial and nuclear genes has been reported in several species (Davis & Wurdack, 2004; Xi *et al.*, 2012; Yoshida *et al.*, 2010). An example is found in parasitic species of *Rafflesia*, flowering plants that express multiple nuclear and mitochondrial genes derived from their hosts, also angiosperms (Xi *et al.*, 2012; Xi *et al.*, 2013). Codon-usage similarities between these host and parasitic plants might have facilitated the fixation of the genes in the latter (Xi *et al.*, 2012).

Viruses often capture sequences from their hosts. During bacteriophage reproduction, particles occasionally capture bacterial DNA sequences. Among animal viruses, nucleocytoplasmatic large DNA viruses, such as poxviruses and herpesviruses, are the most common recipients of host sequences (Haig, 2001; Lalani & McFadden, 1999). These viruses can incorporate foreign genes as long as the total size of their genome is not too large to be encapsidated. Poxviruses (which include the vaccinia and smallpox viruses) have been very successful at incorporating genes from their hosts (Bratke & McLysaght, 2008; Filee, 2009; Hughes & Friedman, 2005; Hughes *et al.*, 2010; Lefkowitz *et al.*, 2006). These comprise several gene families that are present in some viral genera but not others, suggesting that the HTd sequences have contributed to the diversification of poxviruses (Bratke & McLysaght, 2008; Bustos *et al.*, 2009; Filee *et al.*, 2008; Hughes & Friedman, 2005; Lefkowitz *et al.*, 2006; Moss & Shisler, 2001; Odom *et al.*, 2009). Multiple HT events from hosts to herpesviruses have also been reported (Alcami & Lira, 2010; Fu *et al.*, 2008, 2011; Holzerlandt *et al.*, 2002; Lalani & McFadden, 1999).

Viruses often domesticate HTd sequences in order to elude the host immune response (Haig, 2001; Lalani & McFadden, 1999; McFadden *et al.*, 1995; Moss & Shisler, 2001; Seet *et al.*, 2003; Shchelkunov, 2003). Vertebrate viruses have developed diverse strategies aimed to avoid detection and elimination by the host immune response (apoptosis blockage, antigen presentation obstruction, complement cascades disruption, mimicry or modulation of cytokines and their receptors, etc.) (Haig, 2001; Lalani & McFadden, 1999). HTd sequences that have been co-opted for these purposes code for proteins that interact with host ligands or receptors, target cytokines or disrupt elements of the innate immune system (Alcami & Lira, 2010; Lalani & McFadden, 1999; McFadden *et al.*, 1995). Cytokines recruit leukocytes to the sites of infection as part of the antiviral response. Hence, cytokine homologues found in both poxviruses and herpesviruses code for proteins that mimic or interfere with the host copies, counteracting the host defense mechanisms (Alcami & Lira, 2010; Lalani & McFadden, 1999; McFadden *et al.*, 1995; Sin & Dittmer, 2012). For instance, phylogenetic studies have revealed that host Interleukin-10 (*IL-10*) sequences (and other members of the *IL-10* family) have been transferred multiple times to poxviruses by independent HT events (Bratke & McLysaght, 2008; Hughes, 2002; Hughes *et al.*, 2010), as well as to herpesviruses (Kanai *et al.*, 2007; Kotenko *et al.*, 2000; Y. Liu *et al.*, 1997; Sin & Dittmer, 2012; Sunarto *et al.*, 2012; Vieira *et al.*, 1991), suggesting that these sequences provide a selective advantage to the recipients (Hughes, 2002). Indeed, the product of the Epstein-Barr virus IL-10 homologue acts as an agonist of the host IL-10 receptor (Y. Liu *et al.*, 1997); the viral copy has lost the immunomodulatory properties of the host counterpart and its expression diminishes the host immune response during early infection (Kanai *et al.*, 2007; Sin & Dittmer, 2012; Vieira *et al.*, 1991). In poxviruses, the expression of *IL-10* family-derived genes in Orf and vaccinia viruses causes a delay in the development of the acquired immunity in humans and mice, respectively (Chan *et al.*, 2006; Kurilla *et al.*, 1993).

Poxviruses have also domesticated other genes of the host defense machinery, such as those coding for the MHC class I, other interleukins and their receptors (Hughes & Friedman, 2005; Moss & Shisler, 2001). Sometimes the viral copies interfere with the normal functioning of the host proteins, while other HTd genes have acquired novel immunomodulatory roles. In addition, sequences involved in other aspects of the host defenses have been found in poxviruses, such as copies of the glutaredoxin (which has an antiapoptotic function under oxidative stress), serine protease inhibitors (serpins, involved in inflammation regulation) and glutathione peroxidase genes (Bratke & McLysaght, 2008; Hughes & Friedman, 2005; Lefkowitz *et al.*, 2006). Glutathione peroxidases play a protective role against the oxidative stress in the host, while, in viruses, may safeguard both pathogens and infected cells from the oxidative damage derived from the immune response (Moss *et al.*, 2000).

But not all sequences transferred from host to virus play roles that enhance viral survival and propagation: there is evidence that these sequences can also benefit the host by restraining viral propagation and infectivity. Such seems to be the case of a Yaba-like poxvirus homologue of the *interleukin-24* gene, because expression of the viral protein appears to diminish virulence upon infection (Bartlett *et al.*, 2004). Other example is found in poxviral sequences derived from the mammalian *Schlafen* genes. This gene family, which comprises a variable number of genes in diverse mammalian species, is usually transcribed in cells of the host immune system; this expression is stimulated by interferon, a typical feature of genes involved in the innate antiviral defense (Bustos *et al.*, 2009; de la Casa-Esperon, 2011; Li *et al.*, 2012). *Schlafen* sequences of likely rodent origin were transferred to orthopoxviruses; this transfer probably occurred before the divergence of the existing species of this viral group (Bustos *et al.*, 2009; de la Casa-Esperon, 2011). In some viruses, the HTd sequences still conserve an open reading frame, but little is know about their function, the role of the original copies in vertebrates, and the selective forces that drove the fixation of these sequences in poxviruses (Bustos *et al.*, 2009; de la Casa-Esperon, 2011). However, recent studies have shed some light and revealed that expression of one of the human copies (*SLFN11*) restricts the replication of retroviruses; this is achieved through SLFN11-mediated inhibition of viral protein synthesis (Jakobsen *et al.*, 2013; Li *et al.*, 2012). Interestingly, functional studies of a camelpox *Schlafen* copy in a recombinant viral model have suggested that this gene may also contribute to reduce virulence (Gubser *et al.*, 2007).

In view of these findings, the contribution of HT to the evolution of host and pathogens cannot simply be interpreted as part of an arms race: HT can also be instrumental for the co-evolution of both organisms. For instance, herpesviruses remain latent for long periods of time with little cost to their hosts, unless they get reactivated and pathogenic. During latency in mice, they can modulate the animal defenses against secondary infections (Barton *et al.*, 2007; White *et al.*, 2012). Herperviruses themselves can also be the target of the host defenses, but HT of certain vertebrate genes has provided tools to these viruses to evade the immune response (Alcami & Lira, 2010; Kanai *et al.*, 2007; Vieira *et al.*, 1991). Hence, herpesviruses are able to modulate the immune system for self- or host protection, and HT has contributed to the evolution of this dual host-pathogen relationship.

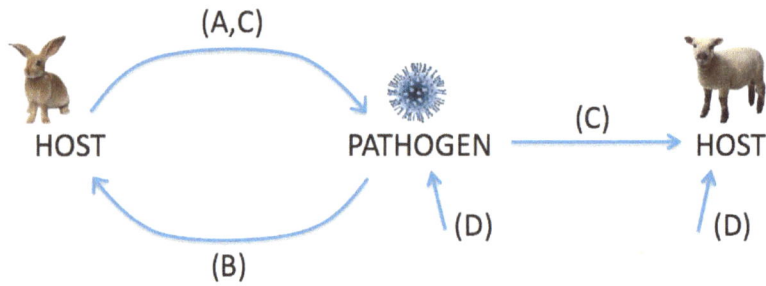

Figure 1: Horizontal transfer of DNA sequences between pathogens and their hosts can occur: A) from hosts to pathogens; B) from pathogens to hosts; C) from one host to other through one or more pathogens. D) Other organisms can also be donors of horizontally transferred genes, especially those that live in close relationship (or have similar lifestyles, *e.g.,* HT from pathogens to pathogens).

5   Pathogens as Vectors of Horizontally Transferred Genes between species

Pathogens can be donors and acceptors of HTd sequences. Hence, they can they serve as vehicles of sequences between organisms (Figure 1). Once transferred, sequences can suffer additional HT events and, in this manner, travel through multiple organisms -especially if they have close relationships, as the ones established between pathogens or endosymbionts with their hosts. For instance, it has been proposed that algal endosymbionts (particularly red algae) could act as vectors of HT between prokaryotes and photosynthetic eukaryotes (Qiu *et al.,* 2013). As previously discussed, sequences derived from the intracellular bacteria *Wolbachia* have been found in a variety of hosts (Dunning Hotopp *et al.,* 2007; Nikoh *et al.,* 2008). Moreover, *Wolbachia* can be infected by bacteriophages, which could mediate HT among these bacteria (Loreto *et al.,* 2008). Viruses may also be the vectors of transposon-derived sequences from lepidopteran hosts to their parasitic wasps (Schaack *et al.,* 2010; Yoshiyama *et al.,* 2001).

In fact, viruses are in a privileged position for transmitting sequences among hosts. As previously discussed, there are many examples of HTd sequences from viruses to hosts and vice versa, representing in some cases a substantial fraction of their genomes (Filee, 2009; Filee *et al.,* 2007; Hughes & Friedman, 2005; Koonin, 2010; Liu *et al.,* 2010; Taylor & Bruenn, 2009). In addition, some of these viruses can infect a variety of hosts or have changed hosts during their evolution, as it is the case of poxviruses (Hughes *et al.,* 2010). This may explain why sequences related to transposons present in reptiles were found in a taterapox virus isolated from a rodent (Piskurek & Okada, 2007). Therefore, viral vectors may mediate the transfer of sequences between distantly related species.

Protozoan and multicellular parasites can also be vectors of HT. As previously discussed, protozoan can capture and donate sequences from/to their hosts. For example, several studies have pointed out to the insect-transmitted *Trypanosoma* as a likely vector; in fact, sequences derived from this parasite have been found in humans (Hecht *et al.,* 2010). Moreover, several observations support the contribution of parasitic arthropods to HT between animals: for instance, a parasitic mite appears to be responsible for the HT of P elements among different species of *Drosophila* (Bartolome *et al.,* 2009; Houck *et al.,* 1991). Arthropod parasites are also the likely vectors of HT of several transposable elements between tetrapods (de Boer *et al.*, 2007; Gilbert *et al.*, 2010; Pace *et al.*, 2008; Silva *et al.*, 2004; Walsh *et al.*, 2013). For example, the BovB long interspersed element (LINE) has been observed in both mammals and reptiles, being very abundant in some species (almost a fourth of the cow genome) while absent in others. It has also been detected in two reptile ticks (but not in other insects) collected from the same host species, although phylogenetic analyses support that the two sequences were independently acquired (Walsh *et al.*, 2013). The authors propose that ticks mediated the HT of BovB sequences between snakes and lizards, and that these parasites also contributed to their transfer to marsupials and ruminants. In cows, one of these sequences acquired a functional role (Iwashita *et al.*, 2006). Therefore, HT of BovB sequences represents a interesting example of the impact that pathogens, as HT vectors, may play in the evolution of their hosts, due to the variety of species affected (both warm- and cold-blooded vertebrates), the success of the HTd sequences in colonizing some genomes (and, hence, their potential for altering the structure and function of such genomes) and their contribution to novel protein-coding genes (Walsh *et al.*, 2013).

6   Conclusions: Horizontal Transfer between Host and Pathogens has Shaped Their Evolution

HT of genetic information between two organisms is facilitated when a close relationship exists between them, such as the host-parasite interaction. After transfer, fixation strongly depends on the selective forces operating on the newly acquired sequences. Pathogens survive at the expense of their hosts, but also depend on them; hosts would be better off without pathogens, but sometimes these provide them with some advantages. Hence, pressures related to both host-pathogen antagonism and mutual benefit can contribute to the evolution of HTd sequences. In the case of pathogens, the adaptation to the pathogenic lifestyle to new hosts can be acquired through HT of sequences from other pathogens. But they can also receive sequences from their hosts; these sequences are often derived from genes involved in host defensive mechanisms and are co-opted, precisely, to elude the host defenses. This can drive rapid diversification of the original copy in the host, in order to counteract the advantageous effect of HT in the pathogen (Murphy, 1993).

Hosts, in turn, can incorporate and co-opt pathogens' sequences to protect themselves against deleterious infections. Moreover, hosts can receive sequences from other hosts through pathogens, allowing for the spreading of sequences between distantly related taxa and, consequently, the emergence of functional novelties in them. Hence, HTd sequences have not only shaped the individual evolution of hosts and pathogens, but also the interactions between them and, therefore, their co-evolution. Moreover, the study of host-pathogen HTd genes, of their original *vs.* co-opted functions in infection or defense has the potential of revealing novel therapeutic targets.

Author

Elena de la Casa-Esperón
Castilla-La Mancha Science and Technology Park (PCTCLM), Regional Center for Biomedical Research (CRIB), University of Castilla-La Mancha, Spain

Acknowledgements

ECE is supported by the INCRECYT Program of the Junta de Comunidades de Castilla-La Mancha and the European Social Funds

References

Acuna, R., Padilla, B. E., Florez-Ramos, C. P., Rubio, J. D., Herrera, J. C., Benavides, P., et al., (2012). *Adaptive horizontal transfer of a bacterial gene to an invasive insect pest of coffee. Proc Natl Acad Sci U S A, 109(11), 4197-4202.*

Alcami, A., & Lira, S. A. (2010). *Modulation of chemokine activity by viruses. Curr Opin Immunol, 22(4), 482-487.*

Anderson, M. T., & Seifert, H. S. (2011). *Opportunity and means: horizontal gene transfer from the human host to a bacterial pathogen. MBio, 2(1), e00005-00011.*

Andersson, J. O. (2005). *Lateral gene transfer in eukaryotes. Cell Mol Life Sci, 62(11), 1182-1197.*

Bartlett, N. W., Dumoutier, L., Renauld, J. C., Kotenko, S. V., McVey, C. E., Lee, H. J., et al., (2004). *A new member of the interleukin 10-related cytokine family encoded by a poxvirus. J Gen Virol, 85(Pt 6), 1401-1412.*

Bartolome, C., Bello, X., & Maside, X. (2009). *Widespread evidence for horizontal transfer of transposable elements across Drosophila genomes. Genome Biol, 10(2), R22.*

Barton, E. S., White, D. W., Cathelyn, J. S., Brett-McClellan, K. A., Engle, M., Diamond, M. S., et al., (2007). *Herpesvirus latency confers symbiotic protection from bacterial infection. Nature, 447(7142), 326-329.*

Bernstein, B. E., Birney, E., Dunham, I., Green, E. D., Gunter, C., & Snyder, M. (2012). *An integrated encyclopedia of DNA elements in the human genome. Nature, 489(7414), 57-74.*

Bock, R. (2010). *The give-and-take of DNA: horizontal gene transfer in plants. Trends Plant Sci, 15(1), 11-22.*

Boschetti, C., Carr, A., Crisp, A., Eyres, I., Wang-Koh, Y., Lubzens, E., et al., (2012). *Biochemical diversification through foreign gene expression in bdelloid rotifers. PLoS Genet, 8(11), e1003035.*

Boto, L. (2010). *Horizontal gene transfer in evolution: facts and challenges. Proc Biol Sci, 277(1683), 819-827.*

Boto, L. (2014). *Horizontal gene transfer in the acquisition of novel traits by metazoans. Proc Biol Sci, 281(1777), 20132450.*

Bratke, K. A., & McLysaght, A. (2008). *Identification of multiple independent horizontal gene transfers into poxviruses using a comparative genomics approach. BMC Evol Biol, 8, 67.*

Bustos, O., Naik, S., Ayers, G., Casola, C., Perez-Lamigueiro, M. A., Chippindale, P. T., et al., (2009). *Evolution of the Schlafen genes, a gene family associated with embryonic lethality, meiotic drive, immune processes and orthopoxvirus virulence. Gene, 447(1), 1-11.*

Chan, A., Baird, M., Mercer, A. A., & Fleming, S. B. (2006). *Maturation and function of human dendritic cells are inhibited by orf virus-encoded interleukin-10. J Gen Virol, 87(Pt 11), 3177-3181.*

Craig, J. P., Bekal, S., Hudson, M., Domier, L., Niblack, T., & Lambert, K. N. (2008). *Analysis of a horizontally transferred pathway involved in vitamin B6 biosynthesis from the soybean cyst nematode Heterodera glycines. Mol Biol Evol, 25(10), 2085-2098.*

Danchin, E. G. (2011). *What Nematode genomes tell us about the importance of horizontal gene transfers in the evolutionary history of animals. Mob Genet Elements, 1(4), 269-273.*

Daniels, S. B., Peterson, K. R., Strausbaugh, L. D., Kidwell, M. G., & Chovnick, A. (1990). *Evidence for horizontal transmission of the P transposable element between Drosophila species. Genetics, 124(2), 339-355.*

Davis, C. C., & Wurdack, K. J. (2004). *Host-to-parasite gene transfer in flowering plants: phylogenetic evidence from Malpighiales. Science, 305(5684), 676-678.*

de Boer, J. G., Yazawa, R., Davidson, W. S., & Koop, B. F. (2007). *Bursts and horizontal evolution of DNA transposons in the speciation of pseudotetraploid salmonids. BMC Genomics, 8, 422.*

de Felipe, K. S., Pampou, S., Jovanovic, O. S., Pericone, C. D., Ye, S. F., Kalachikov, S., et al., (2005). *Evidence for acquisition of Legionella type IV secretion substrates via interdomain horizontal gene transfer. J Bacteriol, 187(22), 7716-7726.*

de la Casa-Esperon, E. (2011). *From mammals to viruses: the Schlafen genes in developmental, proliferative and immune processes. BioMolecular Concepts, 2, 159-169.*

de la Casa-Esperon, E. (2012). *Horizontal transfer and the evolution of host-pathogen interactions. Int J Evol Biol, 2012, 679045.*

Denker, E., Bapteste, E., Le Guyader, H., Manuel, M., & Rabet, N. (2008). *Horizontal gene transfer and the evolution of cnidarian stinging cells. Curr Biol, 18(18), R858-859.*

Du Pasquier, L. (2004). *Speculations on the origin of the vertebrate immune system. Immunol Lett, 92(1-2), 3-9.*

Dunning Hotopp, J. C. (2011). *Horizontal gene transfer between bacteria and animals. Trends Genet, 27(4), 157-163.*

Dunning Hotopp, J. C., Clark, M. E., Oliveira, D. C., Foster, J. M., Fischer, P., Munoz Torres, M. C., et al., (2007). *Widespread lateral gene transfer from intracellular bacteria to multicellular eukaryotes. Science, 317(5845), 1753-1756.*

Filee, J. (2009). *Lateral gene transfer, lineage-specific gene expansion and the evolution of Nucleo Cytoplasmic Large DNA viruses. J Invertebr Pathol, 101(3), 169-171.*

Filee, J., Pouget, N., & Chandler, M. (2008). *Phylogenetic evidence for extensive lateral acquisition of cellular genes by Nucleocytoplasmic large DNA viruses. BMC Evol Biol, 8, 320.*

Filee, J., Siguier, P., & Chandler, M. (2007). *I am what I eat and I eat what I am: acquisition of bacterial genes by giant viruses. Trends Genet, 23(1), 10-15.*

Fu, M., Deng, R., Wang, J., & Wang, X. (2008). *Detection and analysis of horizontal gene transfer in herpesvirus. Virus Res, 131(1), 65-76.*

Fu, M., Deng, R., Wang, J., & Wang, X. (2011). *Horizontal gene transfer in herpesviruses identified by using support vector machine. Acta Virol, 55(3), 203-217.*

Gao, C., Ren, X., Mason, A. S., Liu, H., Xiao, M., Li, J., et al., (2013). *Horizontal gene transfer in plants. Funct Integr Genomics.*

Gilbert, C., Hernandez, S. S., Flores-Benabib, J., Smith, E. N., & Feschotte, C. (2012). *Rampant horizontal transfer of SPIN transposons in squamate reptiles. Mol Biol Evol, 29(2), 503-515.*

Gilbert, C., Schaack, S., Pace, J. K., 2nd, Brindley, P. J., & Feschotte, C. (2010). *A role for host-parasite interactions in the horizontal transfer of transposons across phyla. Nature, 464(7293), 1347-1350.*

Gogarten, J. P., & Townsend, J. P. (2005). *Horizontal gene transfer, genome innovation and evolution. Nat Rev Microbiol, 3(9), 679-687.*

Graham, L. A., Lougheed, S. C., Ewart, K. V., & Davies, P. L. (2008). *Lateral transfer of a lectin-like antifreeze protein gene in fishes. PLoS One, 3(7), e2616.*

Gubser, C., Goodbody, R., Ecker, A., Brady, G., O'Neill, L. A., Jacobs, N., et al., (2007). *Camelpox virus encodes a schlafen-like protein that affects orthopoxvirus virulence. J Gen Virol, 88(Pt 6), 1667-1676.*

Haegeman, A., Jones, J. T., & Danchin, E. G. (2011). *Horizontal gene transfer in nematodes: a catalyst for plant parasitism? Mol Plant Microbe Interact, 24(8), 879-887.*

Haig, D. M. (2001). *Subversion and piracy: DNA viruses and immune evasion. Res Vet Sci, 70(3), 205-219.*

Haring, E., Hagemann, S., & Pinsker, W. (2000). *Ancient and recent horizontal invasions of drosophilids by P elements. J Mol Evol, 51(6), 577-586.*

Haugen, P., Simon, D. M., & Bhattacharya, D. (2005). *The natural history of group I introns. Trends Genet, 21(2), 111-119.*

Hecht, M. M., Nitz, N., Araujo, P. F., Sousa, A. O., Rosa Ade, C., Gomes, D. A., et al., (2010). Inheritance of DNA transferred from American trypanosomes to human hosts. PLoS One, 5(2), e9181.

Holzerlandt, R., Orengo, C., Kellam, P., & Alba, M. M. (2002). Identification of new herpesvirus gene homologs in the human genome. Genome Res, 12(11), 1739-1748.

Horvath, P., & Barrangou, R. (2010). CRISPR/Cas, the immune system of bacteria and archaea. Science, 327(5962), 167-170.

Houck, M. A., Clark, J. B., Peterson, K. R., & Kidwell, M. G. (1991). Possible horizontal transfer of Drosophila genes by the mite Proctolaelaps regalis. Science, 253(5024), 1125-1128.

Huang, J. (2013). Horizontal gene transfer in eukaryotes: the weak-link model. Bioessays, 35(10), 868-875.

Hughes, A. L. (2002). Origin and evolution of viral interleukin-10 and other DNA virus genes with vertebrate homologues. J Mol Evol, 54(1), 90-101.

Hughes, A. L., & Friedman, R. (2005). Poxvirus genome evolution by gene gain and loss. Mol Phylogenet Evol, 35(1), 186-195.

Hughes, A. L., Irausquin, S., & Friedman, R. (2010). The evolutionary biology of poxviruses. Infect Genet Evol, 10(1), 50-59.

Intrieri, M. C., & Buiatti, M. (2001). The horizontal transfer of Agrobacterium rhizogenes genes and the evolution of the genus Nicotiana. Mol Phylogenet Evol, 20(1), 100-110.

Iwashita, S., Ueno, S., Nakashima, K., Song, S. Y., Oshima, K., Tanaka, K., et al., (2006). A tandem gene duplication followed by recruitment of a retrotransposon created the paralogous bucentaur gene (bcntp97) in the ancestral ruminant. Mol Biol Evol, 23(4), 798-806.

Jakobsen, M. R., Mogensen, T. H., & Paludan, S. R. (2013). Caught in translation: innate restriction of HIV mRNA translation by a schlafen family protein. Cell Res, 23(3), 320-322.

Jiang, W., Maniv, I., Arain, F., Wang, Y., Levin, B. R., & Marraffini, L. A. (2013). Dealing with the evolutionary downside of CRISPR immunity: bacteria and beneficial plasmids. PLoS Genet, 9(9), e1003844.

Jordan, I. K., Matyunina, L. V., & McDonald, J. F. (1999). Evidence for the recent horizontal transfer of long terminal repeat retrotransposon. Proc Natl Acad Sci U S A, 96(22), 12621-12625.

Kanai, K., Satoh, Y., Yamanaka, H., Kawaguchi, A., Horie, K., Sugata, K., et al., (2007). The vIL-10 gene of the Epstein-Barr virus (EBV) is conserved in a stable manner except for a few point mutations in various EBV isolates. Virus Genes, 35(3), 563-569.

Keeling, P. J. (2009). Functional and ecological impacts of horizontal gene transfer in eukaryotes. Curr Opin Genet Dev, 19(6), 613-619.

Keeling, P. J., & Palmer, J. D. (2008). Horizontal gene transfer in eukaryotic evolution. Nat Rev Genet, 9(8), 605-618.

Kondo, N., Nikoh, N., Ijicchi, N., & Shimada, M. (2002). Genome frabment of Wolbachia endosymbiont transferred to X chromosome of host insect. Proc Natl Acad Sci U S A, 99, 14280-14285.

Koonin, E. V. (2010). Taming of the shrewd: novel eukaryotic genes from RNA viruses. BMC Biol, 8, 2.

Koonin, E. V., Makarova, K. S., & Aravind, L. (2001). Horizontal gene transfer in prokaryotes: quantification and classification. Annu Rev Microbiol, 55, 709-742.

Kordis, D., & Gubensek, F. (1998). Unusual horizontal transfer of a long interspersed nuclear element between distant vertebrate classes. Proc Natl Acad Sci U S A, 95(18), 10704-10709.

Kotenko, S. V., Saccani, S., Izotova, L. S., Mirochnitchenko, O. V., & Pestka, S. (2000). Human cytomegalovirus harbors its own unique IL-10 homolog (cmvIL-10). Proc Natl Acad Sci U S A, 97(4), 1695-1700.

Kozak, C. A. (2010). The mouse "xenotropic" gammaretroviruses and their XPR1 receptor. Retrovirology, 7, 101.

Kurilla, M. G., Swaminathan, S., Welsh, R. M., Kieff, E., & Brutkiewicz, R. R. (1993). Effects of virally expressed interleukin-10 on vaccinia virus infection in mice. J Virol, 67(12), 7623-7628.

Laha, T., Loukas, A., Wattanasatitarpa, S., Somprakhon, J., Kewgrai, N., Sithithaworn, P., et al., (2007). The bandit, a new DNA transposon from a hookworm -possible horizontal genetic transfer between host and parasite. PLoS Negl Trop Dis, 1(1), e35.

Lalani, A. S., & McFadden, G. (1999). Evasion and exploitation of chemokines by viruses. Cytokine Growth Factor Rev, 10(3-4), 219-233.

Lander, E. S., Linton, L. M., Birren, B., Nusbaum, C., Zody, M. C., Baldwin, J., et al., (2001). Initial sequencing and analysis of the human genome. Nature, 409(6822), 860-921.

Lefkowitz, E. J., Wang, C., & Upton, C. (2006). Poxviruses: past, present and future. Virus Res, 117(1), 105-118.

Li, M., Kao, E., Gao, X., Sandig, H., Limmer, K., Pavon-Eternod, M., et al., (2012). Codon-usage-based inhibition of HIV protein synthesis by human schlafen 11. Nature, 491(7422), 125-128.

Liu, H., Fu, Y., Jiang, D., Li, G., Xie, J., Cheng, J., et al., (2010). Widespread horizontal gene transfer from double-stranded RNA viruses to eukaryotic nuclear genomes. J Virol, 84(22), 11876-11887.

Liu, Y., de Waal Malefyt, R., Briere, F., Parham, C., Bridon, J. M., Banchereau, J., et al., (1997). The EBV IL-10 homologue is a selective agonist with impaired binding to the IL-10 receptor. J Immunol, 158(2), 604-613.

Loreto, E. L., Carareto, C. M., & Capy, P. (2008). Revisiting horizontal transfer of transposable elements in Drosophila. Heredity (Edinb), 100(6), 545-554.

Ma, L. J., van der Does, H. C., Borkovich, K. A., Coleman, J. J., Daboussi, M. J., Di Pietro, A., et al., (2010). Comparative genomics reveals mobile pathogenicity chromosomes in Fusarium. Nature, 464(7287), 367-373.

McClure, M. A., Johnson, M. S., & Doolittle, R. F. (1987). Relocation of a protease-like gene segment between two retroviruses. Proc Natl Acad Sci U S A, 84(9), 2693-2697.

McFadden, G., Graham, K., Ellison, K., Barry, M., Macen, J., Schreiber, M., et al., (1995). Interruption of cytokine networks by poxviruses: lessons from myxoma virus. J Leukoc Biol, 57(5), 731-738.

Mehrabi, R., Bahkali, A. H., Abd-Elsalam, K. A., Moslem, M., Ben M'barek, S., Gohari, A. M., et al., (2011). Horizontal gene and chromosome transfer in plant pathogenic fungi affecting host range. FEMS Microbiol Rev, 35(3), 542-554.

Miller, M. R., White, A., & Boots, M. (2005). The evolution of host resistance: tolerance and control as distinct strategies. J Theor Biol, 236(2), 198-207.

Monier, A., Pagarete, A., de Vargas, C., Allen, M. J., Read, B., Claverie, J. M., et al., (2009). Horizontal gene transfer of an entire metabolic pathway between a eukaryotic alga and its DNA virus. Genome Res, 19(8), 1441-1449.

Moran, N. A., & Jarvik, T. (2010). Lateral transfer of genes from fungi underlies carotenoid production in aphids. Science, 328(5978), 624-627.

Moran, Y., Fredman, D., Szczesny, P., Grynberg, M., & Technau, U. (2012). Recurrent horizontal transfer of bacterial toxin genes to eukaryotes. Mol Biol Evol, 29(9), 2223-2230.

Moriguchi, K., Yamamoto, S., Tanaka, K., Kurata, N., & Suzuki, K. (2013). Trans-kingdom horizontal DNA transfer from bacteria to yeast is highly plastic due to natural polymorphisms in auxiliary nonessential recipient genes. PLoS One, 8(9), e74590.

Moss, B., & Shisler, J. L. (2001). Immunology 101 at poxvirus U: immune evasion genes. Semin Immunol, 13(1), 59-66.

Moss, B., Shisler, J. L., Xiang, Y., & Senkevich, T. G. (2000). Immune-defense molecules of molluscum contagiosum virus, a human poxvirus. Trends Microbiol, 8(10), 473-477.

Mower, J. P., Stefanovic, S., Young, G. J., & Palmer, J. D. (2004). Plant genetics: gene transfer from parasitic to host plants. Nature, 432(7014), 165-166.

Murphy, P. M. (1993). Molecular mimicry and the generation of host defense protein diversity. Cell, 72(6), 823-826.

Nembaware, V., Seoighe, C., Sayed, M., & Gehring, C. (2004). A plant natriuretic peptide-like gene in the bacterial pathogen Xanthomonas axonopodis may induce hyper-hydration in the plant host: a hypothesis of molecular mimicry. BMC Evol Biol, 4, 10.

Nikoh, N., & Nakabachi, A. (2009). Aphids acquired symbiotic genes via lateral gene transfer. BMC Biol, 7, 12.

Nikoh, N., Tanaka, K., Shibata, F., Kondo, N., Hizume, M., Shimada, M., et al., (2008). Wolbachia genome integrated in an insect chromosome: evolution and fate of laterally transferred endosymbiont genes. Genome Res, 18(2), 272-280.

Novick, P., Smith, J., Ray, D., & Boissinot, S. (2010). Independent and parallel lateral transfer of DNA transposons in tetrapod genomes. Gene, 449(1-2), 85-94.

Odom, M. R., Hendrickson, R. C., & Lefkowitz, E. J. (2009). Poxvirus protein evolution: family wide assessment of possible horizontal gene transfer events. Virus Res, 144(1-2), 233-249.

Pace, J. K., 2nd, Gilbert, C., Clark, M. S., & Feschotte, C. (2008). Repeated horizontal transfer of a DNA transposon in mammals and other tetrapods. Proc Natl Acad Sci U S A, 105(44), 17023-17028.

Paganini, J., Campan-Fournier, A., Da Rocha, M., Gouret, P., Pontarotti, P., Wajnberg, E., et al., (2012). Contribution of lateral gene transfers to the genome composition and parasitic ability of root-knot nematodes. PLoS One, 7(11), e50875.

Patel, M. R., Emerman, M., & Malik, H. S. (2011). Paleovirology - ghosts and gifts of viruses past. Curr Opin Virol, 1(4), 304-309.

Piskurek, O., & Okada, N. (2007). Poxviruses as possible vectors for horizontal transfer of retroposons from reptiles to mammals. Proc Natl Acad Sci U S A, 104(29), 12046-12051.

Qiu, H., Yoon, H. S., & Bhattacharya, D. (2013). Algal endosymbionts as vectors of horizontal gene transfer in photosynthetic eukaryotes. Front Plant Sci, 4, 366.

Richards, T. A., Hirt, R. P., Williams, B. A., & Embley, T. M. (2003). Horizontal gene transfer and the evolution of parasitic protozoa. Protist, 154(1), 17-32.

Richards, T. A., Soanes, D. M., Foster, P. G., Leonard, G., Thornton, C. R., & Talbot, N. J. (2009). Phylogenomic analysis demonstrates a pattern of rare and ancient horizontal gene transfer between plants and fungi. Plant Cell, 21(7), 1897-1911.

Richardson, A. O., & Palmer, J. D. (2007). Horizontal gene transfer in plants. J Exp Bot, 58(1), 1-9.

Roy, B. A., & Kirchner, J. W. (2000). Evolutionary dynamics of pathogen resistance and tolerance. Evolution, 54(1), 51-63.

Sanville, B., Dolan, M. A., Wollenberg, K., Yan, Y., Martin, C., Yeung, M. L., et al., (2010). Adaptive evolution of Mus Apobec3 includes retroviral insertion and positive selection at two clusters of residues flanking the substrate groove. PLoS Pathog, 6, e1000974.

Schaack, S., Gilbert, C., & Feschotte, C. (2010). Promiscuous DNA: horizontal transfer of transposable elements and why it matters for eukaryotic evolution. Trends Ecol Evol, 25(9), 537-546.

Schonknecht, G., Weber, A. P., & Lercher, M. J. (2014). Horizontal gene acquisitions by eukaryotes as drivers of adaptive evolution. Bioessays, 36(1), 9-20.

Seet, B. T., Johnston, J. B., Brunetti, C. R., Barrett, J. W., Everett, H., Cameron, C., et al., (2003). Poxviruses and immune evasion. Annu Rev Immunol, 21, 377-423.

Shchelkunov, S. N. (2003). [Immunomodulatory proteins of orthopoxviruses]. Mol Biol (Mosk), 37(1), 41-53.

Silva, J. C., Loreto, E. L., & Clark, J. B. (2004). Factors that affect the horizontal transfer of transposable elements. Curr Issues Mol Biol, 6(1), 57-71.

Sin, S. H., & Dittmer, D. P. (2012). Cytokine homologs of human gammaherpesviruses. J Interferon Cytokine Res, 32(2), 53-59.

Sloan, D. B., Nakabachi, A., Richards, S., Qu, J., Murali, S. C., Gibbs, R. A., et al., (2014). Parallel Histories of Horizontal Gene Transfer Facilitated Extreme Reduction of Endosymbiont Genomes in Sap-Feeding Insects. Mol Biol Evol.

Sorek, R., Kunin, V., & Hugenholtz, P. (2008). CRISPR--a wide-spread system that provides acquired resistance against phages in bacteria and archaea. Nat Rev Microbiol, 6(3), 181-186.

Stern, A., & Sorek, R. (2011). The phage-host arms race: shaping the evolution of microbes. Bioessays, 33(1), 43-51.

Striepen, B., Pruijssers, A. J., Huang, J., Li, C., Gubbels, M. J., Umejiego, N. N., et al., (2004). Gene transfer in the evolution of parasite nucleotide biosynthesis. Proc Natl Acad Sci U S A, 101(9), 3154-3159.

Sun, G., & Huang, J. (2011). Horizontally acquired DAP pathway as a unit of self-regulation. J Evol Biol, 24(3), 587-595.

Sunarto, A., Liongue, C., McColl, K. A., Adams, M. M., Bulach, D., Crane, M. S., et al., (2012). Koi herpesvirus encodes and expresses a functional interleukin-10. J Virol, 86(21), 11512-11520.

Syvanen, M. (2012). Evolutionary Implications of Horizontal Gene Transfer. Annu Rev Genet.

Taylor, D. J., & Bruenn, J. (2009). The evolution of novel fungal genes from non-retroviral RNA viruses. BMC Biol, 7, 88.

Vieira, P., de Waal-Malefyt, R., Dang, M. N., Johnson, K. E., Kastelein, R., Fiorentino, D. F., et al., (1991). Isolation and expression of human cytokine synthesis inhibitory factor cDNA clones: homology to Epstein-Barr virus open reading frame BCRF1. Proc Natl Acad Sci U S A, 88(4), 1172-1176.

Villarreal, L. P. (2009). The source of self: genetic parasites and the origin of adaptive immunity. Ann N Y Acad Sci, 1178, 194-232.

Villarreal, L. P. (2011). Viral ancestors of antiviral systems. Viruses, 3(10), 1933-1958.

Walsh, A. M., Kortschak, R. D., Gardner, M. G., Bertozzi, T., & Adelson, D. L. (2013). Widespread horizontal transfer of re-
trotransposons. Proc Natl Acad Sci U S A, 110(3), 1012-1016.

Wang, X., Kim, Y., Ma, Q., Hong, S. H., Pokusaeva, K., Sturino, J. M., et al., (2010). Cryptic prophages help bacteria cope with
adverse environments. Nat Commun, 1, 147.

White, D. W., Suzanne Beard, R., & Barton, E. S. (2012). Immune modulation during latent herpesvirus infection. Immunol Rev,
245(1), 189-208.

Xi, Z., Bradley, R. K., Wurdack, K. J., Wong, K., Sugumaran, M., Bomblies, K., et al., (2012). Horizontal transfer of expressed
genes in a parasitic flowering plant. BMC Genomics, 13, 227.

Xi, Z., Wang, Y., Bradley, R. K., Sugumaran, M., Marx, C. J., Rest, J. S., et al., (2013). Massive mitochondrial gene transfer in a
parasitic flowering plant clade. PLoS Genet, 9(2), e1003265.

Yan, Y., Buckler-White, A., Wollenberg, K., & Kozak, C. A. (2009). Origin, antiviral function and evidence for positive selection
of the gammaretrovirus restriction gene Fv1 in the genus Mus. Proc Natl Acad Sci U S A, 106(9), 3259-3263.

Yohn, C. T., Jiang, Z., McGrath, S. D., Hayden, K. E., Khaitovich, P., Johnson, M. E., et al., (2005). Lineage-specific expansions
of retroviral insertions within the genomes of African great apes but not humans and orangutans. PLoS Biol, 3(4), e110.

Yoshida, S., Maruyama, S., Nozaki, H., & Shirasu, K. (2010). Horizontal gene transfer by the parasitic plant Striga hermonthica.
Science, 328(5982), 1128.

Yoshiyama, M., Tu, Z., Kainoh, Y., Honda, H., Shono, T., & Kimura, K. (2001). Possible horizontal transfer of a transposable
element from host to parasitoid. Mol Biol Evol, 18(10), 1952-1958.

Yue, J., Hu, X., Sun, H., Yang, Y., & Huang, J. (2012). Widespread impact of horizontal gene transfer on plant colonization of
land. Nat Commun, 3, 1152.

Zhu, S., & Gao, B. (2014). Nematode-derived drosomycin-type antifungal peptides provide evidence for plant-to-ecdysozoan horizontal transfer of a disease resistance gene. Nat Commun, 5, 3154.

Control of Avian Influenza in Poultry with Antivirals and Molecular Manipulation

El-Sayed M. Abdelwhab and Hafez M. Hafez

1   Introduction

Influenza A virus, the only orthomyxovirus known to infect birds, are negative-sense, single-stranded, enveloped viruses contain genomes composed of eight separate ribonucleic acid (RNA) segments encode for at least 10 viral proteins. Two surface glycoproteins; hemagglutinin (HA) and neuraminidase (NA) are playing a vital role in attachment and release of the virus, respectively (Palese & Shaw, 2007). To date, 18 HA and 11 NA subtypes of avian influenza viruses (AIV) have been detected. All AIV subtypes except H17N10 (Tong *et al.*, 2012) and H18N11 (Tong *et al.*, 2013) - which have recently been identified in bats - are known to infect birds. According to their pathogenicity for poultry, AIV are divided into low pathogenic (LPAIV) resulting in mild or asymptomatic infections and highly pathogenic (HPAIV) causing up to 100% morbidity and mortality (Swayne, 2009). Hitherto, only few strains of H5 or H7 subtypes fulfilled the defined criteria of high pathogenicity which potentially evolve from low virulent precursors (Lupiani & Reddy, 2009). Constant genetic and antigenic variation of AIV is an intriguing feature for continuous evolution of the virus in nature (Brown, 2000). Gradual antigenic changes due to acquisition of point mutations known as "antigenic drift" are commonly regarded to be the driving mechanism for influenza virus epidemics from one year to the next. However, possible "antigenic shift or reassortment" of influenza virus occurs by exchange genes from different subtypes is relatively infrequent, however it results in severe pandemics (Ferguson *et al.*, 2003).

HPAIV H5N1 is responsible for magnificent economic losses in poultry industry and poses a serious threat to public health (Webster *et al.*, 1992; Peiris *et al.*, 2007). Measures to control the virus in domestic poultry are the first step to decrease risks of human infections (Mumford *et al.*, 2007). Enhanced biosecurity measures, surveillance, stamping out and movement restriction are the basic principles for control of HPAIV epidemics in poultry (Yee *et al.*, 2009). However, mass depopulation of poultry in the face of an outbreak led to high economic losses for governments, stakeholders and consumers (Capua & Marangon, 2003; Capua & Alexander, 2006; Swayne *et al.*, 2011).

2   Vaccines

The use of vaccines as an option for the control of AI in poultry was not applied in the field until 1995. During the outbreak of HPAI H5N2 in 1994-1995 Mexico applied large-scale vaccination campaign using inactivated homologous H5N2 vaccines (Garcia *et al.*, 1998; Lee *et al.*, 2004). Also, Pakistan used inactivated H7N1 vaccines to control HPAI H7N1 outbreaks in 1995 (Naeem & Hussain, 1995; Naeem *et al.*, 1999; Naeem & Siddique, 2006). Thereafter the use of vaccines as emergency, prophylactic or routine strategy was frequently reported to control H5, H7 and H9 viruses. The inactivated H7N3 and H7N1 vaccines as a part of the intervention plan were used in Italy against H7N1 and H7N3 in 2000-2002, respectively (Capua & Marangon, 2007), in Pakistan against H7N1 in 2003-2004 (Naeem & Siddique, 2006), in USA against LPAIV H7N2 in 2003 (Capua & Alexander, 2004) and in North Korea against H7N7 in 2005 (Swayne, 2012a). Recently, inactivated H7N3 vaccines were used in Mexico to control the ongoing outbreaks of HPAI H7N3 since 2012 (Kapczynski *et al.*, 2013). After the re-emergence of the Asian H5N1 in 2003, vaccines were used in many countries to mitigate the economic and social impact of the disease. Currently, four countries use different H5N1 vaccines in poultry: China since 2004, Indonesia since 2004, Viet Nam since 2005 and Egypt since 2006 (Swayne, 2012a). Occasionally, vaccines for HPAI H5N1 have been used for short periods in Cote d'Ivoire, France, Kazakhstan, Mongolia, Netherlands, Pakistan, Russia and Sudan (Swayne, 2012a). Furthermore, 10 countries used inactivated H9N2 vaccines in poultry. Canada and USA used vaccines to control H1 and H3 swine influenza viruses in turkeys. Germany, South Africa and USA used vaccines to control H6 outbreaks and also USA used H2 and H4 vaccines (Swayne, 2012a). The use of bivalent H5-H7 and H7-H9 inactivated vaccines were used in Italy (Capua & Alexander, 2004) and Pakistan (Capua & Marangon, 2007), respectively.

The conventional inactivated whole virus vaccines are the currently the most used vaccines in poultry and it was expected to continue for the next 10 years (Swayne, 2012a; Spackman & Swayne, 2013). However, using recent molecular techniques a considerable number of vaccines with high efficiency to protect poultry against different AIV infections have been developed. Recombinant viral-vectored vaccines containing the HA and rarely NA of AIV expressed in fowl pox virus (FPV), Newcastle disease virus (NDV), herpes virus of turkeys (HVT), infectious laryngotracheitis virus (ILT), adenovirus or baculovirus have been frequently described (Capua & Marangon, 2007; Abdelwhab *et al.*, 2014). So far, only H5-expressing viral vectored vaccines have been used in the field to control HPAI H5N1 and H5N2 outbreaks in poultry (i.e.: in China, Egypt and Mexico) (Bublot *et al.*, 2007; Swayne, 2012a).

The major advantages of the vaccine to control AIV in poultry are to reduce shedding of the virus, morbidity, mortality, bird-to-bird transmission and to limit decrease in egg production. Moreover, viral-vectored vaccines, can be applied by mass vaccination (e.g. spray, drinking water, etc.) to protect birds simultaneously against several poultry viral pathogens. Also, as a form of live vaccines, the recombinant vaccines elicit not only humoral but also mucosal and cellular immune responses. The generation of recombinant or genetically-modified vaccines can overcome the availability of antigenic match between circulating and vaccine strains as well as providing a tool to differentiate between infected and vaccinated animals "DIVA" (for more information the readers are referred to (Suarez, 2005; Swayne, 2012a; 2012b; Spackman & Swayne, 2013; Abdelwhab *et al.*, 2014).

Nevertheless, several challenges facing the efficiency of the vaccine to control the HPAIV H5N1 outbreaks have been reported: (1) Vaccine is HA subtype specific and in some regions where multiple subtypes are co-circulating (*i.e.*, H5, H7 and H9), vaccination against multiple HA subtypes is required (Suarez & Schultz-Cherry, 2000). (2) Vaccine-induced anti-

bodies hinder routine serological surveillance and differentiation of infected birds from vaccinated ones requires more advanced diagnostic strategies (Suarez, 2005). (3) Vaccination may
prevent the clinical disease but can't prevent the infection of vaccinated birds, thus continuous
"silent" circulation of the virus in vaccinated birds poses a potential risk of virus spread
among poultry flocks and spillover to humans (Savill *et al.*, 2006; Naeem *et al.*, 2007; Capua &
Alexander, 2008; Hafez *et al.*, 2010). (4) Immune pressure induced by vaccination on the circulating virus increases the evolution rate of the virus and accelerates the viral antigenic drift to
evade the host-immune response (Lee *et al.*, 2004; Boni, 2008; Escorcia *et al.*, 2008; Cattoli *et al.*,
2011a; Cattoli *et al.*, 2011b; Park *et al.*, 2011; Lee *et al.*, 2012a; Lee & Song, 2013). (5) After emergence of antigenic variants, the vaccine becomes useless and/or inefficient to protect the birds
and periodical update of the vaccine is required (Lee *et al.*, 2004; Abdelwhab *et al.*, 2011; Grund
et al., 2011; Kilany *et al.*, 2011; Rauw *et al.*, 2011). (6) Vaccine-induced immunity usually peaks
three to four weeks after vaccination and duration of protection following immunization remains to be elucidated (Swayne & Kapczynski, 2008). (7) Maternally acquired immunity induced by vaccination of breeder flocks could interfere with vaccination of young birds (De
Vriese *et al.*, 2010; Kim *et al.*, 2010; Sarfati-Mizrahi *et al.*, 2010; Maas *et al.*, 2011; Abdelwhab *et
al.*, 2012). (8) Other domestic poultry (*i.e.*, ducks, geese, turkeys), zoo and/or exotic birds even
within the same species (*i.e.*, Muscovy *vs.* Pekin ducks) respond differently to vaccination
which have not yet been fully investigated compared to chickens (Oh *et al.*, 2005; Philippa *et
al.*, 2005; Tian *et al.*, 2005; Bertelsen *et al.*, 2007; Kapczynski & Swayne, 2009; Koch *et al.*, 2009;
Lecu *et al.*, 2009; Cagle *et al.*, 2011). (9) Concomitant or prior infection with immunosuppressive pathogens or ingestion of mycotoxins can inhibit the immune response of AIV-vaccinated
birds (Robinson & Easterday, 1979; Hao *et al.*, 2008; Sun *et al.*, 2009; Hegazy *et al.*, 2011). (10)
For the recombinant vaccines, keeping cold-chain is pivotal, it can cause or aggravate respiratory tract infections and reassortment with wild type viruses can not be totally excluded. (11)
And last but not least, factors related to vaccine manufacturing, quality, identity of vaccine
strain, improper handling and/or administration can be decisive for efficiency of any AIV
vaccine (Swayne & Kapczynski, 2008; Swayne, 2009).

Therefore, presence of new alternative and complementary strategies target different AIV
serotypes/subtypes/drift-variants should be encouraged. Insights into possible alternative approaches for control of AIV in poultry particularly against the HPAI (H5N1) subtypes are described below.

3   Antivirals

3.1   Chemotherapy

The use of chemotherapeutic agents for control of AIV in poultry was concurrently studied
just after discovering their anti-microbial effects (Moses *et al.*, 1948; Tolba & Eskarous, 1959). In
the last four decades attention was paid to the M2 blockers and neuraminidase inhibitors
(NAIs), the commonly used antivirals in control of influenza viruses in human, to be used in
eradication of AIV in poultry (Table 1).

On one hand, many antivirals had a potent activity against all subtypes of AIV as
prophylaxis or therapeutic treatment in a wide range of animals including birds. The protection starts relatively rapidly but varies according to the stage of infection. Some of these anti-

influenza drugs are cheap and can be given by mass administration (e.g. feed, water, etc.). On the other hand, the emergence of resistant mutants and subsequently hazards of kicking out cornerstone antivirals in case of pandemic are the most disadvantages. As described below, some antivirals require a long application period to be effective (e.g. Amantadine HCL) or are very expensive in a flock level (e.g. oseltamivir). Moreover, the majority of the novel antivirals were tested only in cell culture and rarely in birds (Table 1). In addition, residues in meat and eggs and compliance with other medical agents are not fully addressed (Table 2).

M2 Blockers (Adamantanes)

Amantadine hydrochloride and rimantadine are two M2 blockers which interrupt virus life cycle by blocking the influx of hydrogen ions through the M2 ion-channel protein and prevent uncoating of the virus in infected host-cells (Kato & Eggers, 1969; Kamps & Hoffman, 2006; Sugrue et al., 2008).

3.1.1   Amantadine

Amantadine is one of the cheapest anti-influenza drugs. The prophylactic activity of amantadine in poultry was firstly studied by Lang et al. (1970) in experimentally infected turkeys with an HPAIV H5N9 isolated in 1966 from Ontario, Canada. Optimum prophylaxis was obtained only when amantadine was administered in an adequate, uninterrupted and sustained amount from at least 2 days pre-infection to 23 days post-infection. During H5N2 outbreaks in Pennsylvania, USA in early 1980s, one of control proposals was the use of amantadine as a therapeutic and/or prophylactic approach. Under experimental condition, amantadine given in drinking water was efficacious to decrease morbidity, mortality, transmissibility and limit decrease in egg production (Webster et al., 1986; Beard et al., 1987). Nonetheless, all recovered birds were susceptible to reinfection (Lang et al., 1970; Webster et al., 1986; Bean et al., 1989) and subclinical infection was reported in most of treated birds (Lang et al., 1970). Importantly, amantadine lost its effectiveness as amantadine-resistant mutants emerged within 2–3 days of treatment and killed all in-contact chickens. Amantadine-resistant strains were irreversible, stable and transmissible with pathogenic potential comparable to the wild-type virus. Even more, the resistant mutants replaced the wild-type virus and became dominant (Scholtissek & Faulkner, 1979; Bean & Webster, 1988; Bean et al., 1989). It is worth pointing out that several subtypes of AIV including the HPAIV H5N1 that currently circulate in both humans and birds around the world are mostly resistant to amantadine (Bright et al., 2005; Ilyushina et al., 2005; Bright et al., 2006; Cheung et al., 2006; Hurt et al., 2007; He et al., 2008; Lan et al., 2010; Tosh et al., 2011). A recent study indicated that the frequency of H5N1 amantadine-resistant variants in humans from 2002 to 2012 was approximately double (62.2%) compared with the number of resistant strains of avian origin (31.6%) (Govorkova et al., 2013), which has been also confirmed in-vitro (Nguyen et al., 2013; Wang et al., 2013). Since the late 1990s, positive selection of amantadine-resistant HPAI H5N1 viruses in poultry in China has been proven to be increased due to extensive illegal application of the relatively inexpensive amantadine by some farmers to control HPAIV H5N1 (and LPAIV H9N2) infections in chickens (Cyranoski, 2005; Parry, 2005; Sipress, 2005; He et al., 2008; Huang et al., 2009). Hence, rapid selection of amantadine-resistant variants threatens the effective use of the drug for control of human influenza epidemics and/or pandemics (Wainright et al., 1991), therefore the extra-label use of amantadine in poultry was banned by all concerned international organizations (WHO, 2005; CDC, 2006).

Antiviral	Experimental host/Model	References
M2 Blockers (Adamantanes)		
Amantadine	Cell culture, humans, mice, ferrets, birds	(Lang et al., 1970; Scholtissek & Faulkner, 1979; Webster et al., 1986; Beard et al., 1987; Bean & Webster, 1988; Bean et al., 1989; Wainright et al., 1991; Bright et al., 2005; Ilyushina et al., 2005; Bright et al., 2006; Cheung et al., 2006; Hurt et al., 2007; He et al., 2008; Lan et al., 2010; Tosh et al., 2011; Nguyen et al., 2013; Wang et al., 2013)
Rimantadine	Cell culture, humans, mice, ferrets, birds	(Webster et al., 1985; Cao et al., 2013; Hai et al., 2013)
Neuraminidase Inhibitors (NAIs)		
Oseltamivir	Cell culture, humans, mice, ferrets, birds	(Leneva et al., 2000; Meijer et al., 2004; de Jong et al., 2005; Ward et al., 2005; Kamps & Hoffman, 2006; Kaleta et al., 2007; McKimm-Breschkin et al., 2007; Yen et al., 2007; Earhart et al., 2009; Hill et al., 2009; Moscona, 2009; Smith, 2010; Kayali et al., 2011; Lee et al., 2011; Orozovic et al., 2011; Brojer et al., 2013; Gillman et al., 2013; Govorkova et al., 2013; Leang et al., 2013; Younan et al., 2013)
Zanamivir	Cell culture, humans, mice, ferrets, birds	(Meijer et al., 2004; Kamps & Hoffman, 2006)
Inhibitors targeting the HA protein		
SA analogs	Cell culture	(Sun, 2007; Waldmann et al., 2014)
Neo6 compound	Computational analysis	(Li et al., 2011)
Synthetic derivatives of pyrazolopyrimidine nucleoside, pyrazole, pyridazinone, oxadiazole, triazole, thiazolidine and thioxopyrimidine	Cell culture	(Rashad et al., 2010a; Rashad et al., 2010b; Flefel et al., 2012)
TBHQ	Cell culture	(Bodian et al., 1993; Hoffman et al., 1997; Russell et al., 2008; Bliu et al., 2012; Antanasijevic et al., 2013; Shen et al., 2013)
FEB	Cell culture	(Bliu et al., 2012)
BMY-27709	Cell culture	(Luo et al., 1996)
MBX2329 & MBX2546	Cell culture	(Basu et al., 2014)
CL-385319	Cell culture	(Liu et al., 2011; Li et al., 2012)

Cyanovirin	Cell culture, mice, ferrets	(O'Keefe et al., 2003; Smee et al., 2007; Smee et al., 2008)
Inhibitors targeting the HA protein		
Laninamivir	Cell culture, humans, mice	(Kiso et al., 2010a; Kubo et al., 2010; Ikematsu & Kawai, 2011; Shobugawa et al., 2012; Ison, 2013; Samson et al., 2013)
Peramivir	Cell culture, humans, mice	(Beigel & Bray, 2008; Udommaneethanakit et al., 2009; Sorbello et al., 2012; Cao et al., 2013; Hai et al., 2013; Hu et al., 2013; Ison et al., 2013; Kamali & Holodniy, 2013; Nguyen et al., 2013; Yen et al., 2013)
Inhibitors targeting the polymerase protein		
Favipiravir	Cell culture, humans, mice	(Furuta et al., 2002; Takahashi et al., 2003; Sidwell et al., 2007; Smee et al., 2009; Boltz et al., 2010; Kiso et al., 2010b; Sleeman et al., 2010; Smee et al., 2010; Furuta et al., 2013)
Ribavirin	Cell culture, humans, mice	(Barnard et al., 2007; De Clercq & Neyts, 2007; Beigel & Bray, 2008; Gilbert & McLeay, 2008; Smee et al., 2008; Boltz et al., 2010; Smee et al., 2010; Samson et al., 2013)
Viramidine	Cell culture, humans, mice	(Sidwell et al., 2005; Boltz et al., 2010)
Inhibitors targeting the NS1 protein		
HENC	Cell culture	(Jablonski et al., 2012)
NSC125044	Cell culture	(Jablonski et al., 2012)
Inhibitors targeting host furin proteases		
Aprotinin	Cell culture, chickens	(Zhirnov et al., 1982)
Inhibitor 15	Cell culture	(Becker et al., 2012)
Inhibitors targeting host sialic acid		
DAS181	Cell culture, humans, mice, ferrets	(Belser et al., 2007; Chan et al., 2009; Triana-Baltzer et al., 2009; Zhang, 2009; Triana-Baltzer et al., 2010; Larson et al., 2011; Moss et al., 2012; Nguyen et al., 2013)
Herbs (Direct effect, targeting the HA protein; RNA synthesis, RNP complex)		
Eugenia jambolana	Cell culture, embryonated chicken eggs	(Sood et al., 2012)
Menthol, eucalyptol and ormosinine	Computational analysis	(Gangopadhyay et al., 2011)
NAS preparation	Chickens	(Shang et al., 2010)
Eucalyptus, peppermint	Chickens	(Barbour et al., 2006; Barbour et al., 2011)

Green tea (Catechins)	Chickens, embryonated chicken eggs	(Shaukat et al., 2011; Lee et al., 2012b)
Statin/caffeine	Cell culture, mice	(Liu et al., 2009; Kumaki et al., 2012)
Stachyflin	Cell culture, mice	(Motohashi et al., 2013; Shen et al., 2013)
Ribes nigrum folium	Cell culture, mice	(Ehrhardt et al., 2013a)
Capparis sinaica Veill	Cell culture	(Ibrahim et al., 2013a; Shen et al., 2013)
Aloe hijazensis	Cell culture	(Abd-Alla et al., 2012)
Red Sea grass Thallasodendron ciliatum	Cell culture	(Ibrahim et al., 2013b)
Phellinus igniarius	Cell culture	(Lee et al., 2013a)
Isatis indigotica	Cell culture	(Yang et al., 2012)
Andrographis paniculata	Cell culture, mice	(Chen et al., 2009)
Lycoris radiata	Cell culture	(Duvauchelle et al., 2013)

Table 1: A list of chemotherapeutic and natural antivirals against influenza viruses and their putative target structure.

Approach		Advantages	Limitations
Vaccines	Inactivated vaccines: Homologous (carrying the same HA and NA genes) or heterologous (carrying different NA genes)	decrease shedding of the virus decrease morbidity and mortality decrease bird-to-bird transmission increase bird resistance to disease reduce virus replication limit drop in egg production	HA subtype specific hinder routine serological surveillance (specially homologous vaccines) individual application (e.g.: by injection) "silent" circulation of the virus in vaccinated birds can't be totally prevented immunity peaks three to four weeks after vaccination duration of protection is variable maternal immunity interferes with vaccination of young birds variable response among domestic poultry species or types elicit humoral immunity only affected by immunosuppression affected by vaccine manufacturing, handling and/or administration increases the antigenic drift of the virus due to immune pressure ineffective against antigenic-drift variants periodical update of the vaccine is required
	Recombinant vaccines: Expression of HA (and NA) genes on FPV, NDV, ILT, HVT, adenovirus or baculovirus	mass administration (e.g. spray, drinking water, etc.) protect birds simultaneously against several poultry viral pathogens immunity peaks quickly after vaccination elicit humoral, mucosal and cellular immune responses overcome the availability of antigenic match between circulating and vaccine strains provide a tool for "DIVA"	HA subtype specific "silent" circulation of the virus in vaccinated birds can't be totally prevented duration of protection is short immunity (due to maternal, prior vaccination or infection) against the vector virus interferes with vaccination of young birds not suitable for all types of birds (e.g.: ILT only for chickens) variable response among domestic poultry species or types affected by immunosuppression keeping cold-chain is critical implication in respiratory illness is not uncommon reassortment with wild type virus can not be totally excluded increases the antigenic drift of the virus due to immune pressure ineffective against antigenic-drift variants periodical update of the vaccine is required

Antivirals	Chemotherapy		
	M2 Blockers (Amantadine and Rimantadine) and Neuraminidase inhibitors (Oseltamivir and Zanamivir)	Rapid protection Mass administration (feed, water) Cost-effective for individual birds (amantadine HCL) Suitable for all types of birds against all types of AIV	Hazards of kicking out cornerstone antivirals in case of pandemic Emergence of resistant mutants Require long application period to be effective Expensive in flock level (Oseltamivir) Residues in meat and eggs was not fully addressed Compliance with other medical agents need to be considered
	Natural Antivirals		
	Herbs	Direct antiviral activity Immunoadjuvant effect Additional effects as antioxidants, anti-inflammatory, etc. No adverse effects on body weight, egg production	Extraction is very expensive Affection with antigenic changes, herb-drug interactions, cytotoxicity and biochemical traits were not fully investigated Extraction methods, preparation, purity of the crude extracts greatly influence the efficacy. Batch-to-batch variations are high due to variable plantations conditions. Animal models of infection are limited
	Probiotics	Direct and indirect antiviral activity Immunoadjuvant effect Dual use as a vaccine-vector and immunomodulator	Efficacy against AIV particularly HPAIV is still questionable
Molecular approaches	Avian Cytokines	Not affected by antigenic changes Broad spectrum antiviral activities	Instability High production costs No mass production Field application limitations
	RNA interference	Inhibition of any influenza subtype/serotype/variant High specificity to particular strain/subtype/variant Do not require intact immune system Use as a prophylactic and/or	Specificity to the viral genome without interference with the host genome and non-specifically inhibition of cellular gene activity is critical. Delivery to the host, costs, mass production, storage and handling of the final products consider questionable aspects. Possibility for arise of mutants with the ability to evade the siRNA activity should not be fully guaranteed Quickly degraded in-vivo

	therapeutic	Induce a transient & short-term protection and multiple-dose is required In-vivo research studies still missing
Naturally resistant birds (Myxovirus Mx resistant gene and other candidate genes)	Few breeds of chickens and ducks can survive challenge with HPAIV in nature	Results on the contribution of the Mx gene to AIV resistant are contradictory Resistant breeds are mostly low producer native breeds. Interrelation of disease-resistance and production should be weighed Studies have been conducted only on a limited number of native breeds in some countries
Transgenic birds	Although all infected transgenic birds succumbed to the infection however the virus did not spread to the in-contact transgenic and non-transgenic cagemates	Replacement of backyard flocks Consumer preferences Food safety Regulatory approval Costs of production Mutations of AIV

Table 2: Advantages and limitations of different approaches for control of avian influenza viruses in poultry.

3.1.2   Rimantadine

The second M2 blocker is rimantadine. Because of the unavailability of rimantadine in most countries, its use in poultry is not reported until now in the field. However, Webster *et al.* (1985) mentioned that rimantadine administered in drinking water was efficacious against HPAIV H5N2 infection in experimentally infected chickens. Nonetheless, the emergence of rimantadine-resistant variants was comparable to amantadine. It is worth mentioning that the most recent LPAIV H7N9 virus which is responsible for the lethality of a considerable number of humans in China since February 2013 is resistant to amantadine and rimantadine (Cao *et al.*, 2013; Hai *et al.*, 2013).

Neuraminidase Inhibitors (NAIs)

Neuraminidase protein, also known as sialidase, is a surface glycoprotein of influenza virus which plays a vital role in the release of the progeny virions from sialic acid (SA) on the infected cells (Gamblin & Skehel, 2010). When exposed to NAIs, influenza virions aggregate on the host cell surface preventing their release and allow the host immune system to eliminate the virus (Dreitlein *et al.*, 2001; McNicholl & McNicholl, 2001). So far, there are two main NAIs, oseltamivir (Tamiflu®) and zanamivir (Relenza®) have been licensed for influenza treatment in human in several countries (Allen *et al.*, 2006) (Table 1).

3.1.3   Oseltamivir

In the early 2000s, oseltamivir was discovered as a potent and selective inhibitor of the NA enzyme of influenza viruses (Kamps & Hoffman, 2006). It is currently the drug of choice for the treatment of influenza virus infections in human and being stockpiled in many countries in anticipation of a pandemic (Ward *et al.*, 2005). Generally, AIV including H5N1 are sensitive to oseltamivir (Leneva *et al.*, 2000) and a small number of H5N1 strains isolated from avian and human origin have been reported to exhibit resistance to oseltamivir (de Jong *et al.*, 2005; McKimm-Breschkin *et al.*, 2007; Earhart *et al.*, 2009; Hill *et al.*, 2009; Smith, 2010; Kayali *et al.*, 2011; Govorkova *et al.*, 2013; Leang *et al.*, 2013; Younan *et al.*, 2013). Oral application of oseltamivir via drinking water reduced the morbidity, mortality, virus excretion and chicken-to-chicken transmission in HPAIV H5N2 experimentally infected chickens (Meijer *et al.*, 2004). Oseltamivir was non-toxic for chicken embryos and prevented the replication of an HPAIV H7N1 in inoculated eggs (Kaleta *et al.*, 2007). An effective prophylactic administration of oseltamivir in experimentally infected chickens and ducks with LPAI H9N2 and H6N2 viruses was also reported (Lee *et al.*, 2011). Although it is very plausible that oseltamivir-resistance mutants emerge after application in poultry as recently reported in wild mallards that previously exposed to oseltamivir (Brojer *et al.*, 2013; Gillman *et al.*, 2013), however none of the few studies conducted to evaluate efficacy of oseltamivir in domestic poultry reported emergence of resistant strains. In nature, oseltamivir-resistant H5N1 viruses isolated from domestic and wild birds emerged probably due to spontaneous mutations rather than exposure to oseltamivir (McKimm-Breschkin *et al.*, 2007; Yen *et al.*, 2007; Moscona, 2009; Orozovic *et al.*, 2011). Administration of oseltamivir during an outbreak in commercial flocks is extremely expensive but it could be useful to protect valuable birds (Kaleta *et al.*, 2007; Lee *et al.*, 2011).

3.1.4   Zanamivir

Zanamivir is currently approved in 19 countries for the treatment and prophylaxis of human influenza (Kamps & Hoffman, 2006). Although, development of zanamivir-resistance in poultry is rare (McKimm-Breschkin *et al.*, 2003), it is not effective in preventing a severe outcome and chicken-to-chicken transmission of an HPAIV H5N2 in experimental chickens (Meijer *et al.*, 2004).

Other Chemotherapeutics
Several chemotherapeutics targeting influenza virus proteins have been designed to target potential vulnerabilities in the life cycle of AIV. The HA, NA, NS1 and polymerase proteins are hotspots for these antivirals in the last decade which has been reviewed in more details elsewhere (Roberts, 2001; Hsieh & Hsu, 2007; Boltz *et al.*, 2010; Xie *et al.*, 2011; Du *et al.*, 2012; Feng *et al.*, 2012; Lee & Yen, 2012; Shen *et al.*, 2013) . So far, none of these studies was done *in-vivo* in birds (Table 1).

3.1.5   Inhibitors targeting the HA protein

Hence the hemagglutinin of AIV contains the receptor binding domain, immunogenic epitopes, glycosylated residues (GS) and proteolytic cleavage site (PCS); it plays vital roles in host-restriction, tropism, immunogenicity, antigenicity and pathogenicity of the virus. It is essential to initiate the virus replication cycle in the host cell via: attachment and entrance of the virus to the host cell, fusion with the plasma membrane and release of the viral ribonucleoproteins inside the infected cells (Luo, 2012; Rumschlag-Booms & Rong, 2013). Influenza virus attaches to the SA on the host cells, where avian and equine influenza viruses bind to the SA-α-2,3 galactose linked receptors and human influenza viruses prefer binding to the SA-α-2,6 galactose linked receptors (Suzuki *et al.*, 2000; Gamblin & Skehel, 2010). In this regard, **SA analogues** showed high inhibitory activity for the binding of human influenza viruses to SA *in-vitro* (Sun, 2007). A chemical synthetic SA analog has successfully inhibited the growth of H5 and the recent Chinese H7N9 in cell culture (Waldmann *et al.*, 2014). Moreover, a number of novel synthetic derivatives of **pyrazolopyrimidine nucleoside, pyrazole, pyridazinone, oxadiazole, triazole, thiazolidine** and **thioxopyrimidine** showed a potent efficacy to reduce HPAIV H5N1 replication *in-vitro*. Some of these derivatives are thought to hinder the interaction of the HA with the host cell receptor (Rashad *et al.*, 2010a; Rashad *et al.*, 2010b; Flefel *et al.*, 2012). Based on docking studies and molecular dynamic simulations, **Neo6 compound** was assumed to bind with receptor binding pocket of the HA of H1N1 virus (Li *et al.*, 2011).

Inhibition of the fusogenic function of the HA has been also frequently described. In *in-vitro* studies, a benzodiazepine derivative known as **TBHQ** which is a widely used food preservative possessed antiviral activity against H1N1 (Bliu *et al.*, 2012), H3N2 (Bodian *et al.*, 1993; Hoffman *et al.*, 1997), H14N5 (Russell *et al.*, 2008), H7 subtype (Antanasijevic *et al.*, 2013) but not H5N1 virus (Shen *et al.*, 2013) through prevention of conformational rearrangements required for membrane fusion. Similarly, benzamide derivative known as **FEB** showed antiviral activity against H1 and H3 viruses in MDCK cells (Bliu *et al.*, 2012). **BMY-27709** inhibited the growth of many H1 and H2 viruses but it was inactive against H3 subtype viruses. It is thought that the drug blocked the membrane fusion function of the HA2 protein. Nevertheless, one single mutation by the virus was sufficient to acquire full resistance to **BMY-27709** of hemagglutinin (Luo *et al.*, 1996). Recently, Basu *et al.* (2014) discovered two novel inhibitors,

MBX2329 and **MBX2546**, that specifically inhibit HA-mediated viral entry via probably inhibition of fusion with the plasma membrane. Both compounds were potent against H1N1 as well as HPAIV H5N1 in MDCK cells. Also a new fusion-inhibitor, **CL-385319**, which hindered the HA mediated fusion of viral and endosomal membranes of HPAIV H5N1 in MDCK cells has been reported by Liu *et al.* (2011) and Li *et al.* (2012).

  Cyanovirin-N was recorded to have a potent anti-influenza virus activity. The drug target the oligosaccharides GS on the HA and is active against different H1N1 and H3N2 strains (O'Keefe *et al.*, 2003). In a second study, the early treatment of H1N1-experimentally infected mice and ferrets resulted in up to 100% survival rate and significantly decreased the virus load in the lungs (Smee *et al.*, 2008). Nonetheless, the mergence of natural Cyanovirin-resistant mutants was reported after passage of H1N1 in MDCK or mice in the presence or absence of the drug (Smee *et al.*, 2007).

3.1.6 Inhibitors targeting the NA protein

During the last decade at least two NAIs have been frequently studied: Laninamivir and peramivir. **Laninamivir** is a promising long acting inhaled NAIs where a high concentration of the drug retained for long period particularly in the lungs after single intranasal administration in mice (Kubo *et al.*, 2010). The drug has been approved for the clinical treatment against human influenza in several countries (Ikematsu & Kawai, 2011; Shobugawa *et al.*, 2012; Ison, 2013). As for AIV, Laninamivir was potent and provided prophylactic and therapeutic long-lasting protection against the Asian HPAIV H5N1 in mice including oseltamivir-resistant strains (Kiso *et al.*, 2010a). Until now, no Laninamivir-resistant mutants have been described (Samson *et al.*, 2013). **Peramivir** showed high efficiency to inhibit the replication of different H5N1 and the recent H7N9 viruses in cell culture (Udommaneethanakit *et al.*, 2009; Cao *et al.*, 2013; Nguyen *et al.*, 2013). Although peramivir has long half-life of binding to the NA active site (Beigel & Bray, 2008), however in humans peramivir has low oral bioavailability and the intravenous route was more effective (Sorbello *et al.*, 2012; Ison *et al.*, 2013; Kamali & Holodniy, 2013) excluding it as an option for the large scale application in poultry industry. In addition, some H7N9 of human origin showed a considerable resistance to peramivir without loss in virulence in mice or transmissibility in experimentally infected Guinea pigs (Hai *et al.*, 2013; Hu *et al.*, 2013; Yen *et al.*, 2013).

3.1.7 Inhibitors targeting the polymerase protein

Influenza virus has three polymerase proteins PB2, PB1 and PA which are essential for virus translation, transcription and replication. Favipiravir, ribavirin and viramidine are three polymerase inhibitors licensed for the treatment of human influenza (Boltz *et al.*, 2010) (Table 1).

  Favipiravir (T-705) is a broadly active small molecule that inhibits a wide range of viruses including seasonal influenza as well as amantadine- and oseltamivir-resistant strains *in-vitro* and *in-vivo* (Furuta *et al.*, 2002; Takahashi *et al.*, 2003; Sleeman *et al.*, 2010; Furuta *et al.*, 2013). In MDCK cells, T-705 inhibited many H5N1 and H7N2 viruses (Sidwell *et al.*, 2007; Smee *et al.*, 2009; Sleeman *et al.*, 2010; Smee *et al.*, 2010). In HPAIV H5N1 infected mice, it was effective to prevent death when given 2 hours before infection or even 4 days post infection, after the onset of clinical signs (Sidwell *et al.*, 2007; Kiso *et al.*, 2010b; Smee *et al.*, 2010). Favipiravir has a high safety margin, long intracellular half-life and can be combined with oseltamivir (Beigel & Bray, 2008; Smee *et al.*, 2010).

The second polymerase inhibitor is **ribavirin** which has multiple mechanisms of action (Beigel & Bray, 2008). Intranasal treatment of influenza H5N1 infected mice with ribavirin resulted in 30% (Smee *et al.*, 2008) to 100% (Barnard *et al.*, 2007; Gilbert & McLeay, 2008) survival rate with a significant decrease in lung virus titers. Resistance of influenza viruses to ribavirin, parental application of the drug as well as severe side effects are the most known disadvantages (De Clercq & Neyts, 2007; Samson *et al.*, 2013). Therefore, the drug was used only in a very limited extent in severe infections (Beigel & Bray, 2008).

The last polymerase inhibitor is **Viramidine** which is a prodrug of ribavirin. It is less toxic than ribavirin with similar activity against H1N1, H3N2 and H5N1 viruses *in-vitro* (Sidwell *et al.*, 2005). *In-vivo*, oral administration of viramidine protected mice from death, lung consolidation and decreased virus titers after infection with H1N1 or H3N2 viruses (Sidwell *et al.*, 2005).

3.1.8   Inhibitors targeting the NS1 protein

The NS1 protein is one of the smallest proteins in influenza virus with diverse functions but mainly acts as a shield against the host innate immune response during the early stage of infection via suppression of the interferon production cascade (Hale *et al.*, 2008; Abdelwhab *et al.*, 2013). Many anti-influenza antivirals aims at restoration of the host innate immune response via inhibition of the NS1 protein has been recently reviewed (Engel, 2013). A hydrazide derivative, designated as **HENC**, had inhibitory effect against H1N1 virus in MDCK cells. Also another inhibitory compound, **NSC125044**, was synthetized using chemical methods with antiviral activity through binding with NS1 protein of H1N1 virus (Jablonski *et al.*, 2012).

3.1.9   Inhibitors targeting the host factors

Cleavage of influenza virus HA into HA1 and HA2 proteins is prerequisite for the infectivity of the virus. The PCS of HA with monobasic amino acid motif characteristic for the LPAI viruses is recognized and cleaved by trypsin like enzymes in the respiratory and digestive tract of humans and birds, respectively. Meanwhile, the multibasic cleavage site of the HPAI viruses is cleaved by the abundant furin proteases in almost all types of cell. Therefore, inhibitors targeting host furin or furin-like enzymes are promising candidates for future drug development against influenza. Many protease inhibitors of human influenza viruses have been reviewed in more details in other literatures (Zhirnov *et al.*, 1982; Zhirnov *et al.*, 1984; Kido *et al.*, 2004; Savarino, 2005; Remacle *et al.*, 2008; Federico, 2011; Zhirnov *et al.*, 2011; Meyer *et al.*, 2013). For avian influenza viruses, scarce data are available. In an early study, intraperitoneal injection of **aprotinin** in experimentally infected chickens with different AIV subtypes including HPAIV H5N3 delayed the time of death and reduced the systemic infection but was not totally effective to protect the birds (Zhirnov *et al.*, 1982). Becker and co-workers (2010) found a highly potent furin inhibitor designated **inhibitor 15** which was able to reduce replication of HPAIV H7N1 in *in-vitro*. The same research team has described potent compound designated **inhibitor 24** that inhibited furin and proprotein convertases and delayed the replication of HPAIV H7N1 in cell culture (Becker *et al.*, 2012).

DAS181, an inhaled bacterial sialidase, is now in phase II development for the treatment of influenza (Moss *et al.*, 2012). DAS181 inhibits the virus-host interaction by removing the SA from the surface of epithelial cells in the respiratory tract (Belser *et al.*, 2007; Chan *et al.*,

2009; Triana-Baltzer *et al.*, 2010; Moss *et al.*, 2012; Nicholls *et al.*, 2013). A safety evaluation study indicated no toxicological, pathological or side effects on rats after administration of DAS181 for 28 days. Additionally, there were no cytotoxic effects on different human and animal primary cells (Larson *et al.*, 2011). Several studies have shown the potent efficacy of DAS181 to inhibit the replication of HPAIV H5N1 *in-vitro*, even the oseltamivir-resistant mutant strains (Chan *et al.*, 2009; Zhang, 2009; Nguyen *et al.*, 2013). *In-vivo*, intranasally infected mice with HPAIV H5N1 was fully protected from clinical disease, viral replication, and spread to the brain. In addition, the infection in over 70% of mice was totally blocked when DAS181 was administered as a therapy or prophylaxis (Belser *et al.*, 2007). Also, it showed high efficiency against H1N1 seasonal and pandemic strains in cell culture, mice and ferrets (Malakhov *et al.*, 2006; Chan *et al.*, 2009; Triana-Baltzer *et al.*, 2010). Moreover, the drug was well tolerated by 177 healthy volunteers and it decreased the viral load and shedding of H1N1 and H3N2 viruses after infection of those volunteers (Moss *et al.*, 2012).

3.2   Natural Antivirals

3.2.1   Herbs

Unlimited herbs products contain polyphenols, flavonoids, alkaloids or lignans, mostly from traditional Chinese medicine, offer promise as adjuncts or alternatives to the current anti-influenza chemotherapy (Guralnik *et al.*, 2007; Kitazato *et al.*, 2007) as shown in Table 1. Generally, complementary medicine for treating or preventing influenza or influenza-like illness in human seems to be cultural practice differs from nation to nation (Wang *et al.*, 2006; Guo *et al.*, 2007; Chen *et al.*, 2011b). Innumerable herbs species with potential inhibitory effects on replication of influenza viruses using *in-vitro* cell culture methods and embryonated eggs or *in-vivo* mouse models were frequently described (Nagai *et al.*, 1992; Nakayama *et al.*, 1993; Kernan *et al.*, 1997; Kurokawa *et al.*, 1998; Mantani *et al.*, 1999; Mantani *et al.*, 2001; Imanishi *et al.*, 2002; Jung *et al.*, 2004; Mak *et al.*, 2004; Kubo & Nishimura, 2007; Miki *et al.*, 2007; Quan *et al.*, 2007; Deryabin *et al.*, 2008; Geng *et al.*, 2009; Pleschka *et al.*, 2009; Kwon *et al.*, 2010; Shin *et al.*, 2010; Sundararajan *et al.*, 2010; Zhang *et al.*, 2010; Garozzo *et al.*, 2011; Glatthaar-Saalmuller *et al.*, 2011; Safronetz *et al.*, 2011; Shaukat *et al.*, 2011; Wu *et al.*, 2011; Mehrbod *et al.*, 2012; Sriwilaijaroen *et al.*, 2012; Zu *et al.*, 2012).

In poultry, antiviral and immunoadjuvant effects of several plants and/or its derivatives have been investigated. Sood *et al.* (2012) found that *Eugenia jambolana* extracts had 100% virucidal activity against HPAIV H5N1 in tissue culture and *in-ovo* inoculated chicken embryonated eggs (ECE). *Menthol, eucalyptol* and *ormosinine* probably have inhibitory effect on H5 viruses due to strong interactions ability with the viral HA protein (Gangopadhyay *et al.*, 2011). *NAS* preparation, a Chinese herbal medicine, prevented H9N2 virus-induced clinical signs in treated chickens; however transmission of the virus to untreated chickens was not interrupted (Shang *et al.*, 2010). Likewise, *eucalyptus* and *peppermint* essential oils preparations protected broilers against H9N2 virus infections (Barbour *et al.*, 2006; Barbour *et al.*, 2011). Moreover, application of lyophilized *green tea* by-product extracts namely catechins in feed or drinking water reduced H9N2 virus replication and excretion in experimentally infected chickens in a dose-dependent manner (Lee *et al.*, 2012b). In addition, green tea extract was comparable to amantadine in protection of chicken embryos against H7N3 subtype (Shaukat *et al.*, 2011). *Catechins* alter the infectivity of influenza viruses probably not only by direct interaction with viral HA but also by inhibition of viral RNA synthesis in cell culture (Song *et al.*,

2005). Furthermore, Liu *et al.* (2009) found that *statin/caffeine* combination was as effective as oseltamivir in reduction HPAIV H5N1-induced lung damage and viral replication in mice. Conversely, Kumaki and colleagues (Kumaki *et al.*, 2012) showed that statin had little antiviral activity against H5N1, H3N2 and H1N1 viruses in mouse-model. *Stachyflin* showed antiviral activity against H1N1, H5N1, H5N2, and H6 viruses in cell cultures as well as in experimentally infected mice (Motohashi *et al.*, 2013). A leave-extract of the wild black currant (*Ribes nigrum folium*) interfered with virus internalization of H1N1 and H7N7 viruses in cell cultures and impaired their replication in mice without evidence for generation of resistant variants (Ehrhardt *et al.*, 2013a). Also, reduced titer of H5N1 viruses in cell culture or ECE was recently described using extracts of *Capparis sinaica Veill* (Ibrahim *et al.*, 2013a), *Aloe hijazensis* (Abd-Alla *et al.*, 2012) and Red Sea grass *Thallasodendron ciliatum* (Ibrahim *et al.*, 2013b). Extracts from *Phellinus igniarius* inhibited replication of H1N1, H3N2 and H9N2 viruses in cell culture probably by preventing virus attachment to the host cells (Lee *et al.*, 2013a). Likewise, roots of *Isatis indigotica* inhibited different subtypes of influenza viruses including H6N2, H7N3 and H9N2 viruses in MDCK cells (Yang *et al.*, 2012). Similar mode of action has been described for a derivative from andrographolide, a bioactive component of the medicinal plant *Andrographis paniculata*, which showed significant inhibitory activity against H9N2 and H5N1 in MDCK cells and in mice by blocking the virus binding to SA receptors (Chen *et al.*, 2009). Moreover, some alkaloids isolated from the bulbs of *Lycoris radiata* had anti-influenza activities against HPAIV H5N1 through inhibition of the nuclear-to-cytoplasmic export of the ribonucleoprotein (RNP) complex in MDCK cells (Duvauchelle *et al.*, 2013). On the contrary, neolignans from leaves of *Miliusa mollis* Pierre (Annonaceae) had no effect on the HPAIV H5N1 in *in-vitro* (Sawasdee *et al.*, 2013). Chickens injected with different doses of Astragalus polysaccharide (APS) at 7 days post hatch for five successive days were protected against H9N2 infection and showed enhanced humoral immune response after vaccination with the same virus (Kallon *et al.*, 2013).

The immunoadjuvant effect of some herbal extracts as feed additives on the humoral immune response induced by inactivated AIV vaccination in poultry has been studied. Oral administration of *ginseng* stem-and-leaf saponins in drinking water or *Hypericum perforatum* L. as a dietary supplement significantly enhanced serum antibody response to inactivated H5N1 or H9N2 vaccines in chickens (Zhai *et al.*, 2011; Jiang *et al.*, 2012; Landy *et al.*, 2012). The *Cochinchina momordica* seed extract, Chinese medicine plant, when combined with an inactivated H5N1 vaccine as adjuvant increased significantly the immune response and daily weight gain of two weeks old chickens (Rajput *et al.*, 2007). On the contrary, herbal extracts of *Radix astragali*, *Radix codonopis*, *Herba epimedii* and *Radix glycyrrizae* in drinking water did not improve chicken immune response to H5-AIV vaccination (Liu *et al.*, 2010), likewise diet supplementation with fresh garlic powder had no effect on the humoral immune response of chickens vaccinated with an inactivated H9N2 vaccine (Jafari *et al.*, 2009).

As reviewed above, many herbs and/or their extracts had direct inhibitory effects on the replication of different AIV subtypes both *in-vitro* and *in-vivo*. In addition to its antiviral activity, these extracts often have immunoadjuvant effect, anti-bacterial, anti-fungal, anti-inflammatory, anti-oxidant and/or analgesic properties which may provide alternative natural broad-spectrum therapy for control of AIV in poultry farms (Garozzo *et al.*, 2009; Hudson, 2009; Krawitz *et al.*, 2011; Sood *et al.*, 2012). To date, no adverse effects on body weight or egg production have been described. Yet, some derivatives (*i.e.*, ginseng saponins) require four to six years to harvest and is very expensive on the market (Zhai *et al.*, 2011). Methods of the extraction and preparation of the crude extracts and its purity greatly influence the inhibition activity of some herbs against AIV (Song *et al.*, 2005; Lee *et al.*, 2012b). Moreover, batch-to-batch variations due to variable growth conditions at the plantations have been considered a limiting factor for treatment of influenza (Garozzo *et al.*, 2009). Evident that mutation in the H5 gene probably affects inhibitor binding of some herbs was reported (Gangopadhyay *et al.*, 2011). In addition, *in-vitro* experiments and animal models to confirm the direct antiviral activities against influenza virus are limited (Kurokawa *et al.*, 2010). Moreover, comprehensive investigations of herb-drug interactions, potential toxicity, heterogeneity of herbs species, plant parts (*i.e.*, aerial *versus* root) and biochemical data identifying the active components are inadequately described (Fusco *et al.*, 2010). To the best of our knowledge, neither field application nor commercial herbal products have been recorded specifically against avian influenza in poultry although some commercial products for human are available (Tao *et al.*, 2013).

3.2.2   Probiotics

A number of studies have reported the efficacy of probiotic lactic acid bacteria such as *Streptococcus thermophiles*, several Lactobacillus and Bifidobacterium species to enhance the immune response and to protect mice against different influenza strains/subtypes (Hori *et al.*, 2001; Yasui *et al.*, 2004; Olivares *et al.*, 2007; Boge *et al.*, 2009; Harata *et al.*, 2010; Davidson *et al.*, 2011; Iwabuchi *et al.*, 2011; Takeda *et al.*, 2011; Kawase *et al.*, 2012; Rizzardini *et al.*, 2012; Goto *et al.*, 2013; Kiso *et al.*, 2013; Lee *et al.*, 2013b; Park *et al.*, 2013; Waki *et al.*, 2014). Although probiotics are widely used in poultry to improve innate and adaptive immunity (Patterson & Burkholder, 2003; Nava *et al.*, 2005; Lutful Kabir, 2009), there is a paucity of information on its ability to ameliorate AIV infections. *Lactobacillus plantarum* KFCC11389P was as effective as oseltamivir to neutralize the H9N2 virus in ECE and slightly reduced amount of tracheal virus excretion in oral-fed experimentally infected chickens (Chon *et al.*, 2008). Out of 220 screened bacterial strains, Seo *et al.* (2012) found that *Leuconostoc mesenteroides* YML003 had highly anti-H9N2 activity in cell culture and ECE. Decrease cloacal excretion of the virus and a significant increase in the cytokine IFN-gamma in experimentally infected chickens were observed. In another study, administration of *Lactobacillus fermentum* via nasal route significantly decreased the viral excretion and chicken-to-chicken transmission of H9N2 virus (Youn *et al.*, 2012). Likewise, oral administration of *Lactobacillus acidophilus* increased immune response to H9N2 vaccination, decreased fecal virus excretion and protected broiler chickens against intranasal challenge with a high dose of H9N2 virus (Poorbaghi *et al.*, 2013). Ghafoor and co-workers (Ghafoor *et al.*, 2005) showed that multi-strains commercial probiotic protexin® (various Lactobacillus spp., *Enterococcus faecium*, *Bifidobacterium bifidum*, *Candida pintolepesii* and *Aspergillus oryzae*) improved immune response of broiler chickens to H9N2 vaccination and prevented the mortality and morbidity. On the other hand, dual use of Lactobacillus spp. or *Lactococcus lactis* as a vector for vaccine production and immunomodulation bacteria has been successfully constructed and protected mice against HPAIV H5N1 (Lei *et al.*, 2010; Wang *et al.*, 2012b), such experiments should be evaluated in poultry.

Together, direct and indirect antiviral and the immune-stimulation effect in addition to dual use as a vaccine-vector and immunomodulator of the probiotics are promising in the control of AIV in poultry; however their efficacy against HPAIV is still questionable.

4   Molecular Approaches for Control of AIV

4.1   Avian Cytokines

Chicken cytokines such as chicken interferon-alpha (ChIFN-α), chicken interleukins (ChIL) and Toll-like receptors (TLR) are essential components of chicken's innate immune system which play a vital role against virus infections (Lukacsi *et al.*, 1985; Sekellick *et al.*, 1994; Suarez & Schultz-Cherry, 2000; Novak *et al.*, 2001). An innovative application of ChIFN-α to antagonize AIV infection in poultry through direct oral feeding or drinking water has received more attention than other components (Wei *et al.*, 2006; Marcus *et al.*, 2007; Song *et al.*, 2008; Reemers *et al.*, 2009; Meng *et al.*, 2011). Sekellick *et al.* (2000) showed that up to 60% of investigated AIV population belonged to the HPAI H5N9 subtype were highly sensitive to the inhibitory effects of ChIFN-α. Interestingly, both IFN-sensitive and -resistant clones were obtained after passage of the resistant clones in the presence of IFN which indicated that resistance to ChIFN-α was transient and did not result from stable genetic changes. Xia *et al.* (2004) cloned the ChIFN-α gene from three different chicken lines and studied their efficacy against H9N2 viruses *in-ovo* and *in-vivo*. Up to 70% of *in-ovo* treated chicken embryos were protected against H9N2 virus infection in dose dependent manner. Moreover, chickens received ChIFN-α by oculonasal inoculation at one day of age were protected from death upon H9N2 virus infection given 24 hours later. Findings of Meng and co-workers (2011) showed that oral administration of exogenous ChIFN-α was effective to prevent and treat chickens experimentally infected with an H9N2 virus. It potentially reduced the viral load in trachea and resulted in rapid recovery of the body weight gain. In another study, White Leghorn (WL) chickens received ChIFN-α in drinking water for 14 successive days augmented detectable humoral anti-influenza antibodies after exposure to a low dose of an LPAIV H7N2 infection (Marcus *et al.*, 2007). Thus, it has been suggested that regular water administration of ChIFN-α can create "super-sentinel" chickens to detect early infections with few amount of LPAIV (Marcus *et al.*, 2007). Interestingly, ChIFN-α had antiviral activity against H1N1 and H5N9 viruses not only in chicken but also in duck and turkey primary cell cultures indicating a promising use in other avian species (Jiang *et al.*, 2011). It has been recently found that ChIFN-α is more potent than the ChIFN-β to inactivate H9N2 virus in chicken fibroblast cell line (DF1) (Qu *et al.*, 2013).Recently, chIFN-λ demonstrated a remarkable inhibitory activity against HPAI H5N1, HPAI H7N7 and H9N2 viruses in ovo as well as in three to four-week-old chickens (Reuter *et al.*, 2013). Intramuscular immunization of four-week-old specific-pathogen-free chickens with the melanoma differentiation-associated gene 5 product (chMDA5) increased resistance of chickens to HPAIV H5N1 infection and reduced virus excretion (Liniger *et al.*, 2012a).

Furthermore, oral administration of live attenuated *Salmonella enterica* serovar Typhimurium expressing ChIFN-α alone or in combination with ChIL-18 significantly reduced clinical signs induced by H9N2 virus and decreased the amount of virus load in cloacal swabs and internal organs (Rahman *et al.*, 2011; Rahman *et al.*, 2012). Likewise, chicken immunized with a recombinant fowl pox virus (rFPV) vaccine expressing both the HA gene of H9N2 virus and ChIL-18 survived challenge with an H9N2 virus and did not excrete any virus in swab samples and/or internal organs in comparison to non-vaccinated birds (Chen *et al.*, 2011a). Also, rFPV expressing the H5, H7 and ChIL-18 genes produced significantly higher humoral and cellular mediated immune response and protected specific pathogen free chickens (SPF) and WL chickens against challenge with an HPAIV H5N1. Vaccinated birds had no virus shedding and showed significant increase in body weight gain (Mingxiao *et al.*, 2006). So far, efficiency of avian-cytokines to limit AIV infection has not been adequately studied in other avian species. The duck IL-18 and IL-2 genes had been identified and shown to have 85% and 55% nucleotide identity to the chicken equivalents, respectively. Intramuscular inoculations of the duck IL-18 or IL-2 enhanced the humoral immune response of ducks vaccinated with H5N1 or H9N2 inactivated vaccines, respectively (Zhou *et al.*, 2005b; Chen *et al.*, 2008a). Likewise, the recombinant goose IL-2 strengthens goose humoral immune responses after vaccination using H9N2 inactivated vaccine (Zhou *et al.*, 2005a). The TLR-3, TLR-7 and TLR9 are other promising chicken cytokines derivatives that showed broad-spectrum anti-influenza virus activity *in-vitro* and *in-ovo* (Jenkins *et al.*, 2009; Wong *et al.*, 2009a; Wong *et al.*, 2009b; Stewart *et al.*, 2012). Recently, goose TLR7 was found to be identical to their mammalian counterpart and was triggered by H5N1 virus at the early stage of infection of geese (Wei *et al.*, 2013b).

The previous literatures have shown that avian cytokines are not affected by antigenic changes and they have broad spectrum antiviral activities. Nevertheless, the cost of mass production of chicken cytokines is still too high to be applied in large-scale in poultry industry (Song *et al.*, 2008). Moreover, protein stability, host-specificity and labor associated with mass administration of chicken cytokines under field conditions require significant improvement (Rahman *et al.*, 2011).

4.2   RNA Interference (RNAi)

RNAi is a natural phenomenon used by many organisms as a defense mechanism against foreign microbial invasion, including viruses, that able to wreak potential genetic havoc of the susceptible host (Stram & Kuzntzova, 2006). Short-interfering RNA (siRNA) is approximately 21–25 nucleotides specific for highly conserved regions of AIV genomes. It effectively mediates the catalytic degradation of complementary viral mRNAs and results in inhibition of a broad spectrum of influenza viruses replication in cell lines, chicken embryos and mice just before or after initiation of an infection (Ge *et al.*, 2003; Ge *et al.*, 2004b; Hui *et al.*, 2004; Zhou *et al.*, 2008; Sui *et al.*, 2009; Betakova & Svancarova, 2013). Tompkins and colleagues (2004) found that siRNA specific for the NP or PA genes induced full protection of mice against lethal challenge with the HPAI H5N1 and H7N7 subtypes and markedly decreased virus titers in lungs. Likewise, prophylactic use of PA-specific siRNA molecule significantly reduced lung H5N1 virus titers and lethality in infected mice (Zhang *et al.*, 2009). Moreover, siRNA targeting M2 or NP genes inhibited replication of H5N1 and H9N2 viruses in canine cell line and partially protected mice against HPAV H5N1 (Zhou *et al.*, 2007). Recently, Jiao and colleagues designed and tested four siRNAs which were to able to inhibit the expression and accumulation of the NS1 protein of an HPAIV H5N1 in human embryonic kidney cell line (Jiao *et al.*, 2013).

In poultry, Li and others (2005) showed that the siRNA targeting NP and/or PA genes inhibited protein expression, RNA transcription and multiplication of HPAIV H5N1 in chicken embryo fibroblasts and ECE as well as prevented apoptosis of infected cells. Likewise, chicken cell line transfected with RNAi molecules specific for the NP or PA of AIV showed decrease the levels of NP mRNA and infective titer of an H10N8 quail virus (Abrahamyan *et al.*, 2009). Also, NP-specific siRNA reduced H5N1 virus replication in cell culture and ECE (Zhou *et al.*, 2008). Moreover, siRNA molecules targeting the NP, PA and PB1 genes interfered with replication of H1N1 virus in ECE (Ge *et al.*, 2003).

One of the most advantages of siRNA application in poultry, in contrast to AIV vaccines, that it might not require an intact immune system (Bennink & Palmore, 2004) which is very important particularly in developing countries where a number of immunosuppressive agents are endemic in poultry. In addition, siRNA molecules targeting the highly conserved regions in influenza genome potentially remain effective regardless of the inter- and intra-subtype genetic and antigenic variations of AIV (Bennink & Palmore, 2004; Suzuki *et al.*, 2009). Moreover, it has also the potential to reduce the emergence of viable resistant variants (Chen *et al.*, 2008b), in this regard combinations of siRNA molecules "cocktail" targeting several genes/regions may be used simultaneously (Ge *et al.*, 2004a; McSwiggen & Seth, 2008). Furthermore, there is no risk of recombination between siRNA nucleotides and circulating influenza viruses, hence siRNA is complementary to the influenza virus genome (Chen *et al.*, 2008b). Moreover, the siRNA dose required for inhibition of AIV is very low (sub-nanomoles) (Ge *et al.*, 2004a). Nevertheless, arise of mutants with the ability to evade the inhibition effect of siRNA are not fully excluded (Bennink & Palmore, 2004). Unfortunately, there is no stretch of conserved nucleotides in the NA and HA genes sufficient to generate specific siRNA due to extensive variations in these genes among AIV from different species (Ge *et al.*, 2004a). The siRNA molecules are quickly degraded *in-vivo* affording a transient short-term protection and multiple-dose is required (Abrahamyan *et al.*, 2009). None of the siRNAs must share any sequence identity with the host genome to avoid non-specific RNAi-induced gene silencing of the host cells (Elbashir *et al.*, 2001; Ge *et al.*, 2004a; Wadhwa *et al.*, 2004; Aigner, 2006). Delivery vehicle of siRNA to the site of infection is a major constraint (Thomas *et al.*, 2005; Morris & Rossi, 2006) remained to be investigated on flock-level in poultry. There is accumulating evidence that siRNA is efficient to inhibit influenza virus replication *in-vitro*, however *in-vivo* studies still missing. Research studies focus on mass application of siRNA in poultry as a spray or via drinking water are highly recommended (O'Neill, 2007).

5   Host Genetic Selection

The host genetics play a pivotal role in susceptibility to influenza including the HPAIV H5N1 which is frequently studied in mice models as reviewed by Horby *et al.* (2012). Indeed, the impact of host genetic selection on resistance to AIV infections in poultry has not yet been fully determined. The on-going H5N1 virus epidemics have raised concerns in respect to influenza-resistant chickens either by selective breeding or genetic modification.

5.1   Natural Resistance

It has been supposed that fast-growing domestic birds have reduced immune competence against several viral diseases and resistant breeds are mostly poor producers (Zekarias *et al.*, 2002). Natural resistance or less susceptibility of some species/breeds of birds to AIV is not uncommon. In an experiment, five chicken lines were infected with an HPAIV H7N1. Three lines showed high susceptibility to the virus while two lines showed some resistance and survived the infection (Sironi *et al.*, 2008). Swayne *et al.* (1994) observed that an LPAIV H4N8 produced more severe lesions in commercial and SPF WL chickens than in 5 week-old commercial broiler chickens suggesting that SPF WL chickens are more susceptible than broilers to this strain. Thomas *et al.* (2008) suggested that WL chickens may be more susceptible to an H3N2 virus of swine origin than White Plymouth Rock broiler-type chickens. On the contrary, severe lesions in commercial broiler chickens compared to SPF was observed after experimental infection with a Jordanian H9N2 isolate (Gharaibeh, 2008). Some wild duck species, particularly mallards, are more resistance to HPAIV H5N1 than others (Keawcharoen *et al.*, 2008). Conversely, dabbling ducks and white fronted goose were more frequently infected with AIV than other wild ducks and geese, respectively (Munster *et al.*, 2007). Wood ducks were the only species to exhibit illness or death between different species of experimentally infected wild ducks in a study conducted by Brown and others (2006).

5.1.1   Myxovirus (Mx) Resistance Gene

Myxovirus resistance gene is an interferon-stimulated gene encodes Mx1 protein that able to interfere with AIV replication by inhibiting viral polymerases in the nucleus and by binding viral components in the cytoplasm. The role of the Mx gene in resistance against influenza viruses including the HPAIV H5N1 in mammals is well defined (Ruff, 1983; Staeheli *et al.*, 1986; Chang *et al.*, 1990; Meier *et al.*, 1990; Pavlovic *et al.*, 1990; Salomon *et al.*, 2007; Haller *et al.*, 2009; Song *et al.*, 2013). However, the contribution of avian Mx proteins as antiviral elements in AIV infection in birds is contradictory and worth further exploration. Although intra- and interbreed/-species Mx variations have been frequently reported (Ko *et al.*, 2002; Li *et al.*, 2006; Li *et al.*, 2007; Watanabe, 2007; Berlin *et al.*, 2008; Sironi *et al.*, 2008; Dillon & Runstadler, 2010; Yin *et al.*, 2010; Sartika *et al.*, 2011), however commercial chicken lines have lower frequencies of the resistant allele compared to the indigenous chicken breeds (Ko *et al.*, 2002; Li *et al.*, 2006; Seyama *et al.*, 2006) probably due to intensive modern breeding techniques (Balkissoon *et al.*, 2007). Duck Mx was the first avian Mx protein to be characterized but no antiviral activity against an HPAIV H7N7 when transfected in chicken and mouse cells was obtained (Bazzigher *et al.*, 1993). On the contrary, chickens have a single Mx1 gene (Schumacher *et al.*, 1994) with multiple alleles (Li *et al.*, 2006) encoding a deduced protein with 705 amino acids in length. Notably, results of anti-influenza activity of the Mx1 protein in chickens are contradictory likely due to using variable experimental setups and different AIV strains. Also, a similar disparity has been noted between *in-vitro* and *in-vivo* experiments (Sironi *et al.*, 2008; Ewald *et al.*, 2011).

Phenotypic variation in the antiviral activity of Mx gene has been linked to a single amino acid substitution of asparagine (Asn) at position 631 in resistant breeds or serine (Ser) in sensitive ones (Ko *et al.*, 2002) probably due to inhibition of the PB2-NP interaction decreasing the viral polymerase activity (Verhelst *et al.*, 2012). The 631Asn identified mostly in Japanese native chicken breeds screened by Ko *et al.* (2002) was associated with enhanced antiviral activity to H5N1 virus in transfected mouse fibroblast 3T3 cells. Conversely, results obtained by Benfield *et al.* (2008); Benfield *et al.* (2010) and Schusser *et al.* (2011) indicated that neither the 631Asn nor the 631Ser genotypes of chicken Mx1 was able to confer protection against several LPAIV and HPAIV including H5N1 subtype in chicken embryo fibroblasts or ECE. Similarly, Mx1 631Asn had no effect on viral replication after *in-vitro* infection of chicken embryo kidney cells with an LPAIV H5N9 (Ewald *et al.*, 2011). Moreover, transfected chicken cells expressing chicken Mx protein did not induce resistance to HPAIV H7N7 (Bernasconi *et al.*, 1995). *In-vivo*, following intranasal infection with an HPAIV H5N2, chickens carry Asn631 allele showed delayed mortality, milder morbidity and lesser virus excretion than 631Ser homozygotes (Ewald *et al.*, 2011). Conversely, no correlation was observed between Mx-631 genotypes and susceptibility of chickens either to an HPAIV H7N1 (Sironi *et al.*, 2008) or after infection with H5N3 (Wang *et al.*, 2012a) as indicated by clinical status and time course of infection. Although, one out of six chicken lines infected with an HPAIV H7N1 had lower mortality, the Mx gene was not involved in this variations among tested chicken lines (Sironi *et al.*, 2011). Additionally, chickens carry the homozygous Mx resistant allele genotype augmented the lowest HI titer after vaccination with an inactivated H5N2 vaccine compared with chickens that carry the sensitive allele (Qu *et al.*, 2009).

Taken together, although few breeds of chickens and ducks can survive challenge with HPAIV in nature, resistance or susceptibility to a disease is usually multifactorial in nature and greatly influenced by both the host and the virus. To elucidate the role of Mx1 gene in the resistance of poultry to AIV more in-depth investigation (Dillon & Runstadler, 2010; Schusser *et al.*, 2011) and *in-vivo* comparative studies using several native breeds from different countries are highly required (Ewald *et al.*, 2011). Also, interrelation of disease-resistance and production should be weighed.

5.1.2   Other Candidate Genes

Apart from the Mx1 gene, resistance or less susceptibility of ducks to AIV infections compared with chickens has been linked to an influenza virus sensor known as retinoic acid-inducible gene I "RIG-I" (a cytoplasmic RNA sensor contribute to AIV detection and IFN production) which is absent in chickens (Barber *et al.*, 2010; Karpala *et al.*, 2011; Liniger *et al.*, 2012b). This RIG-I gene as a natural AIV resistance gene in ducks could be a promising candidate for creation of transgenic chickens (Barber *et al.*, 2010). Likewise, different genes and cytokines have been expressed after infection of chicken and duck cells with several AIV subtypes including HPAIV H5N1 (Sarmento *et al.*, 2008; Adams *et al.*, 2009; Liang *et al.*, 2011; Kuchipudi *et al.*, 2012). Development of new drugs which modulate the expression of those cytokines may be a new target to control AIV replication (Ehrhardt *et al.*, 2013b). Additional genetic candidates that contribute to inhibition of AIV replication such as cyclophilin A (Xu *et al.*, 2010), ISG15 (Hsiang *et al.*, 2009), viperin (Wang *et al.*, 2007), heat shock cognate protein 70 (Hsc70) (Watanabe *et al.*, 2006) or Ebp1 and/or ErbB3-binding protein (Honda *et al.*, 2007) could be useful in creation of genetically modified chickens. It is worth mentioning that genome manipulation technologies have been actively developed and researched in the last decade to design hosts-on-demand. A number of techniques including transcription activator-like effector nucleases (TALENs) and the clustered regularly interspaced palindromic repeats (CRISPR) can modulate desired target genes in poultry in the near future to control AIV infections. For more information the readers are referred to other reviews (Belhaj *et al.*, 2013; Gratz *et al.*, 2013; Pan *et al.*, 2013; Wei *et al.*, 2013a; Daimon *et al.*, 2014; Lisa Li *et al.*, 2014).

5.2   Transgenic Chickens

Current advance in molecular biology and genetic manipulation can facilitate the development of influenza-resistant poultry. Increase resistance of cell lines to influenza virus infection using RNA interfering (RNAi) molecules expressed by a lentiviral vector is more efficient transgenic tool than direct DNA injection or oncoretroviral vectors infection (Harvey *et al.*, 2002; Scott & Lois, 2005; Chen *et al.*, 2008b). Recently, creation of AIV built-in resistant chickens by genetic modification has been experimentally proven by Lyall and colleagues (2011). Chickens equipped with a short-hairpin RNA targets the AIV polymerase binding sites have been created and infected with HPAIV H5N1. Although all infected transgenic birds succumbed to the infection however the virus did not spread to the in-contact transgenic and non-transgenic cagemates (Lyall *et al.*, 2011).

The most important challenges facing the development of genetically modified chickens are the applicability in food production, safety regulations and consumer's preferences (Enserink, 2011; Lyall *et al.*, 2011). Moreover, AIV is a "master of mutability" and global production of the resistant chickens must be equipped with many decoys target different genes to avoid rapid generation of AIV resistance. In addition, replacement of the commercial flocks with the newly flu-resistant birds is expected to occur within short period due to globalization of the poultry industry however replacement of backyard birds seems to be more complicated (Enserink, 2011).

6   Summary and Perspectives

Epidemics of avian influenza in poultry are a real challenge for the scientific community (Capua & Alexander, 2006). Recently, several approaches to control the disease were developed and have yielded promising results. Although beneficial, these approaches face different limitations and restrictions (Table 2). The use of antiviral drugs in poultry could be an ancillary tool to control AIV infections in valuable birds but not in commercial sectors. Fears of kicking out our leading antiviral drugs in control of AIV are increased by adoption of amantadine (and probably oseltamivir) in poultry and transmission of resistant variants to human. On the other hand, limited supply and high costs of oseltamivir preclude its widespread use for poultry. Compliance with other medications, adverse effects and drug residues in eggs, meat and surrounding environment should be investigated. On the other hand, effectiveness of herbal and cytokines-based medications to protect against HPAIV H5N1 should be seriously considered and further investigation *in-vivo* is inevitable.

Molecular approaches including RNAi and transgenic chickens for control of AIV are encouraging. The use of short interfering RNA prevents the replication of AIV seems to be a promising approach; however specificity to the viral genome without interference with the host genome and non-specifically inhibition of cellular gene activity is critical. Delivery to the host, production costs, mass production and application, storage and handling of the final products are important aspects that remain unresolved. Possibility for arise of mutants with the ability to evade the siRNA activity should also be considered. Genetic resistance to AIV determined by only one point mutation in the Mx gene or complex and multigenic host components as recently determined in mice (Boon *et al.*, 2009) should be firstly confirmed and secondly elucidation of its relation to the productivity of birds and other diseases must be considered.

Although a proof-of-principle to produce transgenic chickens has been recently reported, technical, logistic and social constraints are facing development of chicken resistant to AIV. Stable transmission and expression of the transgene from generation to generation require extensive studies. Regulatory approval, mass production, costs and marketing of commercial AIV resistant pedigree lines, consumer preferences and food safety issues need to be carefully and fully addressed. Overall, mutation of the virus in the face of any control approach remains the real challenge. Influenza epidemics and pandemics will likely continue to cause havoc in poultry and human populations, therefore innovative alternative or complementary intervention strategies need to be developed. The ultimate goal of all control (including alternate) strategies must be the eradication of avian influenza. In this context, alternate approaches might be an aid but should not jeopardize surveillance and current control measures.

Authors

El-Sayed M. Abdelwhab

Institute of Poultry Diseases, Faculty of Veterinary Medicine, Free Berlin University, Berlin, Germany

Institute of Molecular Virology and Cell Biology, Federal Research Institute for Animal Health, Friedrich-Loeffler-Institut, Insel Riems, Greifswald, Germany

Hafez M. Hafez

Institute of Poultry Diseases, Faculty of Veterinary Medicine, Free Berlin University, Berlin, Germany

References

Abd-Alla, H. I., Abu-Gabal, N. S., Hassan, A. Z., El-Safty, M. M., & Shalaby, N. M. (2012). Antiviral activity of Aloe hijazensis against some haemagglutinating viruses infection and its phytoconstituents. Archives of pharmacal research, 35(8), 1347-1354.

Abdelwhab, E. M., Grund, C., Aly, M. M., Beer, M., Harder, T. C., & Hafez, H. M. (2011). Multiple dose vaccination with heterologous H5N2 vaccine: immune response and protection against variant clade 2.2.1 highly pathogenic avian influenza H5N1 in broiler breeder chickens. Vaccine, 29(37), 6219-6225.

Abdelwhab, E. M., Grund, C., Aly, M. M., Beer, M., Harder, T. C., & Hafez, H. M. (2012). Influence of maternal immunity on vaccine efficacy and susceptibility of one day old chicks against Egyptian highly pathogenic avian influenza H5N1. Veterinary Microbiology, 155(1), 13-20.

Abdelwhab, E. M., Veits, J., & Mettenleiter, T. C. (2013). Avian influenza virus NS1: A small protein with diverse and versatile functions. Virulence, 4(7), 583-588.

Abdelwhab, E. M., Veits, J., & Mettenleiter, T. C. (2014). Prevalence and control of H7 avian influenza viruses in birds and humans. Epidemiology and Infection, 1-25.

Abrahamyan, A., Nagy, E., & Golovan, S. P. (2009). Human H1 promoter expressed short hairpin RNAs (shRNAs) suppress avian influenza virus replication in chicken CH-SAH and canine MDCK cells. Antiviral Research, 84(2), 159-167.

Adams, S. C., Xing, Z., Li, J., & Cardona, C. J. (2009). Immune-related gene expression in response to H11N9 low pathogenic avian influenza virus infection in chicken and Pekin duck peripheral blood mononuclear cells. Molecular Immunology, 46(8-9), 1744-1749.

Aigner, A. (2006). Gene silencing through RNA interference (RNAi) in vivo: strategies based on the direct application of siRNAs. J Biotechnol, 124(1), 12-25.

Allen, U. D., Aoki, F. Y., & Stiver, H. G. (2006). The use of antiviral drugs for influenza: recommended guidelines for practitioners. Can J Infect Dis Med Microbiol, 17(5), 273-284.

Antanasijevic, A., Cheng, H., Wardrop, D. J., Rong, L., & Caffrey, M. (2013). Inhibition of influenza H7 hemagglutinin-mediated entry. PLoS One, 8(10), e76363.

Balkissoon, D., Staines, K., McCauley, J., Wood, J., Young, J., Kaufman, J., & Butter, C. (2007). Low frequency of the Mx allele for viral resistance predates recent intensive selection in domestic chickens. Immunogenetics, 59(8), 687-691.

Barber, M. R., Aldridge, J. R., Jr., Webster, R. G., & Magor, K. E. (2010). Association of RIG-I with innate immunity of ducks to influenza. Proceedings of the National Academy of Sciences of the United States of America, 107(13), 5913-5918.

Barbour, E. K., El-Hakim, R. G., Kaadi, M. S., Shaib, H. A., Gerges, D. D., & Nehme, P. A. (2006). Evaluation of the histopathology of the respiratory system in essential oil-treated broilers following a challenge with Mycoplasma gallisepticum and/or H9N2 influenza virus. International Journal of Applied Research in Veterinary Medicine, 4(4), 293-300.

Barbour, E. K., Saadé, M. F., Abdel Nour, A. M., Kayali, G., Kidess, S., Bou Ghannam, R., Harakeh, S., & Shaib, H. (2011). Evaluation of essential oils in the treatment of broilers co-infected with multiple respiratory etiologic agents. International Journal of Applied Research in Veterinary Medicine, 9(4), 317-323.

Barnard, D. L., Wong, M. H., Bailey, K., Day, C. W., Sidwell, R. W., Hickok, S. S., & Hall, T. J. (2007). Effect of oral gavage treatment with ZnAL42 and other metallo-ion formulations on influenza A H5N1 and H1N1 virus infections in mice. Antiviral chemistry & chemotherapy, 18(3), 125-132.

Basu, A., Antanasijevic, A., Wang, M., Li, B., Mills, D. M., Ames, J. A., Nash, P. J., Williams, J. D., Peet, N. P., Moir, D. T., Prichard, M. N., Keith, K. A., Barnard, D. L., Caffrey, M., Rong, L., & Bowlin, T. L. (2014). New small molecule entry inhibitors targeting hemagglutinin-mediated influenza a virus fusion. Journal of Virology, 88(3), 1447-1460.

Bazzigher, L., Schwarz, A., & Staeheli, P. (1993). No enhanced influenza virus resistance of murine and avian cells expressing cloned duck Mx protein. Virology, 195(1), 100-112.

Bean, W. J., Threlkeld, S. C., & Webster, R. G. (1989). Biologic potential of amantadine-resistant influenza A virus in an avian model. The Journal of infectious diseases, 159(6), 1050-1056.

Bean, W. J., & Webster, R. G. (1988). Biological properties of amantadine-resistant influenza-virus mutants. Antiviral Research, 9(1-2), 128-128.

Beard, C. W., Brugh, M., & Webster, R. G. (1987). Emergence of amantadine-resistant H5N2 avian influenza virus during a simulated layer flock treatment program. Avian Diseases, 31(3), 533-537.

Becker, G. L., Lu, Y., Hardes, K., Strehlow, B., Levesque, C., Lindberg, I., Sandvig, K., Bakowsky, U., Day, R., Garten, W., & Steinmetzer, T. (2012). Highly potent inhibitors of proprotein convertase furin as potential drugs for treatment of infectious diseases. The Journal of biological chemistry, 287(26), 21992-22003.

Becker, G. L., Sielaff, F., Than, M. E., Lindberg, I., Routhier, S., Day, R., Lu, Y., Garten, W., & Steinmetzer, T. (2010). Potent inhibitors of furin and furin-like proprotein convertases containing decarboxylated P1 arginine mimetics. Journal of medicinal chemistry, 53(3), 1067-1075.

Beigel, J., & Bray, M. (2008). Current and future antiviral therapy of severe seasonal and avian influenza. Antiviral Research, 78(1), 91-102.

Belhaj, K., Chaparro-Garcia, A., Kamoun, S., & Nekrasov, V. (2013). Plant genome editing made easy: targeted mutagenesis in model and crop plants using the CRISPR/Cas system. Plant Methods, 9(1), 39.

Belser, J. A., Lu, X., Szretter, K. J., Jin, X., Aschenbrenner, L. M., Lee, A., Hawley, S., Kim do, H., Malakhov, M. P., Yu, M., Fang, F., & Katz, J. M. (2007). DAS181, a novel sialidase fusion protein, protects mice from lethal avian influenza H5N1 virus infection. Journal of Infectious Diseases, 196(10), 1493-1499.

Benfield, C. T., Lyall, J. W., Kochs, G., & Tiley, L. S. (2008). Asparagine 631 variants of the chicken Mx protein do not inhibit influenza virus replication in primary chicken embryo fibroblasts or in vitro surrogate assays. Journal of Virology, 82(15), 7533-7539.

Benfield, C. T., Lyall, J. W., & Tiley, L. S. (2010). The cytoplasmic location of chicken mx is not the determining factor for its lack of antiviral activity. PLoS One, 5(8), e12151.

Bennink, J. R., & Palmore, T. N. (2004). The promise of siRNAs for the treatment of influenza. Trends in molecular medicine, 10(12), 571-574.

Berlin, S., Qu, L., Li, X., Yang, N., & Ellegren, H. (2008). Positive diversifying selection in avian Mx genes. Immunogenetics, 60(11), 689-697.

Bernasconi, D., Schultz, U., & Staeheli, P. (1995). The interferon-induced Mx protein of chickens lacks antiviral activity. Journal of interferon & cytokine research 15(1), 47-53.

Bertelsen, M. F., Klausen, J., Holm, E., Grondahl, C., & Jorgensen, P. H. (2007). Serological response to vaccination against avian influenza in zoo-birds using an inactivated H5N9 vaccine. Vaccine, 25(22), 4345-4349.

Betakova, T., & Svancarova, P. (2013). Role and application of RNA interference in replication of influenza viruses. Acta Virol, 57(2), 97-104.

Bliu, A., Lemieux, M., Li, C., Li, X., Wang, J., & Farnsworth, A. (2012). Modifying the thermostability of inactivated influenza vaccines. Vaccine, 30(37), 5506-5511.

Bodian, D. L., Yamasaki, R. B., Buswell, R. L., Stearns, J. F., White, J. M., & Kuntz, I. D. (1993). Inhibition of the fusion-inducing conformational change of influenza hemagglutinin by benzoquinones and hydroquinones. Biochemistry, 32(12), 2967-2978.

Boge, T., Remigy, M., Vaudaine, S., Tanguy, J., Bourdet-Sicard, R., & van der Werf, S. (2009). A probiotic fermented dairy drink improves antibody response to influenza vaccination in the elderly in two randomised controlled trials. Vaccine, 27(41), 5677-5684.

Boltz, D. A., Aldridge, J. R., Jr., Webster, R. G., & Govorkova, E. A. (2010). Drugs in development for influenza. Drugs, 70(11), 1349-1362.

Boni, M. F. (2008). Vaccination and antigenic drift in influenza. Vaccine, 26 Suppl 3, C8-14.

Boon, A. C., deBeauchamp, J., Hollmann, A., Luke, J., Kotb, M., Rowe, S., Finkelstein, D., Neale, G., Lu, L., Williams, R. W., & Webby, R. J. (2009). Host genetic variation affects resistance to infection with a highly pathogenic H5N1 influenza A virus in mice. J Virol, 83(20), 10417-10426.

Bright, R. A., Medina, M. J., Xu, X., Perez-Oronoz, G., Wallis, T. R., Davis, X. M., Povinelli, L., Cox, N. J., & Klimov, A. I. (2005). Incidence of adamantane resistance among influenza A (H3N2) viruses isolated worldwide from 1994 to 2005: a cause for concern. Lancet, 366(9492), 1175-1181.

Bright, R. A., Shay, D. K., Shu, B., Cox, N. J., & Klimov, A. I. (2006). Adamantane resistance among influenza A viruses isolated early during the 2005-2006 influenza season in the United States. JAMA, 295(8), 891-894.

Brojer, C., Jarhult, J. D., Muradrasoli, S., Soderstrom, H., Olsen, B., & Gavier-Widen, D. (2013). Pathobiology and virus shedding of low-pathogenic avian influenza virus (A/H1N1) infection in mallards exposed to oseltamivir. Journal of Wildlife Diseases, 49(1), 103-113.

Brown, E. G. (2000). Influenza virus genetics. Biomedicine and Pharmacotherapy, 54(4), 196-209.

Brown, J. D., Stallknecht, D. E., Beck, J. R., Suarez, D. L., & Swayne, D. E. (2006). Susceptibility of North American ducks and gulls to H5N1 highly pathogenic avian influenza viruses. Emerg Infect Dis, 12(11), 1663-1670.

Bublot, M., Pritchard, N., Cruz, J. S., Mickle, T. R., Selleck, P., & Swayne, D. E. (2007). Efficacy of a fowlpox-vectored avian influenza H5 vaccine against Asian H5N1 highly pathogenic avian influenza virus challenge. Avian Diseases, 51(1 Suppl), 498-500.

Cagle, C., To, T. L., Nguyen, T., Wasilenko, J., Adams, S. C., Cardona, C. J., Spackman, E., Suarez, D. L., & Pantin-Jackwood, M. J. (2011). Pekin and Muscovy ducks respond differently to vaccination with a H5N1 highly pathogenic avian influenza (HPAI) commercial inactivated vaccine. Vaccine, 29(38), 6549-6557.

Cao, R. Y., Xiao, J. H., Cao, B., Li, S., Kumaki, Y., & Zhong, W. (2013). Inhibition of novel reassortant avian influenza H7N9 virus infection in vitro with three antiviral drugs, oseltamivir, peramivir and favipiravir. Antivir Chem Chemother.

Capua, I., & Alexander, D. J. (2004). Avian influenza: recent developments. Avian Pathology, 33(4), 393-404.

Capua, I., & Alexander, D. J. (2006). The challenge of avian influenza to the veterinary community. Avian Pathology, 35(3), 189-205.

Capua, I., & Alexander, D. J. (2008). Ecology, epidemiology and human health implications of avian influenza viruses: why do we need to share genetic data? Zoonoses Public Health, 55(1), 2-15.

Capua, I., & Marangon, S. (2003). The use of vaccination as an option for the control of avian influenza. Avian Pathology, 32(4), 335-343.

Capua, I., & Marangon, S. (2007). The use of vaccination to combat multiple introductions of Notifiable Avian Influenza viruses of the H5 and H7 subtypes between 2000 and 2006 in Italy. Vaccine, 25(27), 4987-4995.

Cattoli, G., Fusaro, A., Monne, I., Coven, F., Joannis, T., El-Hamid, H. S., Hussein, A. A., Cornelius, C., Amarin, N. M., Mancin, M., Holmes, E. C., & Capua, I. (2011a). Evidence for differing evolutionary dynamics of A/H5N1 viruses among countries applying or not applying avian influenza vaccination in poultry. Vaccine, 29(50), 9368-9375.

Cattoli, G., Milani, A., Temperton, N., Zecchin, B., Buratin, A., Molesti, E., Aly, M. M., Arafa, A., & Capua, I. (2011b). Antigenic drift in H5N1 avian influenza virus in poultry is driven by mutations in major antigenic sites of the hemagglutinin molecule analogous to those for human influenza virus. J Virol, 85(17), 8718-8724.

CDC. (2006). Centers for Disease Control and Prevention: High levels of adamantane resistance among influenza A (H3N2) viruses and interim guidelines for use of antiviral agents--United States, 2005-06 influenza season. MMWR Morb Mortal Wkly Rep, 55(2), 44-46.

Chan, R. W., Chan, M. C., Wong, A. C., Karamanska, R., Dell, A., Haslam, S. M., Sihoe, A. D., Chui, W. H., Triana-Baltzer, G., Li, Q., Peiris, J. S., Fang, F., & Nicholls, J. M. (2009). DAS181 inhibits H5N1 influenza virus infection of human lung tissues. Antimicrob Agents Chemother, 53(9), 3935-3941.

Chang, K. C., Goldspink, G., & Lida, J. (1990). Studies in the in vivo expression of the influenza resistance gene Mx by in-situ hybridisation. Arch Virol, 110(3-4), 151-164.

Chen, H. Y., Cui, B. A., Xia, P. A., Li, X. S., Hu, G. Z., Yang, M. F., Zhang, H. Y., Wang, X. B., Cao, S. F., Zhang, L. X., Kang, X. T., & Tu, K. (2008a). Cloning, in vitro expression and bioactivity of duck interleukin-18. Vet Immunol Immunopathol, 123(3-4), 205-214.

Chen, H. Y., Shang, Y. H., Yao, H. X., Cui, B. A., Zhang, H. Y., Wang, Z. X., Wang, Y. D., Chao, A. J., & Duan, T. Y. (2011a). Immune responses of chickens inoculated with a recombinant fowlpox vaccine coexpressing HA of H9N2 avain influenza virus and chicken IL-18. Antiviral Res, 91(1), 50-56.

Chen, J., Chen, S. C., Stern, P., Scott, B. B., & Lois, C. (2008b). Genetic strategy to prevent influenza virus infections in animals. J Infect Dis, 197 Suppl 1, S25-28.

Chen, J. X., Xue, H. J., Ye, W. C., Fang, B. H., Liu, Y. H., Yuan, S. H., Yu, P., & Wang, Y. Q. (2009). Activity of andrographolide and its derivatives against influenza virus in vivo and in vitro. Biol Pharm Bull, 32(8), 1385-1391.

Chen, W., Lim, C. E., Kang, H. J., & Liu, J. (2011b). Chinese herbal medicines for the treatment of type A H1N1 influenza: a systematic review of randomized controlled trials. PLoS One, 6(12), e28093.

Cheung, C. L., Rayner, J. M., Smith, G. J., Wang, P., Naipospos, T. S., Zhang, J., Yuen, K. Y., Webster, R. G., Peiris, J. S., Guan, Y., & Chen, H. (2006). Distribution of amantadine-resistant H5N1 avian influenza variants in Asia. J Infect Dis, 193(12), 1626-1629.

Chon, H., Choi, B., Jeong, G., & Mo, I. (2008). Evaluation system for an experimental study of low-pathogenic avian influenza virus (H9N2) infection in specific pathogen free chickens using lactic acid bacteria, Lactobacillus plantarum KFCC11389P. Avian Pathology, 37(6), 593-597.

Cyranoski, D. (2005). China's chicken farmers under fire for antiviral abuse. Nature, 435(7045), 1009.

Daimon, T., Kiuchi, T., & Takasu, Y. (2014). Recent progress in genome engineering techniques in the silkworm, Bombyx mori. Development Growth and Differentiation, 56(1), 14-25.

Davidson, L. E., Fiorino, A. M., Snydman, D. R., & Hibberd, P. L. (2011). Lactobacillus GG as an immune adjuvant for live-attenuated influenza vaccine in healthy adults: a randomized double-blind placebo-controlled trial. Eur J Clin Nutr, 65(4), 501-507.

De Clercq, E., & Neyts, J. (2007). Avian influenza A (H5N1) infection: targets and strategies for chemotherapeutic intervention. Trends in Pharmacological Sciences, 28(6), 280-285.

de Jong, M. D., Tran, T. T., Truong, H. K., Vo, M. H., Smith, G. J., Nguyen, V. C., Bach, V. C., Phan, T. Q., Do, Q. H., Guan, Y., Peiris, J. S., Tran, T. H., & Farrar, J. (2005). Oseltamivir resistance during treatment of influenza A (H5N1) infection. New England Journal of Medicine, 353(25), 2667-2672.

De Vriese, J., Steensels, M., Palya, V., Gardin, Y., Dorsey, K. M., Lambrecht, B., Van Borm, S., & van den Berg, T. (2010). Passive protection afforded by maternally-derived antibodies in chickens and the antibodies' interference with the protection elicited by avian influenza-inactivated vaccines in progeny. Avian Diseases, 54(1 Suppl), 246-252.

Deryabin, P. G., Lvov, D. K., Botikov, A. G., Ivanov, V., Kalinovsky, T., Niedzwiecki, A., & Rath, M. (2008). Effects of a nutrient mixture on infectious properties of the highly pathogenic strain of avian influenza virus A/H5N1. Biofactors, 33(2), 85-97.

Dillon, D., & Runstadler, J. (2010). Mx gene diversity and influenza association among five wild dabbling duck species (Anas spp.) in Alaska. Infect Genet Evol, 10(7), 1085-1093.

Dreitlein, W. B., Maratos, J., & Brocavich, J. (2001). Zanamivir and oseltamivir: two new options for the treatment and prevention of influenza. Clin Ther, 23(3), 327-355.

Du, J., Cross, T. A., & Zhou, H. X. (2012). Recent progress in structure-based anti-influenza drug design. Drug Discov Today, 17(19-20), 1111-1120.

Duvauchelle, A., Huneau-Salaun, A., Balaine, L., Rose, N., & Michel, V. (2013). Risk factors for the introduction of avian influenza virus in breeder duck flocks during the first 24 weeks of laying. Avian Pathol, 42(5), 447-456.

Earhart, K. C., Elsayed, N. M., Saad, M. D., Gubareva, L. V., Nayel, A., Deyde, V. M., Abdelsattar, A., Abdelghani, A. S., Boynton, B. R., Mansour, M. M., Essmat, H. M., Klimov, A., Shuck-Lee, D., Monteville, M. R., & Tjaden, J. A. (2009). Oseltamivir resistance mutation N294S in human influenza A(H5N1) virus in Egypt. J Infect Public Health, 2(2), 74-80.

Ehrhardt, C., Dudek, S. E., Holzberg, M., Urban, S., Hrincius, E. R., Haasbach, E., Seyer, R., Lapuse, J., Planz, O., & Ludwig, S. (2013a). A plant extract of Ribes nigrum folium possesses anti-influenza virus activity in vitro and in vivo by preventing virus entry to host cells. PLoS ONE, 8(5), e63657.

Ehrhardt, C., Ruckle, A., Hrincius, E. R., Haasbach, E., Anhlan, D., Ahmann, K., Banning, C., Reiling, S. J., Kuhn, J., Strobl, S., Vitt, D., Leban, J., Planz, O., & Ludwig, S. (2013b). The NF-kappaB inhibitor SC75741 efficiently blocks influenza virus propagation and confers a high barrier for development of viral resistance. Cell Microbiol, 15(7), 1198-1211.

Elbashir, S. M., Harborth, J., Lendeckel, W., Yalcin, A., Weber, K., & Tuschl, T. (2001). Duplexes of 21-nucleotide RNAs mediate RNA interference in cultured mammalian cells. Nature, 411(6836), 494-498.

Engel, D. A. (2013). The influenza virus NS1 protein as a therapeutic target. Antiviral Research, 99(3), 409-416.

Enserink, M. (2011). Avian influenza. Transgenic chickens could thwart bird flu, curb pandemic risk. Science, 331(6014), 132-133.

Escorcia, M., Vazquez, L., Mendez, S. T., Rodriguez-Ropon, A., Lucio, E., & Nava, G. M. (2008). Avian influenza: genetic evolution under vaccination pressure. Virology Journal, 5, 15.

Ewald, S. J., Kapczynski, D. R., Livant, E. J., Suarez, D. L., Ralph, J., McLeod, S., & Miller, C. (2011). Association of Mx1 Asn631 variant alleles with reductions in morbidity, early mortality, viral shedding, and cytokine responses in chickens infected with a highly pathogenic avian influenza virus. Immunogenetics, 63(6), 363-375.

Federico, M. (2011). HIV-protease inhibitors block the replication of both vesicular stomatitis and influenza viruses at an early post-entry replication step. Virology, 417(1), 37-49.

Feng, E., Ye, D., Li, J., Zhang, D., Wang, J., Zhao, F., Hilgenfeld, R., Zheng, M., Jiang, H., & Liu, H. (2012). Recent advances in neuraminidase inhibitor development as anti-influenza drugs. ChemMedChem, 7(9), 1527-1536.

Ferguson, N. M., Galvani, A. P., & Bush, R. M. (2003). Ecological and immunological determinants of influenza evolution. Nature, 422(6930), 428-433.

Flefel, E. M., Abdel-Mageid, R. E., Tantawy, W. A., Ali, M. A., & Amr Ael, G. (2012). Heterocyclic compounds based on 3-(4-bromophenyl) azo-5-phenyl-2(3H)-furanone: anti-avian influenza virus (H5N1) activity. Acta Pharm, 62(4), 593-606.

Furuta, Y., Gowen, B. B., Takahashi, K., Shiraki, K., Smee, D. F., & Barnard, D. L. (2013). Favipiravir (T-705), a novel viral RNA polymerase inhibitor. Antiviral Res, 100(2), 446-454.

Furuta, Y., Takahashi, K., Fukuda, Y., Kuno, M., Kamiyama, T., Kozaki, K., Nomura, N., Egawa, H., Minami, S., Watanabe, Y., Narita, H., & Shiraki, K. (2002). In vitro and in vivo activities of anti-influenza virus compound T-705. Antimicrob Agents Chemother, 46(4), 977-981.

Fusco, D., Liu, X. Y., Savage, C., Taur, Y., Xiao, W. L., Kennelly, E., Yuan, J. D., Cassileth, B., Salvatore, M., & Papanicolaou, G. A. (2010). Echinacea purpurea aerial extract alters course of influenza infection in mice. Vaccine, 28(23), 3956-3962.

Gamblin, S. J., & Skehel, J. J. (2010). Influenza hemagglutinin and neuraminidase membrane glycoproteins. Journal of Biological Chemistry, 285(37), 28403-28409.

Gangopadhyay, A., Ganguli, S., & Datta, A. (2011). Inhibiting H5N1 hemagglutinin with samll molecule ligands. International Journal of Bioinformatics Research, 3(1), 185-189.

Garcia, A., Johnson, H., Srivastava, D. K., Jayawardene, D. A., Wehr, D. R., & Webster, R. G. (1998). Efficacy of inactivated H5N2 influenza vaccines against lethal A/Chicken/Queretaro/19/95 infection. Avian Dis, 42(2), 248-256.

Garozzo, A., Timpanaro, R., Bisignano, B., Furneri, P. M., Bisignano, G., & Castro, A. (2009). In vitro antiviral activity of Melaleuca alternifolia essential oil. Lett Appl Microbiol, 49(6), 806-808.

Garozzo, A., Timpanaro, R., Stivala, A., Bisignano, G., & Castro, A. (2011). Activity of Melaleuca alternifolia (tea tree) oil on Influenza virus A/PR/8: study on the mechanism of action. Antiviral Res, 89(1), 83-88.

Ge, Q., Eisen, H. N., & Chen, J. (2004a). Use of siRNAs to prevent and treat influenza virus infection. Virus Res, 102(1), 37-42.

Ge, Q., Filip, L., Bai, A., Nguyen, T., Eisen, H. N., & Chen, J. (2004b). *Inhibition of influenza virus production in virus-infected mice by RNA interference.* Proc Natl Acad Sci U S A, 101(23), 8676-8681.

Ge, Q., McManus, M. T., Nguyen, T., Shen, C. H., Sharp, P. A., Eisen, H. N., & Chen, J. (2003). *RNA interference of influenza virus production by directly targeting mRNA for degradation and indirectly inhibiting all viral RNA transcription.* Proc Natl Acad Sci U S A, 100(5), 2718-2723.

Geng, L., Shaozhong, P., Shaohua, Y., Ziren, S., & Xiaoping, L. (2009). *Experimental study on the antivirus effect of Zhongsheng pills on influenza virus H5N1.* World Science and Technology, 11(3), 365-370.

Ghafoor, A., Naseem, S., Younus, M., & Nazir, J. (2005). *Immunomodulatory effects of multistrain probiotics (Protexin™) on broiler chicken vaccinated against avian influenza virus (H9)* International Journal of Poultry Science, 4(10), 777-780.

Gharaibeh, S. (2008). *Pathogenicity of an avian influenza virus serotype H9N2 in chickens.* Avian Diseases, 52(1), 106-110.

Gilbert, B. E., & McLeay, M. T. (2008). *MegaRibavirin aerosol for the treatment of influenza A virus infections in mice.* Antiviral Res, 78(3), 223-229.

Gillman, A., Muradrasoli, S., Soderstrom, H., Nordh, J., Brojer, C., Lindberg, R. H., Latorre-Margalef, N., Waldenstrom, J., Olsen, B., & Jarhult, J. D. (2013). *Resistance mutation R292K is induced in influenza A(H6N2) virus by exposure of infected mallards to low levels of oseltamivir.* PLoS ONE, 8(8), e71230.

Glatthaar-Saalmuller, B., Rauchhaus, U., Rode, S., Haunschild, J., & Saalmuller, A. (2011). *Antiviral activity in vitro of two preparations of the herbal medicinal product Sinupret(R) against viruses causing respiratory infections.* Phytomedicine, 19(1), 1-7.

Goto, H., Sagitani, A., Ashida, N., Kato, S., Hirota, T., Shinoda, T., & Yamamoto, N. (2013). *Anti-influenza virus effects of both live and non-live Lactobacillus acidophilus L-92 accompanied by the activation of innate immunity.* Br J Nutr, 110(10), 1810-1818.

Govorkova, E. A., Baranovich, T., Seiler, P., Armstrong, J., Burnham, A., Guan, Y., Peiris, M., Webby, R. J., & Webster, R. G. (2013). *Antiviral resistance among highly pathogenic influenza A (H5N1) viruses isolated worldwide in 2002-2012 shows need for continued monitoring.* Antiviral Research, 98(2), 297-304.

Gratz, S. J., Wildonger, J., Harrison, M. M., & O'Connor-Giles, K. M. (2013). *CRISPR/Cas9-mediated genome engineering and the promise of designer flies on demand.* Fly (Austin), 7(4).

Grund, C., Abdelwhab el, S. M., Arafa, A. S., Ziller, M., Hassan, M. K., Aly, M. M., Hafez, H. M., Harder, T. C., & Beer, M. (2011). *Highly pathogenic avian influenza virus H5N1 from Egypt escapes vaccine-induced immunity but confers clinical protection against a heterologous clade 2.2.1 Egyptian isolate.* Vaccine, 29(33), 5567-5573.

Guo, R., Pittler, M. H., & Ernst, E. (2007). *Complementary medicine for treating or preventing influenza or influenza-like illness.* Am J Med, 120(11), 923-929 e923.

Guralnik, M., Rosenbloom, R. A., Petteruti, M. P., & Lefante, C. (2007). *Limitations of current prophylaxis against influenza virus infection.* Am J Ther, 14(5), 449-454.

Hafez, M. H., Arafa, A., Abdelwhab, E. M., Selim, A., Khoulosy, S. G., Hassan, M. K., & Aly, M. M. (2010). *Avian influenza H5N1 virus infections in vaccinated commercial and backyard poultry in Egypt.* Poultry Science, 89(8), 1609-1613.

Hai, R., Schmolke, M., Leyva-Grado, V. H., Thangavel, R. R., Margine, I., Jaffe, E. L., Krammer, F., Solorzano, A., Garcia-Sastre, A., Palese, P., & Bouvier, N. M. (2013). *Influenza A(H7N9) virus gains neuraminidase inhibitor resistance without loss of in vivo virulence or transmissibility.* Nat Commun, 4, 2854.

Hale, B. G., Randall, R. E., Ortin, J., & Jackson, D. (2008). *The multifunctional NS1 protein of influenza A viruses.* Journal of General Virology, 89(Pt 10), 2359-2376.

Haller, O., Staeheli, P., & Kochs, G. (2009). *Protective role of interferon-induced Mx GTPases against influenza viruses.* Rev Sci Tech, 28(1), 219-231.

Hao, Y. X., Yang, J. M., He, C., Liu, Q., & McAllister, T. A. (2008). *Reduced serologic response to avian influenza vaccine in specific-pathogen-free chicks inoculated with Cryptosporidium baileyi.* Avian Diseases, 52(4), 690-693.

Harata, G., He, F., Hiruta, N., Kawase, M., Kubota, A., Hiramatsu, M., & Yausi, H. (2010). *Intranasal administration of Lactobacillus rhamnosus GG protects mice from H1N1 influenza virus infection by regulating respiratory immune responses.* Lett Appl Microbiol, 50(6), 597-602.

Harvey, A. J., Speksnijder, G., Baugh, L. R., Morris, J. A., & Ivarie, R. (2002). *Consistent production of transgenic chickens using replication-deficient retroviral vectors and high-throughput screening procedures.* Poult Sci, 81(2), 202-212.

He, G., Qiao, J., Dong, C., He, C., Zhao, L., & Tian, Y. (2008). Amantadine-resistance among H5N1 avian influenza viruses isolated in Northern China. Antiviral Research, 77(1), 72-76.

Hegazy, A. M., Abdallah, F. M., Abd-El Samie, L. K., & Nazim, A. A. (2011). The relation between some immunosuppressive agents and widespread nature of highly pathogenic avian influenza (HPAI) post vaccination. Journal of American Science, 7(9), 66-72.

Hill, A. W., Guralnick, R. P., Wilson, M. J., Habib, F., & Janies, D. (2009). Evolution of drug resistance in multiple distinct lineages of H5N1 avian influenza. Infection, Genetics and Evolution, 9(2), 169-178.

Hoffman, L. R., Kuntz, I. D., & White, J. M. (1997). Structure-based identification of an inducer of the low-pH conformational change in the influenza virus hemagglutinin: irreversible inhibition of infectivity. J Virol, 71(11), 8808-8820.

Honda, A., Okamoto, T., & Ishihama, A. (2007). Host factor Ebp1: selective inhibitor of influenza virus transcriptase. Genes Cells, 12(2), 133-142.

Horby, P., Nguyen, N. Y., Dunstan, S. J., & Baillie, J. K. (2012). The role of host genetics in susceptibility to influenza: a systematic review. PLoS One, 7(3), e33180.

Hori, T., Kiyoshima, J., Shida, K., & Yasui, H. (2001). Effect of intranasal administration of Lactobacillus casei Shirota on influenza virus infection of upper respiratory tract in mice. Clin Diagn Lab Immunol, 8(3), 593-597.

Hsiang, T. Y., Zhao, C., & Krug, R. M. (2009). Interferon-induced ISG15 conjugation inhibits influenza A virus gene expression and replication in human cells. J Virol, 83(12), 5971-5977.

Hsieh, H. P., & Hsu, J. T. (2007). Strategies of development of antiviral agents directed against influenza virus replication. Curr Pharm Des, 13(34), 3531-3542.

Hu, Y., Lu, S., Song, Z., Wang, W., Hao, P., Li, J., Zhang, X., Yen, H. L., Shi, B., Li, T., Guan, W., Xu, L., Liu, Y., Wang, S., Tian, D., Zhu, Z., He, J., Huang, K., Chen, H., Zheng, L., Li, X., Ping, J., Kang, B., Xi, X., Zha, L., Li, Y., Zhang, Z., Peiris, M., & Yuan, Z. (2013). Association between adverse clinical outcome in human disease caused by novel influenza A H7N9 virus and sustained viral shedding and emergence of antiviral resistance. Lancet, 381(9885), 2273-2279.

Huang, Y., Hu, B., Wen, X., Cao, S., Xu, D., Zhang, X., & Khan, M. I. (2009). Evolution analysis of the matrix (M) protein genes of 17 H9N2 chicken influenza viruses isolated in northern China during 1998-2008. Virus Genes, 38(3), 398-403.

Hudson, J. B. (2009). The use of herbal extracts in the control of influenza. Journal of Medicinal Plants Research, 3(13), 1189-1194.

Hui, E. K., Yap, E. M., An, D. S., Chen, I. S., & Nayak, D. P. (2004). Inhibition of influenza virus matrix (M1) protein expression and virus replication by U6 promoter-driven and lentivirus-mediated delivery of siRNA. J Gen Virol, 85(Pt 7), 1877-1884.

Hurt, A. C., Selleck, P., Komadina, N., Shaw, R., Brown, L., & Barr, I. G. (2007). Susceptibility of highly pathogenic A(H5N1) avian influenza viruses to the neuraminidase inhibitors and adamantanes. Antiviral Res, 73(3), 228-231.

Ibrahim, A. K., Youssef, A. I., Arafa, A. S., & Ahmed, S. A. (2013a). Anti-H5N1 virus flavonoids from Capparis sinaica Veill. Nat Prod Res.

Ibrahim, A. K., Youssef, A. I., Arafa, A. S., Foad, R., Radwan, M. M., Ross, S., Hassanean, H. A., & Ahmed, S. A. (2013b). Anti-H5N1 virus new diglyceride ester from the Red Sea grass Thallasodendron ciliatum. Nat Prod Res, 27(18), 1625-1632.

Ikematsu, H., & Kawai, N. (2011). Laninamivir octanoate: a new long-acting neuraminidase inhibitor for the treatment of influenza. Expert Rev Anti Infect Ther, 9(10), 851-857.

Ilyushina, N. A., Govorkova, E. A., & Webster, R. G. (2005). Detection of amantadine-resistant variants among avian influenza viruses isolated in North America and Asia. Virology, 341(1), 102-106.

Imanishi, N., Tuji, Y., Katada, Y., Maruhashi, M., Konosu, S., Mantani, N., Terasawa, K., & Ochiai, H. (2002). Additional inhibitory effect of tea extract on the growth of influenza A and B viruses in MDCK cells. Microbiol Immunol, 46(7), 491-494.

Ison, M. G. (2013). Clinical use of approved influenza antivirals: therapy and prophylaxis. Influenza Other Respir Viruses, 7 Suppl 1, 7-13.

Ison, M. G., Fraiz, J., Heller, B., Jauregui, L., Mills, G., O'Riordan, W., O'Neil, B., Playford, E. G., Rolf, J. D., Sada-Diaz, E., Elder, J., Collis, P., Hernandez, J. E., & Sheridan, W. P. (2013). Intravenous peramivir for treatment of influenza in hospitalized patients. Antiviral Therapy.

Iwabuchi, N., Xiao, J. Z., Yaeshima, T., & Iwatsuki, K. (2011). Oral administration of Bifidobacterium longum ameliorates influenza virus infection in mice. Biol Pharm Bull, 34(8), 1352-1355.

Jablonski, J. J., Basu, D., Engel, D. A., & Geysen, H. M. (2012). Design, synthesis, and evaluation of novel small molecule inhibitors of the influenza virus protein NS1. Bioorg Med Chem, 20(1), 487-497.

Jafari, R. A., Ghorbanpoor, M., & Hoshmand Diarjan, S. (2009). Study on immunomodulatory activity of dietary garlic in chickens vaccinated against avian influenza virus (subtype H9N2). International Journal of Poultry Science, 8(4), 401-403.

Jenkins, K. A., Lowenthal, J. W., Kimpton, W., & Bean, A. G. (2009). The in vitro and in ovo responses of chickens to TLR9 subfamily ligands. Dev Comp Immunol, 33(5), 660-667.

Jiang, H., Yang, H., & Kapczynski, D. R. (2011). Chicken interferon alpha pretreatment reduces virus replication of pandemic H1N1 and H5N9 avian influenza viruses in lung cell cultures from different avian species. Virology Journal, 8, 447.

Jiang, W., Liu, Y., Zheng, H., Zheng, Y., Xu, H., & Lu, H. (2012). Immune regulation of avian influenza vaccine in hens using Hypericum perforatum L. methanol extraction. Plant Omics Journal, 5(1), 40 - 45.

Jiao, H., Du, L., Hao, Y., Cheng, Y., Luo, J., Kuang, W., Zhang, D., Lei, M., Jia, X., Zhang, X., Qi, C., He, H., & Wang, F. (2013). Effective inhibition of mRNA accumulation and protein expression of H5N1 avian influenza virus NS1 gene in vitro by small interfering RNAs. Folia Microbiologica, 58(4), 335-342.

Jung, K., Ha, Y., Ha, S. K., Han, D. U., Kim, D. W., Moon, W. K., & Chae, C. (2004). Antiviral effect of Saccharomyces cerevisiae beta-glucan to swine influenza virus by increased production of interferon-gamma and nitric oxide. J Vet Med B Infect Dis Vet Public Health, 51(2), 72-76.

Kaleta, E. F., Blanco Pena, K. M., Yilmaz, A., Redmann, T., & Hofheinz, S. (2007). Avian influenza A viruses in birds of the order Psittaciformes: reports on virus isolations, transmission experiments and vaccinations and initial studies on innocuity and efficacy of oseltamivir in ovo. Dtsch Tierarztl Wochenschr, 114(7), 260-267.

Kallon, S., Li, X., Ji, J., Chen, C., Xi, Q., Chang, S., Xue, C., Ma, J., Xie, Q., & Zhang, Y. (2013). Astragalus polysaccharide enhances immunity and inhibits H9N2 avian influenza virus in vitro and in vivo. J Anim Sci Biotechnol, 4(1), 22.

Kamali, A., & Holodniy, M. (2013). Influenza treatment and prophylaxis with neuraminidase inhibitors: a review. Infect Drug Resist, 6, 187-198.

Kamps, B. S., & Hoffman, C. (2006). Drug profiles. In B. S. Kamps, C. Hoffman & W. Preiser (Eds.), Influenza report 2006 (pp. 188 - 221). Paris, Cagliari, Wuppertal, Sevilla: Flying Publisher.

Kapczynski, D. R., Pantin-Jackwood, M., Guzman, S. G., Ricardez, Y., Spackman, E., Bertran, K., Suarez, D. L., & Swayne, D. E. (2013). Characterization of the 2012 highly pathogenic avian influenza H7N3 virus isolated from poultry in an outbreak in Mexico: pathobiology and vaccine protection. Journal of Virology, 87(16), 9086-9096.

Kapczynski, D. R., & Swayne, D. E. (2009). Influenza vaccines for avian species. Current Topics in Microbiology and Immunology, 333, 133-152.

Karpala, A. J., Stewart, C., McKay, J., Lowenthal, J. W., & Bean, A. G. (2011). Characterization of chicken Mda5 activity: regulation of IFN-beta in the absence of RIG-I functionality. J Immunol, 186(9), 5397-5405.

Kato, N., & Eggers, H. J. (1969). Inhibition of uncoating of fowl plague virus by l-adamantanamine hydrochloride. Virology, 37(4), 632-641.

Kawase, M., He, F., Kubota, A., Yoda, K., Miyazawa, K., & Hiramatsu, M. (2012). Heat-killed Lactobacillus gasseri TMC0356 protects mice against influenza virus infection by stimulating gut and respiratory immune responses. FEMS Immunol Med Microbiol, 64(2), 280-288.

Kayali, G., Webby, R. J., Ducatez, M. F., El Shesheny, R. A., Kandeil, A. M., Govorkova, E. A., Mostafa, A., & Ali, M. A. (2011). The epidemiological and molecular aspects of influenza H5N1 viruses at the human-animal interface in Egypt. PLoS One, 6(3), e17730.

Keawcharoen, J., van Riel, D., van Amerongen, G., Bestebroer, T., Beyer, W. E., van Lavieren, R., Osterhaus, A. D., Fouchier, R. A., & Kuiken, T. (2008). Wild ducks as long-distance vectors of highly pathogenic avian influenza virus (H5N1). Emerging Infectious Diseases, 14(4), 600-607.

Kernan, M. R., Sendl, A., Chen, J. L., Jolad, S. D., Blanc, P., Murphy, J. T., Stoddart, C. A., Nanakorn, W., Balick, M. J., & Rozhon, E. J. (1997). Two new lignans with activity against influenza virus from the medicinal plant Rhinacanthus nasutus. J Nat Prod, 60(6), 635-637.

Kido, H., Okumura, Y., Yamada, H., Mizuno, D., Higashi, Y., & Yano, M. (2004). Secretory leukoprotease inhibitor and pulmonary surfactant serve as principal defenses against influenza A virus infection in the airway and chemical agents up-regulating their levels may have therapeutic potential. Biol Chem, 385(11), 1029-1034.

Kilany, W. H., Abdelwhab, E. M., Arafa, A. S., Selim, A., Safwat, M., Nawar, A. A., Erfan, A. M., Hassan, M. K., Aly, M. M., & Hafez, H. M. (2011). Protective efficacy of H5 inactivated vaccines in meat turkey poults after challenge with Egyptian variant highly pathogenic avian influenza H5N1 virus. Veterinary Microbiology, 150(1-2), 28-34.

Kim, J. K., Kayali, G., Walker, D., Forrest, H. L., Ellebedy, A. H., Griffin, Y. S., Rubrum, A., Bahgat, M. M., Kutkat, M. A., Ali, M. A., Aldridge, J. R., Negovetich, N. J., Krauss, S., Webby, R. J., & Webster, R. G. (2010). Puzzling inefficiency of H5N1 influenza vaccines in Egyptian poultry. Proceedings of the National Academy of Sciences of the United States of America, 107(24), 11044-11049.

Kiso, M., Kubo, S., Ozawa, M., Le, Q. M., Nidom, C. A., Yamashita, M., & Kawaoka, Y. (2010a). Efficacy of the new neuraminidase inhibitor CS-8958 against H5N1 influenza viruses. PLoS Pathog, 6(2), e1000786.

Kiso, M., Takahashi, K., Sakai-Tagawa, Y., Shinya, K., Sakabe, S., Le, Q. M., Ozawa, M., Furuta, Y., & Kawaoka, Y. (2010b). T-705 (favipiravir) activity against lethal H5N1 influenza A viruses. Proceedings of the National Academy of Sciences of the United States of America, 107(2), 882-887.

Kiso, M., Takano, R., Sakabe, S., Katsura, H., Shinya, K., Uraki, R., Watanabe, S., Saito, H., Toba, M., Kohda, N., & Kawaoka, Y. (2013). Protective efficacy of orally administered, heat-killed Lactobacillus pentosus b240 against influenza A virus. Sci Rep, 3, 1563.

Kitazato, K., Wang, Y., & Kobayashi, N. (2007). Viral infectious disease and natural products with antiviral activity. Drug Discov Ther, 1(1), 14-22.

Ko, J. H., Jin, H. K., Asano, A., Takada, A., Ninomiya, A., Kida, H., Hokiyama, H., Ohara, M., Tsuzuki, M., Nishibori, M., Mizutani, M., & Watanabe, T. (2002). Polymorphisms and the differential antiviral activity of the chicken Mx gene. Genome Res, 12(4), 595-601.

Koch, G., Steensels, M., & van den Berg, T. (2009). Vaccination of birds other than chickens and turkeys against avian influenza. Revue Scientifique et Technique, Office International des Epizooties, 28(1), 307-318.

Krawitz, C., Mraheil, M. A., Stein, M., Imirzalioglu, C., Domann, E., Pleschka, S., & Hain, T. (2011). Inhibitory activity of a standardized elderberry liquid extract against clinically-relevant human respiratory bacterial pathogens and influenza A and B viruses. BMC Complement Altern Med, 11, 16.

Kubo, S., Tomozawa, T., Kakuta, M., Tokumitsu, A., & Yamashita, M. (2010). Laninamivir prodrug CS-8958, a long-acting neuraminidase inhibitor, shows superior anti-influenza virus activity after a single administration. Antimicrobial agents and chemotherapy, 54(3), 1256-1264.

Kubo, T., & Nishimura, H. (2007). Antipyretic effect of Mao-to, a Japanese herbal medicine, for treatment of type A influenza infection in children. Phytomedicine, 14(2-3), 96-101.

Kuchipudi, S. V., Dunham, S. P., Nelli, R., White, G. A., Coward, V. J., Slomka, M. J., Brown, I. H., & Chang, K. C. (2012). Rapid death of duck cells infected with influenza: a potential mechanism for host resistance to H5N1. Immunol Cell Biol, 90(1), 116-123.

Kumaki, Y., Morrey, J. D., & Barnard, D. L. (2012). Effect of statin treatments on highly pathogenic avian influenza H5N1, seasonal and H1N1pdm09 virus infections in BALB/c mice. Future Virology, 7(8), 801-818.

Kurokawa, M., Kumeda, C. A., Yamamura, J., Kamiyama, T., & Shiraki, K. (1998). Antipyretic activity of cinnamyl derivatives and related compounds in influenza virus-infected mice. Eur J Pharmacol, 348(1), 45-51.

Kurokawa, M., Watanabe, W., Shimizu, T., Sawamura, R., & Shiraki, K. (2010). Modulation of cytokine production by 7-hydroxycoumarin in vitro and its efficacy against influenza infection in mice. Antiviral Res, 85(2), 373-380.

Kwon, H. J., Kim, H. H., Yoon, S. Y., Ryu, Y. B., Chang, J. S., Cho, K. O., Rho, M. C., Park, S. J., & Lee, W. S. (2010). In vitro inhibitory activity of Alpinia katsumadai extracts against influenza virus infection and hemagglutination. Virol J, 7, 307.

Lan, Y., Zhang, Y., Dong, L., Wang, D., Huang, W., Xin, L., Yang, L., Zhao, X., Li, Z., Wang, W., Li, X., Xu, C., Guo, J., Wang, M., Peng, Y., Gao, Y., Guo, Y., Wen, L., Jiang, T., & Shu, Y. (2010). A comprehensive surveillance of adamantane resistance among human influenza A virus isolated from mainland China between 1956 and 2009. Antiviral Therapy, 15(6), 853-859.

Landy, N., Ghalamkari, G. H., & Toghyani, M. (2012). Evaluation of St John's Wort (Hypericum perforatum L.) as an antibiotic growth promoter substitution on performance, carcass characteristics, some of the immune responses, and serum biochemical parameters of broiler chicks. Journal of Medicinal Plants Research, 6(3), 510-515.

Lang, G., Narayan, O., & Rouse, B. T. (1970). Prevention of malignant avian influenza by 1-adamantanamine hydrochloride. Arch Gesamte Virusforsch, 32(2), 171-184.

Larson, J. L., Kang, S. K., Choi, B. I., Hedlund, M., Aschenbrenner, L. M., Cecil, B., Machado, G., Nieder, M., & Fang, F. (2011). A safety evaluation of DAS181, a sialidase fusion protein, in rodents. Toxicol Sci, 122(2), 567-578.

Leang, S. K., Deng, Y. M., Shaw, R., Caldwell, N., Iannello, P., Komadina, N., Buchy, P., Chittaganpitch, M., Dwyer, D. E., Fagan, P., Gourinat, A. C., Hammill, F., Horwood, P. F., Huang, Q. S., Ip, P. K., Jennings, L., Kesson, A., Kok, T., Kool, J. L., Levy, A., Lin, C., Lindsay, K., Osman, O., Papadakis, G., Rahnamal, F., Rawlinson, W., Redden, C., Ridgway, J., Sam, I. C., Svobodova, S., Tandoc, A., Wickramasinghe, G., Williamson, J., Wilson, N., Yusof, M. A., Kelso, A., Barr, I. G., & Hurt, A. C. (2013). Influenza antiviral resistance in the Asia-Pacific region during 2011. Antiviral Res, 97(2), 206-210.

Lecu, A., De Langhe, C., Petit, T., Bernard, F., & Swam, H. (2009). Serologic response and safety to vaccination against avian influenza using inactivated H5N2 vaccine in zoo birds. J Zoo Wildl Med, 40(4), 731-743.

Lee, C. H., Byun, S. H., Lee, Y. J., & Mo, I. P. (2012a). Genetic evolution of the H9N2 avian influenza virus in Korean poultry farms. Virus Genes, 45(1), 38-47.

Lee, C. W., Senne, D. A., & Suarez, D. L. (2004). Effect of vaccine use in the evolution of Mexican lineage H5N2 avian influenza virus. Journal of Virology, 78(15), 8372-8381.

Lee, D. H., Lee, Y. N., Park, J. K., Yuk, S. S., Lee, J. W., Kim, J. I., Han, J. S., Lee, J. B., Park, S. Y., Choi, I. S., & Song, C. S. (2011). Antiviral efficacy of oseltamivir against avian influenza virus in avian species. Avian Diseases, 55(4), 677-679.

Lee, D. H., & Song, C. S. (2013). H9N2 avian influenza virus in Korea: evolution and vaccination. Clin Exp Vaccine Res, 2(1), 26-33.

Lee, H. J., Lee, Y. N., Youn, H. N., Lee, D. H., Kwak, J. H., Seong, B. L., Lee, J. B., Park, S. Y., Choi, I. S., & Song, C. S. (2012b). Anti-influenza virus activity of green tea by-products in vitro and efficacy against influenza virus infection in chickens. Poult Sci, 91(1), 66-73.

Lee, S., Kim, J. I., Heo, J., Lee, I., Park, S., Hwang, M. W., Bae, J. Y., Park, M. S., & Park, H. J. (2013a). The anti-influenza virus effect of Phellinus igniarius extract. J Microbiol, 51(5), 676-681.

Lee, S. M., & Yen, H. L. (2012). Targeting the host or the virus: current and novel concepts for antiviral approaches against influenza virus infection. Antiviral Res, 96(3), 391-404.

Lee, Y. N., Youn, H. N., Kwon, J. H., Lee, D. H., Park, J. K., Yuk, S. S., Erdene-Ochir, T. O., Kim, K. T., Lee, J. B., Park, S. Y., Choi, I. S., & Song, C. S. (2013b). Sublingual administration of Lactobacillus rhamnosus affects respiratory immune responses and facilitates protection against influenza virus infection in mice. Antiviral Res, 98(2), 284-290.

Lei, H., Xu, Y., Chen, J., Wei, X., & Lam, D. M. (2010). Immunoprotection against influenza H5N1 virus by oral administration of enteric-coated recombinant Lactococcus lactis mini-capsules. Virology, 407(2), 319-324.

Leneva, I. A., Roberts, N., Govorkova, E. A., Goloubeva, O. G., & Webster, R. G. (2000). The neuraminidase inhibitor GS4104 (oseltamivir phosphate) is efficacious against A/Hong Kong/156/97 (H5N1) and A/Hong Kong/1074/99 (H9N2) influenza viruses. Antiviral Res, 48(2), 101-115.

Li, R., Song, D., Zhu, Z., Xu, H., & Liu, S. (2012). An induced pocket for the binding of potent fusion inhibitor CL-385319 with H5N1 influenza virus hemagglutinin. PLoS One, 7(8), e41956.

Li, X. B., Wang, S. Q., Xu, W. R., Wang, R. L., & Chou, K. C. (2011). Novel inhibitor design for hemagglutinin against H1N1 influenza virus by core hopping method. PLoS One, 6(11), e28111.

Li, X. Y., Qu, L. J., Hou, Z. C., Yao, J. F., Xu, G. Y., & Yang, N. (2007). Genomic structure and diversity of the chicken Mx gene. Poult Sci, 86(4), 786-789.

Li, X. Y., Qu, L. J., Yao, J. F., & Yang, N. (2006). Skewed allele frequencies of an Mx gene mutation with potential resistance to avian influenza virus in different chicken populations. Poult Sci, 85(7), 1327-1329.

Li, Y. C., Kong, L. H., Cheng, B. Z., & Li, K. S. (2005). Construction of influenza virus siRNA expression vectors and their inhibitory effects on multiplication of influenza virus. Avian Dis, 49(4), 562-573.

Liang, Q. L., Luo, J., Zhou, K., Dong, J. X., & He, H. X. (2011). Immune-related gene expression in response to H5N1 avian influenza virus infection in chicken and duck embryonic fibroblasts. Molecular Immunology, 48(6-7), 924-930.

Liniger, M., Summerfield, A., & Ruggli, N. (2012a). MDA5 can be exploited as efficacious genetic adjuvant for DNA vaccination against lethal H5N1 influenza virus infection in chickens. PLoS One, 7(12), e49952.

Liniger, M., Summerfield, A., Zimmer, G., McCullough, K. C., & Ruggli, N. (2012b). Chicken cells sense influenza A virus infection through MDA5 and CARDIF signaling involving LGP2. J Virol, 86(2), 705-717.

Lisa Li, H., Nakano, T., & Hotta, A. (2014). Genetic correction using engineered nucleases for gene therapy applications. Development Growth and Differentiation, 56(1), 63-77.

Liu, F. X., Sun, S., & Cui, Z. Z. (2010). Analysis of immunological enhancement of immunosuppressed chickens by Chinese herbal extracts. J Ethnopharmacol, 127(2), 251-256.

Liu, S., Li, R., Zhang, R., Chan, C. C., Xi, B., Zhu, Z., Yang, J., Poon, V. K., Zhou, J., Chen, M., Munch, J., Kirchhoff, F., Pleschka, S., Haarmann, T., Dietrich, U., Pan, C., Du, L., Jiang, S., & Zheng, B. (2011). CL-385319 inhibits H5N1 avian influenza A virus infection by blocking viral entry. European Journal of Pharmacology, 660(2-3), 460-467.

Liu, Z., Guo, Z., Wang, G., Zhang, D., He, H., Li, G., Liu, Y., Higgins, D., Walsh, A., Shanahan-Prendergast, L., & Lu, J. (2009). Evaluation of the efficacy and safety of a statin/caffeine combination against H5N1, H3N2 and H1N1 virus infection in BALB/c mice. Eur J Pharm Sci, 38(3), 215-223.

Lukacsi, K., Molnar, M., Siroki, O., & Rosztoczy, I. (1985). Combined effects of amantadine and interferon on influenza virus replication in chicken and human embryo trachea organ culture. Acta Microbiol Hung, 32(4), 357-362.

Luo, G., Colonno, R., & Krystal, M. (1996). Characterization of a hemagglutinin-specific inhibitor of influenza A virus. Virology, 226(1), 66-76.

Luo, M. (2012). Influenza virus entry. Advances in Experimental Medicine and Biology, 726, 201-221.

Lupiani, B., & Reddy, S. M. (2009). The history of avian influenza. Comp Immunol Microbiol Infect Dis, 32(4), 311-323.

Lutful Kabir, S. M. (2009). The role of probiotics in the poultry industry. Int J Mol Sci, 10(8), 3531-3546.

Lyall, J., Irvine, R. M., Sherman, A., McKinley, T. J., Nunez, A., Purdie, A., Outtrim, L., Brown, I. H., Rolleston-Smith, G., Sang, H., & Tiley, L. (2011). Suppression of avian influenza transmission in genetically modified chickens. Science, 331(6014), 223-226.

Maas, R., Rosema, S., van Zoelen, D., & Venema, S. (2011). Maternal immunity against avian influenza H5N1 in chickens: limited protection and interference with vaccine efficacy. Avian Pathology, 40(1), 87-92.

Mak, N. K., Leung, C. Y., Wei, X. Y., Shen, X. L., Wong, R. N., Leung, K. N., & Fung, M. C. (2004). Inhibition of RANTES expression by indirubin in influenza virus-infected human bronchial epithelial cells. Biochem Pharmacol, 67(1), 167-174.

Malakhov, M. P., Aschenbrenner, L. M., Smee, D. F., Wandersee, M. K., Sidwell, R. W., Gubareva, L. V., Mishin, V. P., Hayden, F. G., Kim, D. H., Ing, A., Campbell, E. R., Yu, M., & Fang, F. (2006). Sialidase fusion protein as a novel broad-spectrum inhibitor of influenza virus infection. Antimicrob Agents Chemother, 50(4), 1470-1479.

Mantani, N., Andoh, T., Kawamata, H., Terasawa, K., & Ochiai, H. (1999). Inhibitory effect of Ephedrae herba, an oriental traditional medicine, on the growth of influenza A/PR/8 virus in MDCK cells. Antiviral Res, 44(3), 193-200.

Mantani, N., Imanishi, N., Kawamata, H., Terasawa, K., & Ochiai, H. (2001). Inhibitory effect of (+)-catechin on the growth of influenza A/PR/8 virus in MDCK cells. Planta Med, 67(3), 240-243.

Marcus, P. I., Girshick, T., van der Heide, L., & Sekellick, M. J. (2007). Super-sentinel chickens and detection of low-pathogenicity influenza virus. Emerg Infect Dis, 13(10), 1608-1610.

McKimm-Breschkin, J., Trivedi, T., Hampson, A., Hay, A., Klimov, A., Tashiro, M., Hayden, F., & Zambon, M. (2003). Neuraminidase sequence analysis and susceptibilities of influenza virus clinical isolates to zanamivir and oseltamivir. Antimicrob Agents Chemother, 47(7), 2264-2272.

McKimm-Breschkin, J. L., Selleck, P. W., Usman, T. B., & Johnson, M. A. (2007). Reduced sensitivity of influenza A (H5N1) to oseltamivir. Emerg Infect Dis, 13(9), 1354-1357.

McNicholl, I. R., & McNicholl, J. J. (2001). Neuraminidase inhibitors: Zanamivir and oseltamivir. Annals of Pharmacotherapy, 35(1), 57-70.

McSwiggen, J. A., & Seth, S. (2008). A potential treatment for pandemic influenza using siRNAs targeting conserved regions of influenza A. Expert Opin Biol Ther, 8(3), 299-313.

Mehrbod, P., Ideris, A., Omar, A. R., Hair-Bejo, M., Tan, S. W., Kheiri, M. T., & Tabatabaian, M. (2012). Attenuation of influenza virus infectivity with herbal-marine compound (HESA-A): an in vitro study in MDCK cells. Virol J, 9, 44.

Meier, E., Kunz, G., Haller, O., & Arnheiter, H. (1990). Activity of rat Mx proteins against a rhabdovirus. J Virol, 64(12), 6263-6269.

Meijer, A., van der Goot, A. J., Koch, G., van Bovenc, M., & Kimman, T. G. (2004). Oseltamivir reduces transmission, morbidity, and mortality of highly pathogenic avian influenza in chickens. International Congress Series, 1263, 495-498.

Meng, S., Yang, L., Xu, C., Qin, Z., Xu, H., Wang, Y., Sun, L., & Liu, W. (2011). Recombinant chicken interferon-alpha inhibits H9N2 avian influenza virus replication in vivo by oral administration. Journal of Interferon and Cytokine Research, 31(7), 533-538.

Meyer, D., Sielaff, F., Hammami, M., Bottcher-Friebertshauser, E., Garten, W., & Steinmetzer, T. (2013). Identification of the first synthetic inhibitors of the type II transmembrane serine protease TMPRSS2 suitable for inhibition of influenza virus activation. Biochem J, 452(2), 331-343.

Miki, K., Nagai, T., Suzuki, K., Tsujimura, R., Koyama, K., Kinoshita, K., Furuhata, K., Yamada, H., & Takahashi, K. (2007). Anti-influenza virus activity of biflavonoids. Bioorg Med Chem Lett, 17(3), 772-775.

Mingxiao, M., Ningyi, J., Zhenguo, W., Ruilin, W., Dongliang, F., Min, Z., Gefen, Y., Chang, L., Leili, J., Kuoshi, J., & Yingjiu, Z. (2006). Construction and immunogenicity of recombinant fowlpox vaccines coexpressing HA of AIV H5N1 and chicken IL18. Vaccine, 24(20), 4304-4311.

Morris, K. V., & Rossi, J. J. (2006). Lentivirus-mediated RNA interference therapy for human immunodeficiency virus type 1 infection. Hum Gene Ther, 17(5), 479-486.

Moscona, A. (2009). Global transmission of oseltamivir-resistant influenza. N Engl J Med, 360(10), 953-956.

Moses, H. E., Brandly, C. A., Jones, E. E., & Jungherr, E. L. (1948). The Isolation and Identification of Fowl Plague Virus. Am J Vet Res, 9(32), 314-328.

Moss, R. B., Hansen, C., Sanders, R. L., Hawley, S., Li, T., & Steigbigel, R. T. (2012). A phase II study of DAS181, a novel host directed antiviral for the treatment of influenza infection. J Infect Dis, 206(12), 1844-1851.

Motohashi, Y., Igarashi, M., Okamatsu, M., Noshi, T., Sakoda, Y., Yamamoto, N., Ito, K., Yoshida, R., & Kida, H. (2013). Antiviral activity of stachyflin on influenza A viruses of different hemagglutinin subtypes. Virol J, 10, 118.

Mumford, E., Bishop, J., Hendrickx, S., Embarek, P. B., & Perdue, M. (2007). Avian influenza H5N1: risks at the human-animal interface. Food Nutr Bull, 28(2 Suppl), S357-363.

Munster, V. J., Baas, C., Lexmond, P., Waldenstrom, J., Wallensten, A., Fransson, T., Rimmelzwaan, G. F., Beyer, W. E., Schutten, M., Olsen, B., Osterhaus, A. D., & Fouchier, R. A. (2007). Spatial, temporal, and species variation in prevalence of influenza A viruses in wild migratory birds. PLoS Pathog, 3(5), e61.

Naeem, K., & Hussain, M. (1995). An outbreak of avian influenza in poultry in Pakistan. Vet Rec, 137(17), 439.

Naeem, K., & Siddique, N. (2006). Use of strategic vaccination for the control of avian influenza in Pakistan. Dev Biol (Basel), 124, 145-150.

Naeem, K., Siddique, N., Ayaz, M., & Jalalee, M. A. (2007). Avian influenza in Pakistan: outbreaks of low- and high-pathogenicity avian influenza in Pakistan during 2003-2006. Avian Dis, 51(1 Suppl), 189-193.

Naeem, K., Ullah, A., Manvell, R. J., & Alexander, D. J. (1999). Avian influenza A subtype H9N2 in poultry in Pakistan. Vet Rec, 145(19), 560.

Nagai, T., Miyaichi, Y., Tomimori, T., Suzuki, Y., & Yamada, H. (1992). In vivo anti-influenza virus activity of plant flavonoids possessing inhibitory activity for influenza virus sialidase. Antiviral Res, 19(3), 207-217.

Nakayama, M., Suzuki, K., Toda, M., Okubo, S., Hara, Y., & Shimamura, T. (1993). Inhibition of the infectivity of influenza virus by tea polyphenols. Antiviral Res, 21(4), 289-299.

Nava, G. M., Bielke, L. R., Callaway, T. R., & Castaneda, M. P. (2005). Probiotic alternatives to reduce gastrointestinal infections: the poultry experience. Anim Health Res Rev, 6(1), 105-118.

Nguyen, H. T., Nguyen, T., Mishin, V. P., Sleeman, K., Balish, A., Jones, J., Creanga, A., Marjuki, H., Uyeki, T. M., Nguyen, D. H., Nguyen, D. T., Do, H. T., Klimov, A. I., Davis, C. T., & Gubareva, L. V. (2013). Antiviral susceptibility of highly pathogenic avian influenza A(H5N1) viruses isolated from poultry, Vietnam, 2009-2011. Emerg Infect Dis, 19(12), 1963-1971.

Nicholls, J. M., Moss, R. B., & Haslam, S. M. (2013). The use of sialidase therapy for respiratory viral infections. Antiviral Res, 98(3), 401-409.

Novak, R., Ester, K., Savic, V., Sekellick, M. J., Marcus, P. I., Lowenthal, J. W., Vainio, O., & Ragland, W. L. (2001). Immune status assessment by abundance of IFN-alpha and IFN-gamma mRNA in chicken blood. J Interferon Cytokine Res, 21(8), 643-651.

O'Keefe, B. R., Smee, D. F., Turpin, J. A., Saucedo, C. J., Gustafson, K. R., Mori, T., Blakeslee, D., Buckheit, R., & Boyd, M. R. (2003). Potent anti-influenza activity of cyanovirin-N and interactions with viral hemagglutinin. Antimicrob Agents Chemother, 47(8), 2518-2525.

O'Neill, G. (2007). Australia tackles bird flu using RNAi. Nat Biotechnol, 25(6), 605-606.

Oh, S., Martelli, P., Hock, O. S., Luz, S., Furley, C., Chiek, E. J., Wee, L. C., & Keun, N. M. (2005). Field study on the use of inactivated H5N2 vaccine in avian species. Vet Rec, 157(10), 299-300.

Olivares, M., Diaz-Ropero, M. P., Sierra, S., Lara-Villoslada, F., Fonolla, J., Navas, M., Rodriguez, J. M., & Xaus, J. (2007). Oral intake of Lactobacillus fermentum CECT5716 enhances the effects of influenza vaccination. Nutrition, 23(3), 254-260.

Orozovic, G., Orozovic, K., Lennerstrand, J., & Olsen, B. (2011). Detection of resistance mutations to antivirals oseltamivir and zanamivir in avian influenza A viruses isolated from wild birds. PLoS ONE, 6(1), e16028.

Palese, P., & Shaw, M. L. (2007). Orthomyxoviridae: The viruses and their replication. In D. M. Knipe & P. M. Howley (Eds.), Fields Virology (5th ed., pp. 1647-1689). Philadelphia: Lippincott Williams & Wilkins.

Pan, Y., Xiao, L., Li, A. S., Zhang, X., Sirois, P., Zhang, J., & Li, K. (2013). Biological and biomedical applications of engineered nucleases. Molecular Biotechnology, 55(1), 54-62.

Park, K. J., Kwon, H. I., Song, M. S., Pascua, P. N., Baek, Y. H., Lee, J. H., Jang, H. L., Lim, J. Y., Mo, I. P., Moon, H. J., Kim, C. J., & Choi, Y. K. (2011). Rapid evolution of low-pathogenic H9N2 avian influenza viruses following poultry vaccination programmes. J Gen Virol, 92(Pt 1), 36-50.

Park, M. K., Ngo, V., Kwon, Y. M., Lee, Y. T., Yoo, S., Cho, Y. H., Hong, S. M., Hwang, H. S., Ko, E. J., Jung, Y. J., Moon, D. W., Jeong, E. J., Kim, M. C., Lee, Y. N., Jang, J. H., Oh, J. S., Kim, C. H., & Kang, S. M. (2013). Lactobacillus plantarum DK119 as a Probiotic Confers Protection against Influenza Virus by Modulating Innate Immunity. PLoS ONE, 8(10), e75368.

Parry, J. (2005). Use of antiviral drug in poultry is blamed for drug resistant strains of avian flu. BMJ, 331(7507), 10.

Patterson, J. A., & Burkholder, K. M. (2003). Application of prebiotics and probiotics in poultry production. Poult Sci, 82(4), 627-631.

Pavlovic, J., Zurcher, T., Haller, O., & Staeheli, P. (1990). Resistance to influenza virus and vesicular stomatitis virus conferred by expression of human MxA protein. J Virol, 64(7), 3370-3375.

Peiris, J. S., de Jong, M. D., & Guan, Y. (2007). Avian influenza virus (H5N1): a threat to human health. Clinical Microbiology Reviews, 20(2), 243-267.

Philippa, J. D., Munster, V. J., Bolhuis, H., Bestebroer, T. M., Schaftenaar, W., Beyer, W. E., Fouchier, R. A., Kuiken, T., & Osterhaus, A. D. (2005). Highly pathogenic avian influenza (H7N7): vaccination of zoo birds and transmission to non-poultry species. Vaccine, 23(50), 5743-5750.

Pleschka, S., Stein, M., Schoop, R., & Hudson, J. B. (2009). Anti-viral properties and mode of action of standardized Echinacea purpurea extract against highly pathogenic avian influenza virus (H5N1, H7N7) and swine-origin H1N1 (S-OIV). Virol J, 6, 197.

Poorbaghi, S. L., Dadras, H., Gheisari, H. R., Mosleh, N., Firouzi, S., & Roohallazadeh, H. (2013). Effects of Lactobacillus acidophilus and inulin on fecal viral shedding and immunization against H N Avian influenza virus. J Appl Microbiol.

Qu, H., Yang, L., Meng, S., Xu, L., Bi, Y., Jia, X., Li, J., Sun, L., & Liu, W. (2013). The differential antiviral activities of chicken interferon alpha (ChIFN-alpha) and ChIFN-beta are related to distinct interferon-stimulated gene expression. PLoS One, 8(3), e59307.

Qu, L. J., Li, X. Y., Xu, G. Y., Ning, Z. H., & Yang, N. (2009). Lower antibody response in chickens homozygous for the Mx resistant allele to avian influenza. Asian-Aust J Anim Sci, 22(4), 465 - 470.

Quan, F. S., Compans, R. W., Cho, Y. K., & Kang, S. M. (2007). Ginseng and Salviae herbs play a role as immune activators and modulate immune responses during influenza virus infection. Vaccine, 25(2), 272-282.

Rahman, M. M., Uyangaa, E., Han, Y. W., Kim, S. B., Kim, J. H., Choi, J. Y., & Eo, S. K. (2012). Oral co-administration of live attenuated Salmonella enterica serovar Typhimurium expressing chicken interferon-alpha and interleukin-18 enhances the *alleviation of clinical signs caused by respiratory infection with avian influenza virus H9N2. Veterinary Microbiology, 157(3-4), 448-455.*

Rahman, M. M., Uyangaa, E., Han, Y. W., Kim, S. B., Kim, J. H., Choi, J. Y., Yoo, D. J., Hong, J. T., Han, S. B., Kim, B., Kim, K., & Eo, S. K. (2011). *Oral administration of live attenuated Salmonella enterica serovar Typhimurium expressing chicken interferon-alpha alleviates clinical signs caused by respiratory infection with avian influenza virus H9N2. Veterinary Microbiology, 154(1-2), 140-151.*

Rajput, Z. I., Xiao, C. W., Hu, S. H., Arijo, A. G., & Soomro, N. M. (2007). *Improvement of the efficacy of influenza vaccination (H5N1) in chicken by using extract of Cochinchina momordica seed (ECMS). J Zhejiang Univ Sci B, 8(5), 331-337.*

Rashad, A. E., Shamroukh, A. H., Abdel-Megeid, R. E., Mostafa, A., Ali, M. A., & Banert, K. (2010a). *A facile synthesis and anti-avian influenza virus (H5N1) screening of some novel pyrazolopyrimidine nucleoside derivatives. Nucleosides, Nucleotides and Nucleic Acids, 29(11), 809-820.*

Rashad, A. E., Shamroukh, A. H., Abdel-Megeid, R. E., Mostafa, A., el-Shesheny, R., Kandeil, A., Ali, M. A., & Banert, K. (2010b). *Synthesis and screening of some novel fused thiophene and thienopyrimidine derivatives for anti-avian influenza virus (H5N1) activity. Eur J Med Chem, 45(11), 5251-5257.*

Rauw, F., Palya, V., Van Borm, S., Welby, S., Tatar-Kis, T., Gardin, Y., Dorsey, K. M., Aly, M. M., Hassan, M. K., Soliman, M. A., Lambrecht, B., & van den Berg, T. (2011). *Further evidence of antigenic drift and protective efficacy afforded by a recombinant HVT-H5 vaccine against challenge with two antigenically divergent Egyptian clade 2.2.1 HPAI H5N1 strains. Vaccine, 29(14), 2590-2600.*

Reemers, S. S., van Haarlem, D. A., Groot Koerkamp, M. J., & Vervelde, L. (2009). *Differential gene-expression and host-response profiles against avian influenza virus within the chicken lung due to anatomy and airflow. Journal of General Virology, 90(Pt 9), 2134-2146.*

Remacle, A. G., Shiryaev, S. A., Oh, E. S., Cieplak, P., Srinivasan, A., Wei, G., Liddington, R. C., Ratnikov, B. I., Parent, A., Desjardins, R., Day, R., Smith, J. W., Lebl, M., & Strongin, A. Y. (2008). *Substrate cleavage analysis of furin and related proprotein convertases. A comparative study. J Biol Chem, 283(30), 20897-20906.*

Reuter, A., Soubies, S., Hartle, S., Schusser, B., Kaspers, B., Staeheli, P., & Rubbenstroth, D. (2013). *Antiviral activity of interferon-lambda in chickens. J Virol.*

Rizzardini, G., Eskesen, D., Calder, P. C., Capetti, A., Jespersen, L., & Clerici, M. (2012). *Evaluation of the immune benefits of two probiotic strains Bifidobacterium animalis ssp. lactis, BB-12(R) and Lactobacillus paracasei ssp. paracasei, L. casei 431(R) in an influenza vaccination model: a randomised, double-blind, placebo-controlled study. Br J Nutr, 107(6), 876-884.*

Roberts, N. A. (2001). *Anti-influenza drugs and neuraminidase inhibitors. Prog Drug Res, Spec No, 35-77.*

Robinson, J. H., & Easterday, B. C. (1979). *Avian influenza virus infection of the immunosuppressed turkey. Am J Vet Res, 40(9), 1219-1222.*

Ruff, M. (1983). *Interferon-mediated development of influenza virus resistance in hybrids between Mx gene-bearing and control mouse embryo fibroblasts. J Gen Virol, 64 (Pt 6), 1291-1300.*

Rumschlag-Booms, E., & Rong, L. (2013). *Influenza a virus entry: implications in virulence and future therapeutics. Adv Virol, 2013, 121924.*

Russell, R. J., Kerry, P. S., Stevens, D. J., Steinhauer, D. A., Martin, S. R., Gamblin, S. J., & Skehel, J. J. (2008). *Structure of influenza hemagglutinin in complex with an inhibitor of membrane fusion. Proc Natl Acad Sci U S A, 105(46), 17736-17741.*

Safronetz, D., Rockx, B., Feldmann, F., Belisle, S. E., Palermo, R. E., Brining, D., Gardner, D., Proll, S. C., Marzi, A., Tsuda, Y., Lacasse, R. A., Kercher, L., York, A., Korth, M. J., Long, D., Rosenke, R., Shupert, W. L., Aranda, C. A., Mattoon, J. S., Kobasa, D., Kobinger, G., Li, Y., Taubenberger, J. K., Richt, J. A., Parnell, M., Ebihara, H., Kawaoka, Y., Katze, M. G., & Feldmann, H. (2011). *Pandemic swine-origin H1N1 influenza A virus isolates show heterogeneous virulence in macaques. J Virol, 85(3), 1214-1223.*

Salomon, R., Staeheli, P., Kochs, G., Yen, H. L., Franks, J., Rehg, J. E., Webster, R. G., & Hoffmann, E. (2007). *Mx1 gene protects mice against the highly lethal human H5N1 influenza virus. Cell Cycle, 6(19), 2417-2421.*

Samson, M., Pizzorno, A., Abed, Y., & Boivin, G. (2013). *Influenza virus resistance to neuraminidase inhibitors. Antiviral Res, 98(2), 174-185.*

Sarfati-Mizrahi, D., Lozano-Dubernard, B., Soto-Priante, E., Castro-Peralta, F., Flores-Castro, R., Loza-Rubio, E., & Gay-Gutierrez, M. (2010). Protective dose of a recombinant Newcastle disease LaSota-avian influenza virus H5 vaccine against H5N2 highly pathogenic avian influenza virus and velogenic viscerotropic Newcastle disease virus in broilers with high maternal antibody levels. Avian Diseases, 54(1 Suppl), 239-241.

Sarmento, L., Afonso, C. L., Estevez, C., Wasilenko, J., & Pantin-Jackwood, M. (2008). Differential host gene expression in cells infected with highly pathogenic H5N1 avian influenza viruses. Veterinary Immunology and Immunopathology, 125(3-4), 291-302.

Sartika, T., Sulandari, S., & Zein, M. S. (2011). Selection of Mx gene genotype as genetic marker for Avian Influenza resistance in Indonesian native chicken. BMC Proc, 5 Suppl 4, S37.

Savarino, A. (2005). Expanding the frontiers of existing antiviral drugs: possible effects of HIV-1 protease inhibitors against SARS and avian influenza. J Clin Virol, 34(3), 170-178.

Savill, N. J., St Rose, S. G., Keeling, M. J., & Woolhouse, M. E. (2006). Silent spread of H5N1 in vaccinated poultry. Nature, 442(7104), 757.

Sawasdee, K., Chaowasku, T., Lipipun, V., Dufat, T. H., Michel, S., & Likhitwitayawuid, K. (2013). Neolignans from leaves of Miliusa mollis. Fitoterapia, 85, 49-56.

Scholtissek, C., & Faulkner, G. P. (1979). Amantadine-resistant and -sensitive influenza A strains and recombinants. J Gen Virol, 44(3), 807-815.

Schumacher, B., Bernasconi, D., Schultz, U., & Staeheli, P. (1994). The chicken Mx promoter contains an ISRE motif and confers interferon inducibility to a reporter gene in chick and monkey cells. Virology, 203(1), 144-148.

Schusser, B., Reuter, A., von der Malsburg, A., Penski, N., Weigend, S., Kaspers, B., Staeheli, P., & Hartle, S. (2011). Mx is dispensable for interferon-mediated resistance of chicken cells against influenza A virus. J Virol, 85(16), 8307-8315.

Scott, B. B., & Lois, C. (2005). Generation of tissue-specific transgenic birds with lentiviral vectors. Proc Natl Acad Sci U S A, 102(45), 16443-16447.

Sekellick, M. J., Carra, S. A., Bowman, A., Hopkins, D. A., & Marcus, P. I. (2000). Transient resistance of influenza virus to interferon action attributed to random multiple packaging and activity of NS genes. J Interferon Cytokine Res, 20(11), 963-970.

Sekellick, M. J., Ferrandino, A. F., Hopkins, D. A., & Marcus, P. I. (1994). Chicken interferon gene: cloning, expression, and analysis. J Interferon Res, 14(2), 71-79.

Seo, B. J., Rather, I. A., Kumar, V. J., Choi, U. H., Moon, M. R., Lim, J. H., & Park, Y. H. (2012). Evaluation of Leuconostoc mesenteroides YML003 as a probiotic against low-pathogenic avian influenza (H9N2) virus in chickens. J Appl Microbiol.

Seyama, T., Ko, J. H., Ohe, M., Sasaoka, N., Okada, A., Gomi, H., Yoneda, A., Ueda, J., Nishibori, M., Okamoto, S., Maeda, Y., & Watanabe, T. (2006). Population research of genetic polymorphism at amino acid position 631 in chicken Mx protein with differential antiviral activity. Biochem Genet, 44(9-10), 437-448.

Shang, R.-f., Liang, J.-p., Na, Z.-y., Yang, H.-j., Lu, Y., Hua, L.-y., Guo, W.-z., Cui, Y., & Wang, L. (2010). In vivo inhibition of NAS preparation on H9N2 subtype AIV. Virologica Sinica, 25(2), 145-150.

Shaukat, T. M., Ashraf, M., Omer, M. O., Rasheed, M. A., Muhammad, K., Shaukat, T. M., Younus, M., & Shahzad, M. K. (2011). Comparative efficacy of various antiviral agents against avian influenza virus (Type H7N3/Pakistan/2003). Pakistan J. Zool, 43(5), 849-854.

Shen, X., Zhang, X., & Liu, S. (2013). Novel hemagglutinin-based influenza virus inhibitors. J Thorac Dis, 5(Suppl 2), S149-159.

Shin, W. J., Lee, K. H., Park, M. H., & Seong, B. L. (2010). Broad-spectrum antiviral effect of Agrimonia pilosa extract on influenza viruses. Microbiol Immunol, 54(1), 11-19.

Shobugawa, Y., Saito, R., Sato, I., Kawashima, T., Dapat, C., Dapat, I. C., Kondo, H., Suzuki, Y., Saito, K., & Suzuki, H. (2012). Clinical effectiveness of neuraminidase inhibitors--oseltamivir, zanamivir, laninamivir, and peramivir--for treatment of influenza A(H3N2) and A(H1N1)pdm09 infection: an observational study in the 2010-2011 influenza season in Japan. J Infect Chemother, 18(6), 858-864.

Sidwell, R. W., Bailey, K. W., Wong, M. H., Barnard, D. L., & Smee, D. F. (2005). In vitro and in vivo influenza virus-inhibitory effects of viramidine. Antiviral Res, 68(1), 10-17.

Sidwell, R. W., Barnard, D. L., Day, C. W., Smee, D. F., Bailey, K. W., Wong, M. H., Morrey, J. D., & Furuta, Y. (2007). Efficacy of orally administered T-705 on lethal avian influenza A (H5N1) virus infections in mice. Antimicrob Agents Chemother, 51(3), 845-851.

Sipress, A. (2005). Bird flu drug rendered useless. Washington Post, A01. Retrieved from http://www.washingtonpost.com/wpdyn/content/article/2005/06/17/AR2005061701214.html

Sironi, L., Williams, J. L., Moreno-Martin, A. M., Ramelli, P., Stella, A., Jianlin, H., Weigend, S., Lombardi, G., Cordioli, P., & Mariani, P. (2008). Susceptibility of different chicken lines to H7N1 highly pathogenic avian influenza virus and the role of Mx gene polymorphism coding amino acid position 631. Virology, 380(1), 152-156.

Sironi, L., Williams, J. L., Stella, A., Minozzi, G., Moreno, A., Ramelli, P., Han, J., Weigend, S., Wan, J., Lombardi, G., Cordioli, P., & Mariani, P. (2011). Genomic study of the response of chicken to highly pathogenic avian influenza virus. BMC Proc, 5 Suppl 4, S25.

Sleeman, K., Mishin, V. P., Deyde, V. M., Furuta, Y., Klimov, A. I., & Gubareva, L. V. (2010). In vitro antiviral activity of favipiravir (T-705) against drug-resistant influenza and 2009 A(H1N1) viruses. Antimicrob Agents Chemother, 54(6), 2517-2524.

Smee, D. F., Bailey, K. W., Wong, M. H., O'Keefe, B. R., Gustafson, K. R., Mishin, V. P., & Gubareva, L. V. (2008). Treatment of influenza A (H1N1) virus infections in mice and ferrets with cyanovirin-N. Antiviral Res, 80(3), 266-271.

Smee, D. F., Hurst, B. L., Egawa, H., Takahashi, K., Kadota, T., & Furuta, Y. (2009). Intracellular metabolism of favipiravir (T-705) in uninfected and influenza A (H5N1) virus-infected cells. J Antimicrob Chemother, 64(4), 741-746.

Smee, D. F., Hurst, B. L., Wong, M. H., Bailey, K. W., Tarbet, E. B., Morrey, J. D., & Furuta, Y. (2010). Effects of the combination of favipiravir (T-705) and oseltamivir on influenza A virus infections in mice. Antimicrob Agents Chemother, 54(1), 126-133.

Smee, D. F., Wandersee, M. K., Checketts, M. B., O'Keefe, B. R., Saucedo, C., Boyd, M. R., Mishin, V. P., & Gubareva, L. V. (2007). Influenza A (H1N1) virus resistance to cyanovirin-N arises naturally during adaptation to mice and by passage in cell culture in the presence of the inhibitor. Antivir Chem Chemother, 18(6), 317-327.

Smith, J. R. (2010). Oseltamivir in human avian influenza infection. Journal of Antimicrobial Chemotherapy, 65 Suppl 2, ii25-ii33.

Song, J. M., Lee, K. H., & Seong, B. L. (2005). Antiviral effect of catechins in green tea on influenza virus. Antiviral Res, 68(2), 66-74.

Song, L., Zhao, D. G., Wu, Y. J., & Li, Y. (2008). Transient expression of chicken alpha interferon gene in lettuce. J Zhejiang Univ Sci B, 9(5), 351-355.

Song, M. S., Cho, Y. H., Park, S. J., Pascua, P. N., Baek, Y. H., Kwon, H. I., Lee, O. J., Kong, B. W., Kim, H., Shin, E. C., Kim, C. J., & Choi, Y. K. (2013). Early regulation of viral infection reduces inflammation and rescues mx-positive mice from lethal avian influenza infection. American Journal of Pathology, 182(4), 1308-1321.

Sood, R., Swarup, D., Bhatia, S., Kulkarni, D. D., Dey, S., Saini, M., & Dubey, S. C. (2012). Antiviral activity of crude extracts of Eugenia jambolana Lam. against highly pathogenic avian influenza (H5N1) virus. Indian Journal of Experimental Biology, 50(3), 179-186.

Sorbello, A., Jones, S. C., Carter, W., Struble, K., Boucher, R., Truffa, M., Birnkrant, D., Gada, N., Camilli, S., Chan, I., Dallas, S., Scales, T., Kosko, R., Thompson, E., Goodman, J., Francis, H., & Dal Pan, G. (2012). Emergency use authorization for intravenous peramivir: evaluation of safety in the treatment of hospitalized patients infected with 2009 H1N1 influenza A virus. Clinical Infectious Diseases, 55(1), 1-7.

Spackman, E., & Swayne, D. E. (2013). Vaccination of gallinaceous poultry for H5N1 highly pathogenic avian influenza: current questions and new technology. Virus Res, 178(1), 121-132.

Sriwilaijaroen, N., Fukumoto, S., Kumagai, K., Hiramatsu, H., Odagiri, T., Tashiro, M., & Suzuki, Y. (2012). Antiviral effects of Psidium guajava Linn. (guava) tea on the growth of clinical isolated H1N1 viruses: Its role in viral hemagglutination and neuraminidase inhibition. Antiviral Res, 94(2), 139-146.

Staeheli, P., Haller, O., Boll, W., Lindenmann, J., & Weissmann, C. (1986). Mx protein: constitutive expression in 3T3 cells transformed with cloned Mx cDNA confers selective resistance to influenza virus. Cell, 44(1), 147-158.

Stewart, C. R., Bagnaud-Baule, A., Karpala, A. J., Lowther, S., Mohr, P. G., Wise, T. G., Lowenthal, J. W., & Bean, A. G. (2012). Toll-like receptor 7 ligands inhibit influenza A infection in chickens. J Interferon Cytokine Res, 32(1), 46-51.

Stram, Y., & Kuzntzova, L. (2006). Inhibition of viruses by RNA interference. Virus Genes, 32(3), 299-306.

Suarez, D. L. (2005). Overview of avian influenza DIVA test strategies. Biologicals, 33(4), 221-226.

Suarez, D. L., & Schultz-Cherry, S. (2000). Immunology of avian influenza virus: a review. Dev Comp Immunol, 24(2-3), 269-283.

Sugrue, R. J., Tan, B. H., Yeo, D. S., & Sutejo, R. (2008). Antiviral drugs for the control of pandemic influenza virus. Ann Acad Med Singapore, 37(6), 518-524.

Sui, H. Y., Zhao, G. Y., Huang, J. D., Jin, D. Y., Yuen, K. Y., & Zheng, B. J. (2009). Small interfering RNA targeting m2 gene induces effective and long term inhibition of influenza A virus replication. PLoS One, 4(5), e5671.

Sun, S., Cui, Z., Wang, J., & Wang, Z. (2009). Protective efficacy of vaccination against highly pathogenic avian influenza is dramatically suppressed by early infection of chickens with reticuloendotheliosis virus. Avian Pathology, 38(1), 31-34.

Sun, X. L. (2007). Recent anti-influenza strategies in multivalent sialyloligosaccharides and sialylmimetics approaches. Curr Med Chem, 14(21), 2304-2313.

Sundararajan, A., Ganapathy, R., Huan, L., Dunlap, J. R., Webby, R. J., Kotwal, G. J., & Sangster, M. Y. (2010). Influenza virus variation in susceptibility to inactivation by pomegranate polyphenols is determined by envelope glycoproteins. Antiviral Res, 88(1), 1-9.

Suzuki, H., Saitoh, H., Suzuki, T., & Takaku, H. (2009). Inhibition of influenza virus by baculovirus-mediated shRNA. Nucleic Acids Symp Ser (Oxf)(53), 287-288.

Suzuki, Y., Ito, T., Suzuki, T., Holland, R. E., Jr., Chambers, T. M., Kiso, M., Ishida, H., & Kawaoka, Y. (2000). Sialic acid species as a determinant of the host range of influenza A viruses. J Virol, 74(24), 11825-11831.

Swayne, D. E. (2009). Avian influenza vaccines and therapies for poultry. Comparative Immunology, Microbiology and Infectious Diseases, 32(4), 351-363.

Swayne, D. E. (2012a). Impact of vaccines and vaccination on global control of avian influenza. Avian Diseases, 56(4 Suppl), 818-828.

Swayne, D. E. (2012b). The role of vaccines and vaccination in high pathogenicity avian influenza control and eradication. Expert Review of Vaccines, 11(8), 877-880.

Swayne, D. E., & Kapczynski, D. (2008). Strategies and challenges for eliciting immunity against avian influenza virus in birds. Immunological Reviews, 225, 314-331.

Swayne, D. E., Pavade, G., Hamilton, K., Vallat, B., & Miyagishima, K. (2011). Assessment of national strategies for control of high-pathogenicity avian influenza and low-pathogenicity notifiable avian influenza in poultry, with emphasis on vaccines and vaccination. Revue Scientifique et Technique, Office International des Epizooties, 30(3), 839-870.

Swayne, D. E., Radin, M. J., Hoepf, T. M., & Slemons, R. D. (1994). Acute renal failure as the cause of death in chickens following intravenous inoculation with avian influenza virus A/chicken/Alabama/7395/75 (H4N8). Avian Dis, 38(1), 151-157.

Takahashi, K., Furuta, Y., Fukuda, Y., Kuno, M., Kamiyama, T., Kozaki, K., Nomura, N., Egawa, H., Minami, S., & Shiraki, K. (2003). In vitro and in vivo activities of T-705 and oseltamivir against influenza virus. Antivir Chem Chemother, 14(5), 235-241.

Takeda, S., Takeshita, M., Kikuchi, Y., Dashnyam, B., Kawahara, S., Yoshida, H., Watanabe, W., Muguruma, M., & Kurokawa, M. (2011). Efficacy of oral administration of heat-killed probiotics from Mongolian dairy products against influenza infection in mice: alleviation of influenza infection by its immunomodulatory activity through intestinal immunity. Int Immunopharmacol, 11(12), 1976-1983.

Tao, Z., Yang, Y., Shi, W., Xue, M., Yang, W., Song, Z., Yao, C., Yin, J., Shi, D., Zhang, Y., Cai, Y., Tong, C., & Yuan, Y. (2013). Complementary and alternative medicine is expected to make greater contribution in controlling the prevalence of influenza. Biosci Trends, 7(5), 253-256.

Thomas, C., Manin, T. B., Andriyasov, A. V., & Swayne, D. E. (2008). Limited susceptibility and lack of systemic infection by an H3N2 swine influenza virus in intranasally inoculated chickens. Avian Dis, 52(3), 498-501.

Thomas, M., Ge, Q., Lu, J. J., Klibanov, A. M., & Chen, J. (2005). Polycation-mediated delivery of siRNAs for prophylaxis and treatment of influenza virus infection. Expert Opin Biol Ther, 5(4), 495-505.

Tian, G., Zhang, S., Li, Y., Bu, Z., Liu, P., Zhou, J., Li, C., Shi, J., Yu, K., & Chen, H. (2005). *Protective efficacy in chickens, geese and ducks of an H5N1-inactivated vaccine developed by reverse genetics. Virology, 341(1), 153-162.*

Tolba, M. K., & Eskarous, J. K. (1959). *Response of some strains of Newcastle disease and fowl-plague viruses to two quinones. Arch Mikrobiol, 34, 325-332.*

Tompkins, S. M., Lo, C. Y., Tumpey, T. M., & Epstein, S. L. (2004). *Protection against lethal influenza virus challenge by RNA interference in vivo. Proc Natl Acad Sci U S A, 101(23), 8682-8686.*

Tong, S., Li, Y., Rivailler, P., Conrardy, C., Castillo, D. A., Chen, L. M., Recuenco, S., Ellison, J. A., Davis, C. T., York, I. A., Turmelle, A. S., Moran, D., Rogers, S., Shi, M., Tao, Y., Weil, M. R., Tang, K., Rowe, L. A., Sammons, S., Xu, X., Frace, M., Lindblade, K. A., Cox, N. J., Anderson, L. J., Rupprecht, C. E., & Donis, R. O. (2012). *A distinct lineage of influenza A virus from bats. Proceedings of the National Academy of Sciences of the United States of America, 109(11), 4269-4274.*

Tong, S., Zhu, X., Li, Y., Shi, M., Zhang, J., Bourgeois, M., Yang, H., Chen, X., Recuenco, S., Gomez, J., Chen, L. M., Johnson, A., Tao, Y., Dreyfus, C., Yu, W., McBride, R., Carney, P. J., Gilbert, A. T., Chang, J., Guo, Z., Davis, C. T., Paulson, J. C., Stevens, J., Rupprecht, C. E., Holmes, E. C., Wilson, I. A., & Donis, R. O. (2013). *New world bats harbor diverse influenza a viruses. PLoS Pathogens, 9(10), e1003657.*

Tosh, C., Murugkar, H. V., Nagarajan, S., Tripathi, S., Katare, M., Jain, R., Khandia, R., Syed, Z., Behera, P., Patil, S., Kulkarni, D. D., & Dubey, S. C. (2011). *Emergence of amantadine-resistant avian influenza H5N1 virus in India. Virus Genes, 42(1), 10-15.*

Triana-Baltzer, G. B., Babizki, M., Chan, M. C., Wong, A. C., Aschenbrenner, L. M., Campbell, E. R., Li, Q. X., Chan, R. W., Peiris, J. S., Nicholls, J. M., & Fang, F. (2010). *DAS181, a sialidase fusion protein, protects human airway epithelium against influenza virus infection: an in vitro pharmacodynamic analysis. J Antimicrob Chemother, 65(2), 275-284.*

Triana-Baltzer, G. B., Gubareva, L. V., Klimov, A. I., Wurtman, D. F., Moss, R. B., Hedlund, M., Larson, J. L., Belshe, R. B., & Fang, F. (2009). *Inhibition of neuraminidase inhibitor-resistant influenza virus by DAS181, a novel sialidase fusion protein. PLoS One, 4(11), e7838.*

Udommaneethanakit, T., Rungrotmongkol, T., Bren, U., Frecer, V., & Stanislav, M. (2009). *Dynamic behavior of avian influenza A virus neuraminidase subtype H5N1 in complex with oseltamivir, zanamivir, peramivir, and their phosphonate analogues. Journal of Chemical Information and Modeling, 49(10), 2323-2332.*

Verhelst, J., Parthoens, E., Schepens, B., Fiers, W., & Saelens, X. (2012). *Interferon-inducible protein Mx1 inhibits influenza virus by interfering with functional viral ribonucleoprotein complex assembly. J Virol, 86(24), 13445-13455.*

Wadhwa, R., Kaul, S. C., Miyagishi, M., & Taira, K. (2004). *Know-how of RNA interference and its applications in research and therapy. Mutat Res, 567(1), 71-84.*

Wainright, P. O., Perdue, M. L., Brugh, M., & Beard, C. W. (1991). *Amantadine resistance among hemagglutinin subtype 5 strains of avian influenza virus. Avian Dis, 35(1), 31-39.*

Waki, N., Yajima, N., Suganuma, H., Buddle, B. M., Luo, D., Heiser, A., & Zheng, T. (2014). *Oral administration of Lactobacillus brevis KB290 to mice alleviates clinical symptoms following influenza virus infection. Lett Appl Microbiol, 58(1), 87-93.*

Waldmann, M., Jirmann, R., Hoelscher, K., Wienke, M., Niemeyer, F. C., Rehders, D., & Meyer, B. (2014). *A nanomolar multivalent ligand as entry inhibitor of the hemagglutinin of avian influenza. J Am Chem Soc, 136(2), 783-788.*

Wang, J., Ma, C., Jo, H., Canturk, B., Fiorin, G., Pinto, L. H., Lamb, R. A., Klein, M. L., & DeGrado, W. F. (2013). *Discovery of novel dual inhibitors of the wild-type and the most prevalent drug-resistant mutant, S31N, of the M2 proton channel from influenza A virus. Journal of Medicinal Chemistry, 56(7), 2804-2812.*

Wang, X., Hinson, E. R., & Cresswell, P. (2007). *The interferon-inducible protein viperin inhibits influenza virus release by perturbing lipid rafts. Cell Host Microbe, 2(2), 96-105.*

Wang, X., Jia, W., & Zhao, A. (2006). *Anti-influenza agents from plants and traditional Chinese medicine. Phytother Res, 20(5), 335-341.*

Wang, Y., Brahmakshatriya, V., Lupiani, B., Reddy, S., Okimoto, R., Li, X., Chiang, H., & Zhou, H. (2012a). *Associations of chicken Mx1 polymorphism with antiviral responses in avian influenza virus infected embryos and broilers. Poultry Science, 91(12), 3019-3024.*

Wang, Z., Yu, Q., Gao, J., & Yang, Q. (2012b). *Mucosal and systemic immune responses induced by recombinant Lactobacillus spp. expressing the hemagglutinin of the avian influenza virus H5N1. Clinical and Vaccine Immunology, 19(2), 174-179.*

Ward, P., Small, I., Smith, J., Suter, P., & Dutkowski, R. (2005). Oseltamivir (Tamiflu) and its potential for use in the event of an influenza pandemic. J Antimicrob Chemother, 55 Suppl 1, i5-i21.

Watanabe, K., Fuse, T., Asano, I., Tsukahara, F., Maru, Y., Nagata, K., Kitazato, K., & Kobayashi, N. (2006). Identification of Hsc70 as an influenza virus matrix protein (M1) binding factor involved in the virus life cycle. FEBS Lett, 580(24), 5785-5790.

Watanabe, T. (2007). Polymorphisms of the chicken antiviral MX gene. Cytogenet Genome Res, 117(1-4), 370-375.

Webster, R. G., Bean, W. J., Gorman, O. T., Chambers, T. M., & Kawaoka, Y. (1992). Evolution and ecology of influenza A viruses. Microbiological Reviews, 56(1), 152-179.

Webster, R. G., Kawaoka, Y., & Bean, W. J. (1986). Vaccination as a strategy to reduce the emergence of amantadine- and rimantadine-resistant strains of A/Chick/Pennsylvania/83 (H5N2) influenza virus. J Antimicrob Chemother, 18 Suppl B, 157-164.

Webster, R. G., Kawaoka, Y., Bean, W. J., Beard, C. W., & Brugh, M. (1985). Chemotherapy and vaccination: a possible strategy for the control of highly virulent influenza virus. J Virol, 55(1), 173-176.

Wei, C., Liu, J., Yu, Z., Zhang, B., Gao, G., & Jiao, R. (2013a). TALEN or Cas9 - rapid, efficient and specific choices for genome modifications. J Genet Genomics, 40(6), 281-289.

Wei, L., Jiao, P., Yuan, R., Song, Y., Cui, P., Guo, X., Zheng, B., Jia, W., Qi, W., Ren, T., & Liao, M. (2013b). Goose Toll-like receptor 7 (TLR7), myeloid differentiation factor 88 (MyD88) and antiviral molecules involved in anti-H5N1 highly pathogenic avian influenza virus response. Veterinary Immunology and Immunopathology, 153(1-2), 99-106.

Wei, Q., Peng, G. Q., Jin, M. L., Zhu, Y. D., Zhou, H. B., Guo, H. Y., & Chen, H. C. (2006). [Cloning, prokaryotic expression of chicken interferon-alpha gene and study on antiviral effect of recombinant chicken interferon-alpha]. Sheng Wu Gong Cheng Xue Bao, 22(5), 737-743.

WHO. (2005). World Health Organisation: Use of antiviral drugs in poultry, a threat to their effectiveness for the treatment of human avian influenza http://www.who.int/foodsafety/micro/avian_antiviral/en/print.html. Retrieved from

Wong, J. P., Christopher, M. E., Viswanathan, S., Dai, X., Salazar, A. M., Sun, L. Q., & Wang, M. (2009a). Antiviral role of toll-like receptor-3 agonists against seasonal and avian influenza viruses. Current Pharmaceutical Design, 15(11), 1269-1274.

Wong, J. P., Christopher, M. E., Viswanathan, S., Karpoff, N., Dai, X., Das, D., Sun, L. Q., Wang, M., & Salazar, A. M. (2009b). Activation of toll-like receptor signaling pathway for protection against influenza virus infection. Vaccine, 27(25-26), 3481-3483.

Wu, Y., Li, J. Q., Kim, Y. J., Wu, J., Wang, Q., & Hao, Y. (2011). In vivo and in vitro antiviral effects of berberine on influenza virus. Chin J Integr Med, 17(6), 444-452.

Xia, C., Liu, J., Wu, Z. G., Lin, C. Y., & Wang, M. (2004). The interferon-alpha genes from three chicken lines and its effects on H9N2 influenza viruses. Anim Biotechnol, 15(1), 77-88.

Xie, Y., Gong, J., Li, M., Fang, H., & Xu, W. (2011). The medicinal potential of influenza virus surface proteins: hemagglutinin and neuraminidase. Curr Med Chem, 18(7), 1050-1066.

Xu, C., Meng, S., Liu, X., Sun, L., & Liu, W. (2010). Chicken cyclophilin A is an inhibitory factor to influenza virus replication. Virol J, 7(1), 372.

Yang, Z., Wang, Y., Zhong, S., Zhao, S., Zeng, X., Mo, Z., Qin, S., Guan, W., Li, C., & Zhong, N. (2012). In vitro inhibition of influenza virus infection by a crude extract from Isatis indigotica root resulting in the prevention of viral attachment. Mol Med Rep, 5(3), 793-799.

Yasui, H., Kiyoshima, J., & Hori, T. (2004). Reduction of influenza virus titer and protection against influenza virus infection in infant mice fed Lactobacillus casei Shirota. Clin Diagn Lab Immunol, 11(4), 675-679.

Yee, K. S., Carpenter, T. E., & Cardona, C. J. (2009). Epidemiology of H5N1 avian influenza. Comparative Immunology, Microbiology and Infectious Diseases, 32(4), 325-340.

Yen, H. L., Ilyushina, N. A., Salomon, R., Hoffmann, E., Webster, R. G., & Govorkova, E. A. (2007). Neuraminidase inhibitor-resistant recombinant A/Vietnam/1203/04 (H5N1) influenza viruses retain their replication efficiency and pathogenicity in vitro and in vivo. J Virol, 81(22), 12418-12426.

Yen, H. L., McKimm-Breschkin, J. L., Choy, K. T., Wong, D. D., Cheung, P. P., Zhou, J., Ng, I. H., Zhu, H., Webby, R. J., Guan, Y., Webster, R. G., & Peiris, J. S. (2013). Resistance to neuraminidase inhibitors conferred by an R292K mutation in a human influenza virus H7N9 isolate can be masked by a mixed R/K viral population. MBio, 4(4).

Yin, C. G., Zhang, C. S., Zhang, A. M., Qin, H. W., Wang, X. Q., Du, L. X., & Zhao, G. P. (2010). Expression analyses and antiviral properties of the Beijing-You and White Leghorn myxovirus resistance gene with different amino acids at position 631. Poult Sci, 89(10), 2259-2264.

Youn, H. N., Lee, Y. N., Lee, D. H., Park, J. K., Yuk, S. S., Lee, H. J., Yeo, J. M., Yang, S. Y., Lee, J. B., Park, S. Y., Choi, I. S., & Song, C. S. (2012). Effect of intranasal administration of Lactobacillus fermentum CJL-112 on horizontal transmission of influenza virus in chickens. Poult Sci, 91(10), 2517-2522.

Younan, M., Poh, M. K., Elassal, E., Davis, T., Rivailler, P., Balish, A. L., Simpson, N., Jones, J., Deyde, V., Loughlin, R., Perry, I., Gubareva, L., ElBadry, M. A., Truelove, S., Gaynor, A. M., Mohareb, E., Amin, M., Cornelius, C., Pimentel, G., Earhart, K., Naguib, A., Abdelghani, A. S., Refaey, S., Klimov, A. I., Donis, R. O., & Kandeel, A. (2013). Microevolution of highly pathogenic avian influenza A(H5N1) viruses isolated from humans, Egypt, 2007-2011. Emerg Infect Dis, 19(1), 43-50.

Zekarias, B., Ter Huurne, A. A., Landman, W. J., Rebel, J. M., Pol, J. M., & Gruys, E. (2002). Immunological basis of differences in disease resistance in the chicken. Vet Res, 33(2), 109-125.

Zhai, L., Li, Y., Wang, W., & Hu, S. (2011). Enhancement of humoral immune responses to inactivated Newcastle disease and avian influenza vaccines by oral administration of ginseng stem-and-leaf saponins in chickens. Poultry Science, 90(9), 1955-1959.

Zhang, H. (2009). DAS181 and H5N1 virus infection. J Infect Dis, 199(8), 1250, author reply 1250-1251.

Zhang, L., Cheng, Y. X., Liu, A. L., Wang, H. D., Wang, Y. L., & Du, G. H. (2010). Antioxidant, anti-inflammatory and anti-influenza properties of components from Chaenomeles speciosa. Molecules, 15(11), 8507-8517.

Zhang, W., Wang, C. Y., Yang, S. T., Qin, C., Hu, J. L., & Xia, X. Z. (2009). Inhibition of highly pathogenic avian influenza virus H5N1 replication by the small interfering RNA targeting polymerase A gene. Biochemical and Biophysical Research Communications, 390(3), 421-426.

Zhirnov, O. P., Klenk, H. D., & Wright, P. F. (2011). Aprotinin and similar protease inhibitors as drugs against influenza. Antiviral Res, 92(1), 27-36.

Zhirnov, O. P., Ovcharenko, A. V., & Bukrinskaya, A. G. (1982). Protective effect of protease inhibitors in influenza virus infected animals. Arch Virol, 73(3-4), 263-272.

Zhirnov, O. P., Ovcharenko, A. V., & Bukrinskaya, A. G. (1984). Suppression of influenza virus replication in infected mice by protease inhibitors. J Gen Virol, 65 (Pt 1), 191-196.

Zhou, H., Jin, M., Yu, Z., Xu, X., Peng, Y., Wu, H., Liu, J., Liu, H., Cao, S., & Chen, H. (2007). Effective small interfering RNAs targeting matrix and nucleocapsid protein gene inhibit influenza A virus replication in cells and mice. Antiviral Res, 76(2), 186-193.

Zhou, J. Y., Chen, J. G., Wang, J. Y., Wu, J. X., & Gong, H. (2005a). cDNA cloning and functional analysis of goose interleukin-2. Cytokine, 30(6), 328-338.

Zhou, J. Y., Wang, J. Y., Chen, J. G., Wu, J. X., Gong, H., Teng, Q. Y., Guo, J. Q., & Shen, H. G. (2005b). Cloning, in vitro expression and bioactivity of duck interleukin-2. Mol Immunol, 42(5), 589-598.

Zhou, K., He, H., Wu, Y., & Duan, M. (2008). RNA interference of avian influenza virus H5N1 by inhibiting viral mRNA with siRNA expression plasmids. Journal of Biotechnology, 135(2), 140-144.

Zu, M., Yang, F., Zhou, W., Liu, A., Du, G., & Zheng, L. (2012). In vitro anti-influenza virus and anti-inflammatory activities of theaflavin derivatives. Antiviral Res, 94(3), 217-224.

Survey and Molecular Analysis of *Babesia microti* Group Parasites in Japan: Strategy and Surveying for Identification of Tick Vectors

Aya Zamoto-Niikura, Masayoshi Tsuji, Rui Nakajima, Haruyuki Hirata,
Chiaki Ishihara, Qiang Wei, Shigeru Morikawa, Patricia J. Holman

1   Background

Babesia is a genus of protozoan parasites that infect erythrocytes and cause a hemolytic disease known as babesiosis. In nature *Babesia* parasites are transmitted to vertebrate animals by Ixodid ticks, then invade and asexually multiply in the erythrocytes of the host (Figure 1). *Babesia microti* (*B. microti* sensu stricto or *B. microti* U.S. lineage) is the most common causative agent of human babesiosis and its detailed life cycle is well documented (Hu & Hyland, 1997; Vannier & Krause, 2012). Since the first human case caused by *B. microti* was reported in the United States on Nantucket Island, Massachusetts in 1970, patients have been almost exclusively reported in the Northeastern and upper Midwestern United States (Vannier & Krause, 2012; Western *et al.*, 1970). There were about 850 confirmed human babesiosis cases in 2011 with 97% occurring in seven *B. microti*-endemic states - Connecticut, Massachusetts, Minnesota, New Jersey, New York, Rhode Island, and Wisconsin (CDC, 2012). More recently, a number of cases attributed to *B. microti* were reported involving international travelers from the United States (Holler *et al.*, 2013; Poisnel *et al.*, 2013; Ramharter *et al.*, 2010), and presumably locally acquired cases were reported in Germany and Australia (Hildebrandt *et al.*, 2007; Senanayake *et al.*, 2012). In China, a case of human babesiosis was attributed to a pathogen that at this time cannot be differentiated from *B. microti* (Saito-Ito *et al.*, 2008; Yao *et al.*, 2012). Moreover, serologic evidence suggests human exposure to *B. microti* or closely related species outside the United States as well (Foppa *et al.*, 2002; Hunfeld *et al.*, 2002; Meer-Scherrer *et al.*, 2004; Pancewicz *et al.*, 2011). Thus human babesiosis is increasingly recognized as an emerging disease.

In an endemic area, such as in the United States on Nantucket Island, Massachusetts, the ecology of *B. microti* has been well established by extensive epidemiological surveys (Piesman & Spielman, 1980; Spielman, 1976; Spielman *et al.*, 1981). The white-footed mouse (*Peromyscus leucopus*) and blacklegged tick (*Ixodes scapularis*; formerly *Ixodes dammini*) are the reservoir host and vector, respectively. The larval tick acquires *B. microti* from an infected mouse and, after molting, the nymphal tick transmits *B. microti* to the human. Coincidentally, the number of human cases increases during the months of May and October during which the nymphs are most active (CDC, 2012; Main *et al.*, 1982; Piesman *et al.*, 1987; Piesman &

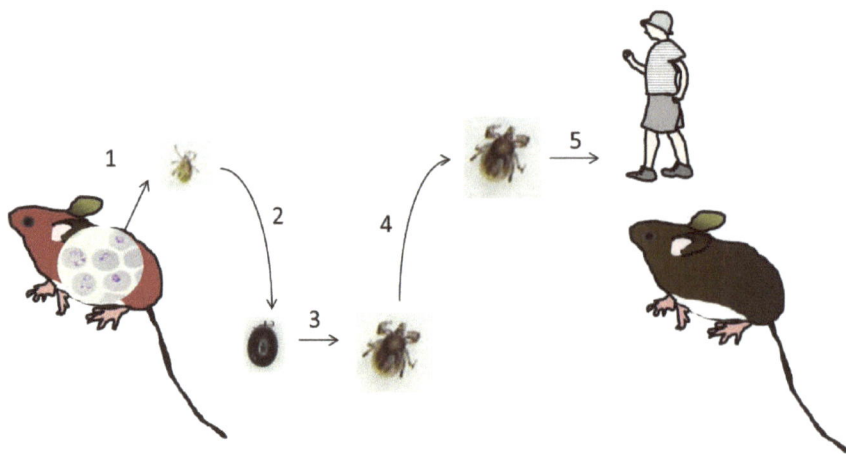

Figure 1: Life cycle of *Babesia microti* group parasites. 1. Larval or nymphal tick obtains *B. microti* by feeding on an infected reservoir. 2. Engorged tick detaches and drops to ground. 3. Tick molts into next stage (larva to nymph or nymph to adult which then overwinter in most cases) retaining *B. microti* in competent vector (transstadial transmission). 4. Tick matures and seeks host for feeding. 5. *B. microti* group parasites are transmitted to naïve reservoir host or human during feeding by infected tick.

Spielman, 1980, 1982; Spielman, 1976; Spielman *et al.*, 1981). The expanded distribution of adult vector ticks in association with the burgeoning deer population is often attributed to the increased incidence of cases. Deer aid in maintaining the tick populations, but are not competent hosts for *B. microti* (Vannier & Krause, 2009).

Another aspect of *Babesia* parasites as agents of emerging disease is that parasites closely related to *B. microti* or *Babesia divergens,* another main causative agent of human babesiosis, as well as novel species were increasingly discovered to infect humans in the last decade (Beattie *et al.*, 2002; Haselbarth *et al.*, 2007; Herwaldt *et al.*, 1996, 2003, 2004; Kim *et al.*, 2007; Persing *et al.*, 1995; Qi *et al.*, 2011; Quick *et al.*, 1993; Rios *et al.*, 2003; Shih *et al.*, 1997). In Japan, the first case occurred in 1999, and the *18S rRNA* gene sequence of the *Babesia* parasite (Kobe524; AB032434) isolated from the patient was closely related (99.2% identical in 1,767 base pair sequence) but distinguishable from that of *B. microti* (Gray and GI strains) in the United States (Saito-Ito *et al.*, 2000, referred as Kobe strain). Antibody cross-reactivity as examined by the indirect immunofluorescent-antibody (IFA) test and western blot analysis between these isolates was very low, demonstrating that Kobe strain is antigenically distinct from the *B. microti* (Saito-Ito *et al.*, 2000; Tsuji *et al.*, 2001). Furthermore, the reservoir host for indigenous human babesiosis in Japan was identified when parasites with the identical *18S rRNA* gene sequence were identified in blood from the rodent *Apodemus speciosus* (Wei *et al.*, 2001).

Extensive field and molecular surveys over the past 10 years have revealed that *B. microti* is a complex of genetically diverse parasites which is comprised of at least four distinct lineages - Kobe, U.S., Hobetsu, and Munich (Nakajima *et al.*, 2009; Tsuji *et al.*, 2001; Zamoto *et al.*, 2004a; Zamoto *et al.*, 2004b) (Figure 2). The Kobe and U.S. lineages include Kobe524 and *B. microti* sensu stricto GI and Gray strains (Figure 2), respectively.

Distribution of *B. microti* in Japan is unique in that as many as three lineages, (Kobe, U.S. and Hobetsu) of the *B. microti* group exist and have been detected from various rodents and/or shrews (Figure 3 and Table 1). Among them, the large Japanese field mouse, *A. specio-*

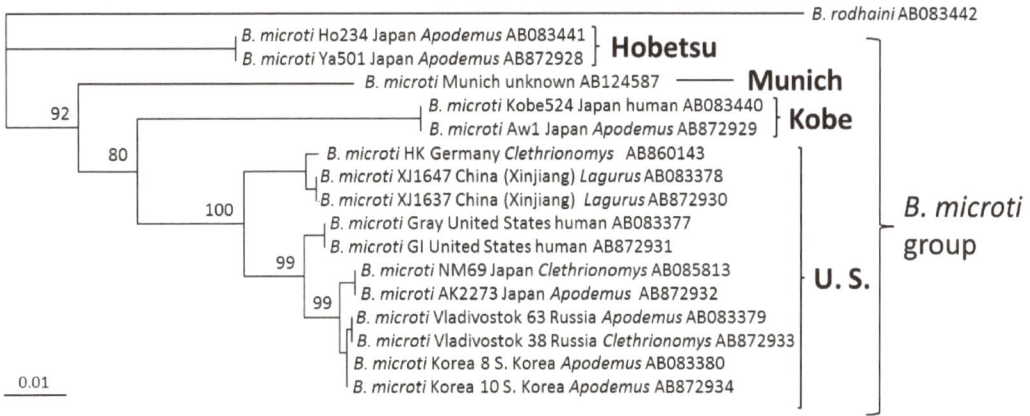

Figure 2: Neighbor joining phylogenetic tree of *Babesia microti* group parasites based on partial *β-tubulin* gene sequences (1,120 bp). Bootstrap support based on 1,000 replicates is shown at branch nodes. Accession numbers for the sequences are shown with each strain. Scale bar indicates number of nucleotide changes per site.

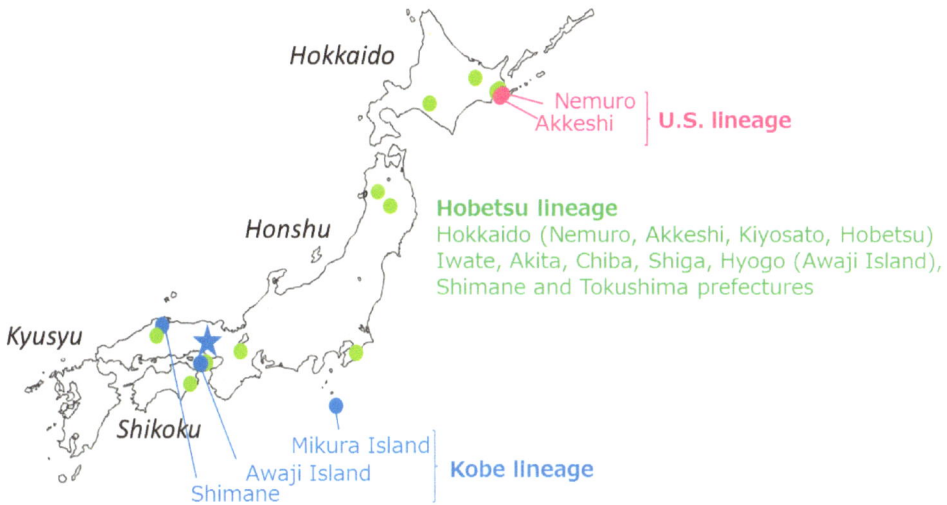

Figure 3: Distribution of hosts carrying *Babesia microti* group parasites in Japan. Reservoir (circles) and human (star) hosts in Japan infected by U.S. (pink), Hobetsu (green), and Kobe (blue) lineages of *B. microti* identified by molecular testing.

sus, which is a common rodent found only in Japan, harbors all three lineages with higher infection rates than found in other small animals. This suggests that *A. speciosus* is a main reservoir for parasites in the *B. microti* group. In contrast to the Kobe and Hobetsu lineages, which have been isolated exclusively in Japan, the U.S. and Munich lineages are widely distributed in rodents and shrews over Holarctic regions of the Eurasia and North America, and Europe, respectively (Table 1 and Figure 4). The U.S. lineage has been detected in both old and new world rodents, including *Apodemus, Myodes, Microtus, Lagurus, Sicista, Sigmodon,* and *Peromyscus,* and in *Sorex* shrews. Some rodent species and shrews are shared by different lineages. *Apodemus,* which is an old world rodent distributed in the Palearctic region, carries all

Country (area)	Host species (common name)	Babesia microti group					References
		U.S.	Hobetsu	Kobe	Munich	Unclassified	
Japan	*Apodemus speciosus* (mouse)[1]	1/204[2]	51/204	7/204			Zamoto et al. 2004a
	A. argenteus (mouse)[1]		1/51				Tsuji et al. 2001
	Myodes rufocanus (vole)[1]	1/25	3/25				Wei et al. 2001
	My. rutilus (vole)[1]	1/12	1/12				Tabara et al. 2007
	Microtus montebelli (vole)[1]		1/1				
	Sorex unguiculatus (shrew)[1]		1/7				
	So. caecutiens (shrew)[1]		1/2				
	Rattus sp. (rat)			1			Fujisawa et al. 2011
	Sciurus vulgaris orientis (squirrel)					1	Tsuji et al. 2006
	Macaca fuscata (macaque)					1	Hirata et al. 2011
South Korea	*A. agrarius* (mouse)	16/146					Zamoto et al. 2004b
	A. peninsulae (mouse)	1/2					
Russia (Vladivostok)	*A. peninsulae* (mouse)	1/32					Zamoto et al. 2004b
	My. rufocanus (vole)	1/4					
Xinjiang	*Lagurus luteus* (lemming)	2/3					Zamoto et al. 2004b
Russia (Novosibirsk region)	*My. rutilus* (vole)	5/50					Rar et al. 2011
	My. rufocanus (vole)	2/62					
	A. agrarius (mouse)	1/17					
	Microtus spp. (vole)	4/44					
	Sicista betulina (mouse)	1/35					
	So. araneus (shrew)	2/60					
Russia (Sverdlovsk region)	*My. rutilus* (vole)				41/99		Rar et al. 2011
	My. rufocanus (vole)				4/7		
	My. glareolus (vole)				14/37		
	Si. betulina (mouse)				1/1		
	So. araneus (shrew)				8/47		
	Sorex spp. (shrew)				4/5		
Slovenia	*My. glareolus* (vole)	11/69					Duh D et al. 2003
	A. flavicollis (mouse)	15/127					
Croatia	*My. glareolus* (vole)	1/33			1/33		Beck et al. 2011
	A. flavicollis (mouse)	5/37			1/37		
Poland	*Mi. arvalis* (vole)				38/53		Sinski et al. 2006
	Mi. oeconomus (vole)				2/5		
United States (Florida)	*Sigmodon hispidus* (rat)	21/31					Clark et al. 2012
United States (Maine)	*My. gapperi* (vole)	1/2					Goethert et al. 2003
	Blarina brevicauda (shrew)	1/1					

Table 1: Molecular detection and lineage classification of *Babesia microti* group DNA from various reservoir hosts. [1]Total numbers from 4 field surveys (Zamoto et al. 2004a, Tsuji et al. 2001, Wei et al. 2001, Tabara et al. 2007). [2]Number of positives isolated or detected/number of samples examined.

four lineages. *Myodes* rodents (former *Clethrionomys*), which are found in North America, Europe and Asia carry three lineages - U.S., Hobetsu, and Munich. *Sorex* shrews also carry the same three lineages. These observations suggest that there is no specific relationship between reservoir species and the *B. microti* group lineage, regardless of the typical geographical distribution of each lineage (Figures 3 and 4).

By sequencing the full length *18S rRNA* gene (approximately 1.6 kbp), four lineages, U.S., Hobetsu, Kobe and Munich, of the *B. microti* group can be identified by comparing nucleotide substitutions (Table 2) or constructing phylogenetic trees (Tsuji *et al.*, 2006). The *18S rRNA* gene has evolved slowly as evidenced by the estimated mutation rate of 0.85 to 2% in 100 million years in this gene from another apicomplexan, *Plasmodium* (Escalante & Ayala, 1995). If this is the case, 14 to 33 base pair changes would accumulate during 100 million years

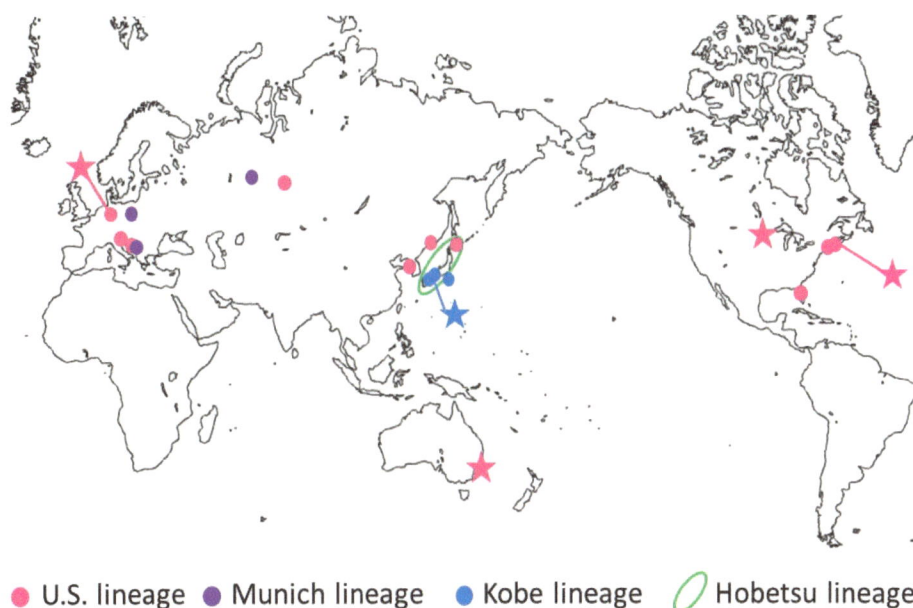

● U.S. lineage ● Munich lineage ● Kobe lineage ⬭ Hobetsu lineage

Figure 4: Global distribution of hosts with *Babesia microti* group parasites of confirmed lineage. Reservoir (circles) and human (star) origins of confirmed U.S. (pink), Munich (purple), Kobe (blue), and Hobetsu (green) lineages of *B. microti*.

Lineage	Reference strain	Gray	Ho234[1]	Kobe524	Munich	*B. rodhaini*
U.S.	Gray	100	91.6%	92.2%	91.8%	82.1%
		0	99	92	96	210
Hobetsu	Ho226[1]	99.3%	100	89.8%	91.0%	83.7%
		22	0	120	106	191
Kobe	Kobe524	99.2%	99.4%	100	89.2%	82.7%
		15	22	0	127	203
Munich	Munich	98.8%	98.5%	98.5%	100	82.1%
		22	26	26	0	210
Babesia rodhaini		96.1%	96.1%	96.0%	95.5%	100
		78	81	84	82	0

Table 2: *Babesia microti* group lineage *rRNA* (lower matrix, light color) and *β-tubulin* gene (upper matrix, dark color) comparisons as percentage identity (top value) and number of substitutions (bottom value). Partial *18S rRNA* genes were compared; 1,762 bp, Gray (AY693840); 1,763 bp, Ho226 (AB050732); 1,767 bp, Kobe524 (AB032434); 1,769 bp, Munich (AB071177); 1,750 bp, *B. rodhaini* (AB049999). Partial *β-tubulin* genes (*B. microti* group, 1,175 bp; *B. rodhaini*, 1,173 bp) were compared; Gray, AB083377; Ho234, AB083441; Kobe524, AB083440; Munich, AB124587; *B. rodhaini*, AB083442. *B. rodhaini* served as out group. [1]*rRNA* and *β-tubulin* gene sequences among isolates in Hobetsu lineage, including Ho234 and Ho226, are identical.

in the *B. microti 18S rRNA* gene. Although the order Piroplasmida is thought to be very ancient, perhaps instead it emerged as early as 550-600 million years ago (Nguyen *et al.*, 2007). Regardless, the high degree of *18S rRNA* gene sequence conservation would indicate that this is not an appropriate genetic marker to investigate further inter- and intra-group genetic variations in this species complex. In fact, there is more than 98% similarity between the *18S rRNA* gene sequences among the four lineages (Table 2).

The search for gene(s) which evolved more quickly than the *18S rRNA* gene and which might serve as a tool for population genetic research led to investigation of the *β-tubulin* gene (Goethert & Telford, 2003; Zamoto *et al.*, 2004b). The *β-tubulin* genes from the three different lineages (Hobetsu, Kobe and Munich) are similar in structure to the gene from *B. microti* Gray strain (U.S. lineage) (AB083377), where the gene is 1,651 bp in length and comprised of 3 exons and 2 small introns of 21 and 23 bp (Zamoto *et al.*, 2004b). *B. microti* strains from a single survey area in Japan and other areas are shown to have identical *β-tubulin* gene sequences, whereas numerous nucleotide substitutions exist among the four lineages (Tsuji *et al.*, 2006; Zamoto *et al.*, 2004b) (Figure 2, Table 2). There are 4 to 6 times as many differences in 1,175 bp of the *β-tubulin* gene as in 1,770 bp of *18S rRNA* gene (Table 2). In a phylogenetic tree based on the *β-tubulin* gene sequences (Figure 2), branching of each lineage is supported by strong bootstrap values (80-100% in 1,000 replicates). Furthermore, within the U.S. lineage, the *18S rRNA* sequences are identical, whereas 1 to 34 nucleotides of the *β-tubulin* gene are substituted between parasites from South Korea, Vladivostok, Japan, Xinjiang, Germany and United States (Table 3), indicating geographical variations within this lineage (Figure 2). It is obvious that the parasites which have long been designated "*B. microti*" are convincingly a genetically diverse group of parasites and that *β-tubulin* gene is a suitable gene to analyze inter- as well as intra-species variations (Goethert & Telford, 2003; Tsuji *et al.*, 2006; Zamoto *et al.*, 2004b). In the past decade, *β-tubulin* gene sequences from members of the *B. microti* group and closely related parasites have been accumulated in genetic data banks, and phylogenetic trees can be constructed using available sequences. As detailed above, the *B. microti* group is comprised of at least four named lineages, U.S., Kobe, Munich, and Hobetsu (Figure 5).

Sample ID (region)	No. of differences or % identity for:					
	Gray	Korea8	VL63	NM69	XJ1647	HK
Gray (U.S.A)	-	99.0	98.9	98.8	97.74	97.74
Korea8 (S. Korea)	11	-	99.9	99.6	97.1	97.1
VL63 (Vladivostok, Russia)	12	1	-	99.5	97.0	97.0
NM69 (Japan)	13	4	5	-	97.1	96.9
XJ1647 (Xinjiang, China)	25	32	33	32	-	99.6
HK (Germany)	25	32	33	34	4	-

Table 3: Percent identity (upper matrix, dark color) and number of nucleotide substitutions (lower matrix, light color) between *β-tubulin* sequences from *Babesia microti* U.S. lineage from different geographical regions. Accession numbers; Gray, AB083377; Korea8, AB083380; VL63, AB083379; NM69, AB085813; XJ1647, AB083378; HK, AB860143. Partial *β-tubulin* genes (1,105 bp) were compared.

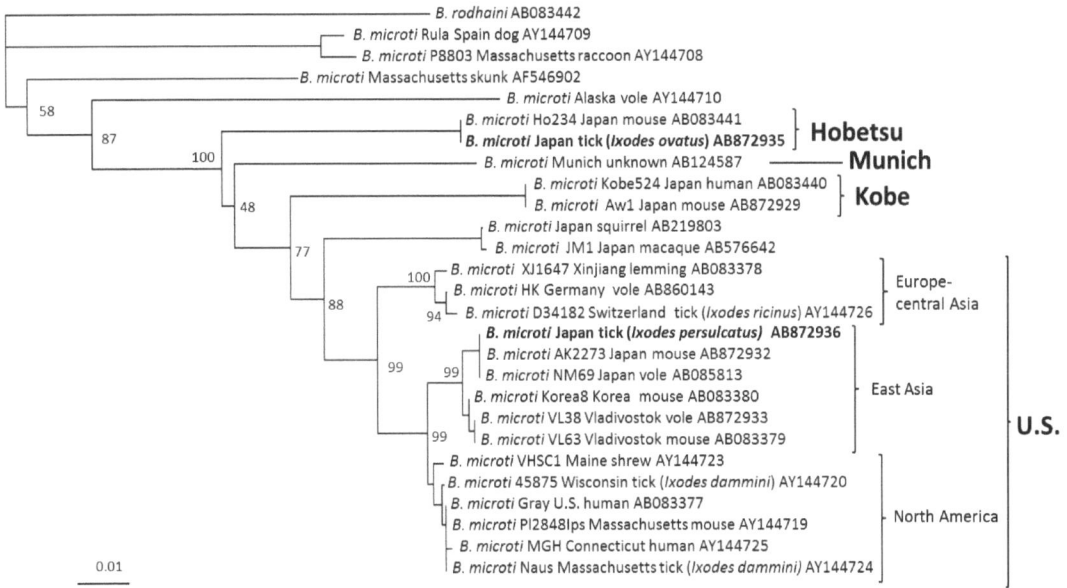

Figure 5: Neighbor joining phylogenetic tree of *Babesia microti* group parasites based on *β-tubulin* gene exons 2 and 3 (885 bp). Bootstrap support based on 1,000 replicates is shown at branch nodes. Accession numbers for the sequences are shown with each strain. Scale bar indicates number of nucleotide change per site. Sequences determined in this study are shown in bold font.

Additionally, unnamed lineages of parasites from squirrel (Tsuji *et al.*, 2006) and monkey (Hirata *et al.*, 2011) are phylogenetically placed between the U.S. and Kobe lineages. Outside of these lineages, *Babesia* isolates also named *B. microti* from the Alaskan vole, skunk, raccoon, and dog (clades 2 and 3 in Goethert & Telford, 2003) independently branch (Figure 5). The U.S. lineage is further divided into three sub-lineages, which are composed of parasites from Europe-central Asia (Europe and Xinjiang), East Asia (Japan, Korea and Vladivostok) and North America (the United States), indicating parasites in the U.S. lineage are genetically diverse in concordance with their geographical distribution.

2   Identification of *B. microti* Vector Tick in Japan

To investigate whether U.S., Hobetsu and Kobe *B. microti* lineages share tick vectors, and whether various tick species carry the parasites, we selected particular areas to survey. Furthermore, to investigate a large number of samples at the molecular level, a convenient and accurate classification-specific PCR system for the *B. microti* group lineages was developed and used for vector surveillance (Figures 7, 8 and Table 4) (Zamoto *et al.*, 2004b).

2.1   Selection of Survey Areas

Field surveys of reservoir hosts revealed that two different lineages co-exist in several areas of Japan (Figure 3) (Tsuji *et al.*, 2001; Wei *et al.*, 2001; Zamoto *et al.*, 2004a). At Nemuro, both U.S. and Hobetsu lineages were isolated from the vole *Myodes*, as either single or mixed infections.

On Awaji Island, Kobe and Hobetsu lineages were isolated from *A. speciosus*, but as single infections. On the basis of these findings, Awaji Island, Nemuro and surrounding areas were selected for surveying ticks. The survey areas were grouped based on geographical features (Figure 6): 1) Nemuro and adjacent areas in Hokkaido (eastern Hokkaido), which are surrounded by mountains of Hidaka and Ishikari, 2) other areas in Hokkaido outside of the mountains, and 3) Awaji Island. We then conducted surveys at 5 study sites in eastern Hokkaido including Nemuro, 9 study sites in the other areas in Hokkaido, and 1 site on Awaji Island, for a total of 15 study sites.

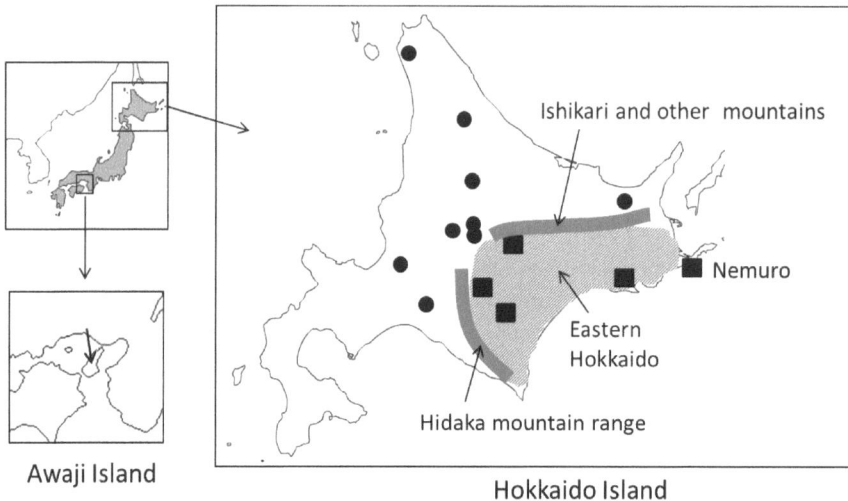

Figure 6: Survey areas of ticks in Japan. The study areas for tick collections are shown as squares in eastern Hokkaido (shaded in gray) and as circles in the other areas of Hokkaido Island. Awaji Island is also shown.

2.2   Detection of *B. microti* Group by Classification-specific PCR

Host seeking (questing) adult ticks were collected by flagging vegetation, on the premise that such ticks would not have taken in any blood infected with *B. microti* group since molting. To maximize the amount of DNA obtained from ticks, DNA extraction was performed by a standard phenol precipitation method. Briefly, ticks were homogenized and digested in TNE buffer containing 0.1% SDS and 10mg/ml proteinase K, then DNA was phenol extracted and ethanol precipitated (Zamoto-Niikura *et al.*, 2012). To detect *B. microti* group DNA, classification-specific PCR was performed as described below (see Figures 7 and 8) using pooled DNA, typically from 5 ticks. Because the tick DNA was pooled for testing, a minimum infection rate (MIR, %) was calculated by comparing the number of pools that were PCR positive to the total number of ticks examined. The calculation was based on the assumption that each PCR-positive pool contained at least one tick with a detectable *B. microti* group parasite(s). Thus the highest possible MIR should be 20%.

The sequence diversity observed in the *β-tubulin* genes among the four lineages enabled us to design 4 sets of specific nested PCR primers (Figure 7, Table 4), each of which annealed to lineage-specific sequences in variable regions of the gene (Zamoto *et al.*, 2004b). A nested PCR was utilized in which the first primer pair, BmTubu111F/BmTubu897R, was designed to

Primers	Oligonucleotide sequences (5'-3')	Purpose
BmTubu111F	GATTCCRGTAAGTAGTTMAACATTCAGAC	Universal 1st
BmTubu897R	CGRTCGAACATTTGTTGHGTCARTTC	Universal 1st
BmTubu93F	GAYAGYCCCTTRCAACTAGAAAGAGC	Universal nested
BmTubu782R	GGGAADGGDATRAGATTCACAGC	Universal nested
Tubu-US5'[1]	GCAAAYGTTTTYTATAACCAGTTTAGTG	U.S. specific, nested
Tubu-US3'[1]	GAAATGCAATCTCGGGAAGGTAATGA	U.S. specific, nested
Tubu-Ho5'[1]	AAGAGCTAACGTTTTTTACAATCTATCAAG	Hobetsu specific, nested
Tubu-Ho3'[1]	CGCAAATCCAATCATAAAAAAGTTTAGTC	Hobetsu specific, nested
Tubu-Ko5'[1]	CAAATGTTTTTTATAACCAGACGAGCG	Kobe specific, nested
Tubu-Ko3'[1]	GAAAGGAATAAGATTCACAGTGAGCT	Kobe specific, nested
Tubu-Mu5'[1]	CAGAGGGAGCG_AACTTATAGACACTGTG	Munich specific, nested
Tubu-Mu3'[1]	AGTTAAGGGCGCGAACCACGA	Munich specific, nested

Table 4. Oligonucleotide primers used for amplification of *β-tubulin* genes from *Babesia microti* group parasite. [1]A single base mismatch indicated by underline was introduced to enhance type specificity (Zamoto *et al.*, 2004b).

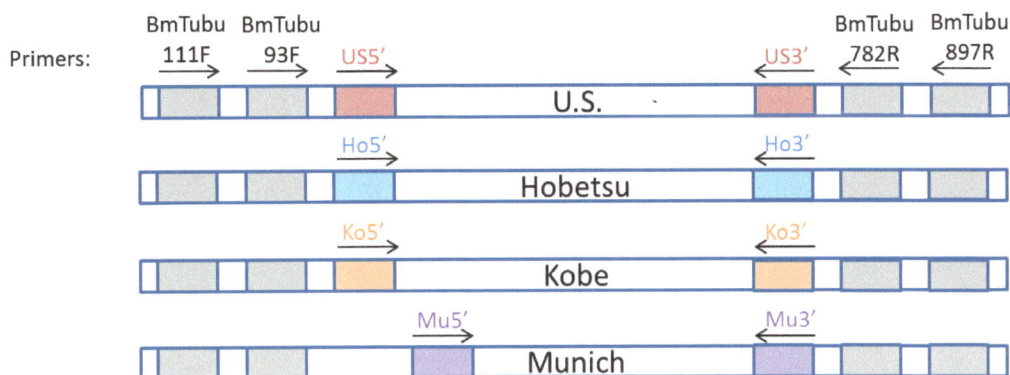

Figure 7: Schematic diagram of the *β-tubulin* gene primers used for the lineage classification-specific PCR system and RFLP for *Babesia microti* group parasites. Each bar represents the *β-tubulin* gene of one of the four *B. microti* lineages with boxes showing the annealing sites for the universal and specific primers as indicated. Conserved gene regions are shown in gray for the universal primary PCR primer pair BmTubu111F and BmTubu897R used for both classification-specific PCR and RFLP, and the universal nested primer pair BmTubu93F/BmTubu782R used for RFLP. The lineage specific primers, used in nested PCR of the primary products, are depicted in various colors.

anneal with conserved *β-tubulin* gene regions and amplify the gene from any lineage. Nested primers specific for each lineage, Tubu-US5' and -US3', Tubu-Ho5' and -Ho3', Tubu-Ko5' and -Ko3', and Tubu-Mu5' and -Mu3' (Table 4, Figure 7), were designed to anneal with variable regions and specifically amplify only the specified lineage. Therefore, PCR amplicons were observed only when the specific primers matched the corresponding lineages (Figure 8A).

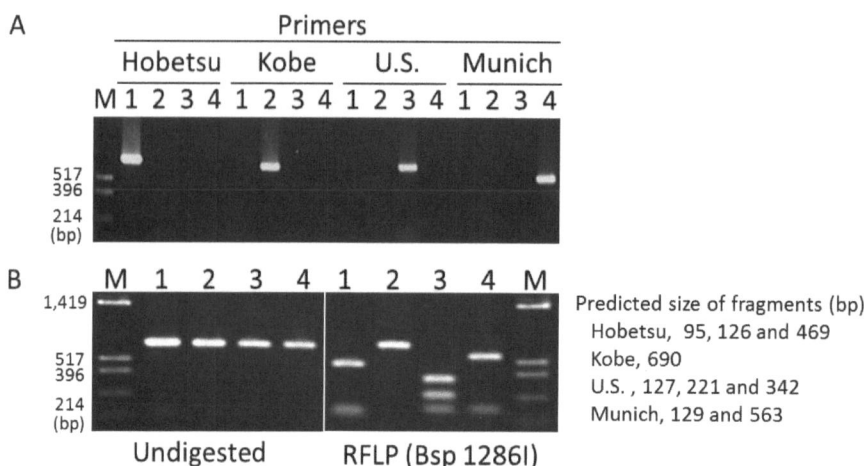

Figure 8: Classification-specific nested PCR (A) and RFLP (B) targeting *β-tubulin* genes of Hobetsu, Kobe, U.S., and Munich lineage parasites. Lanes: 1, Hobetsu lineage (Ho234 strain); 2, Kobe lineage (Kobe524 strain); 3, U.S. lineage (Gray strain); 4, Munich lineage (Munich strain); M, DNA size markers.

To further confirm the lineage identified by PCR, a restriction fragment length polymorphism assay (RFLP) was also designed. Primary PCR was performed with the universal primers BmTubu111F/BmTubu897R, and then nested PCR using the primers BmTubu93F/BmTubu782R (Figures 7 and 8B, left), which were also designed to amplify all lineages, was performed. These nested PCR products were subjected to digestion with the restriction enzyme Bsp1286I. Classification as to lineage was then made based on specific length and number of fragments that characterized each lineage (Figure 8B, right).

In our field survey, *Ixodes persulcatus*, *I. ovatus* (Figure 9A and B) and *Haemaphysalis flava* were predominantly collected. Results obtained from this and previous studies (Zamoto-Niikura *et al.*, 2012) by using specific PCR are summarized in Table 5. In eastern Hokkaido, of 546 *I. persulcatus* examined, 18 pools were positive for *B. microti* group DNA and were all classified into the U.S. lineage. *I. persulcatus* carrying *B. microti* were distributed in all 4 study sites in eastern Hokkaido where minimum infection rates (MIR) ranged from 1.4 to 6.5%. In the same study sites, 285 *I. ovatus* ticks were examined and 13 pools of these from 3 sites were found positive for *B. microti* that was classified as Hobetsu lineage. The MIR of *I. ovatus* carrying Hobetsu lineage ranged from 4.3 to 8.3%.

In the other areas of Hokkaido, Hobetsu lineage was also detected in *I. ovatus* collected at 4 of 9 study sites, with an MIR ranging from 2.0 to 12.3% (Zamoto-Niikura *et al.*, 2012). However, in contrast to the findings in eastern Hokkaido, the U.S. lineage was not detected in any ticks examined even though 481 *I. persulcatus* were tested. Furthermore, although the 481 *I. persulcatus* samples included 200 that were collected at the study sites where *I. ovatus* carrying the Hobetsu lineage were detected, they were negative for this lineage as well. Thus, the results from the survey in Hokkaido strongly indicated specific lineage-tick relationship in nature where U.S. and Hobetsu lineages were independently carried by *I. persulcatus* and *I. ovatus*, respectively. Because the U.S. lineage was isolated from rodents only in Nemuro and Akkeshi (Figure 3), the lineage was thought to be restricted to the east end of Hokkaido. The

				Babesia microti group					
Species	**Area**		**N**	**U.S.**	**(MIR)**[1]	**Hobetsu**	**(MIR)**	**Kobe**	**(MIR)**
I. persulca-	Hokkaido	eastern [2]	546	18	(3.3%)[3]	0	-	0	-
tus		others[4]	481	0	-	0	-	0	-
	Awaji Island		0	0	-	0	-	0	-
I. ovatus	Hokkaido	eastern[2]	285	0	-	13	(4.6%)[5]	0	-
		others[4]	609	0	-	23	(3.7%)[6]	0	-
	Awaji Island		180	0	-	11	(6.1%)	0	-
H. flava	Hokkaido	others[4]	27	0	-	0	-	0	-
	Awaji Island		897	0	-	0	-	0	-

Table 5: Detection of *Babesia microti* group parasites from field collected adult *Ixodes persulcatus, I. ovatus,* and *Haemaphysalis flava* ticks. [1]Minimum infection rate. [2]Five areas are included. [3]U.S. lineages in *I. persulcatus* were detected in 4 study sites with MIR of 1.4-6.5%. [4]Nine areas included. [5]Hobetsu lineage in *I. ovatus* was detected in 3 areas with MIR of 4.3-8.3%. [6]Hobetsu lineage in *I. ovatus* was detected in 4 areas with MIR of 2.0-12.3%.

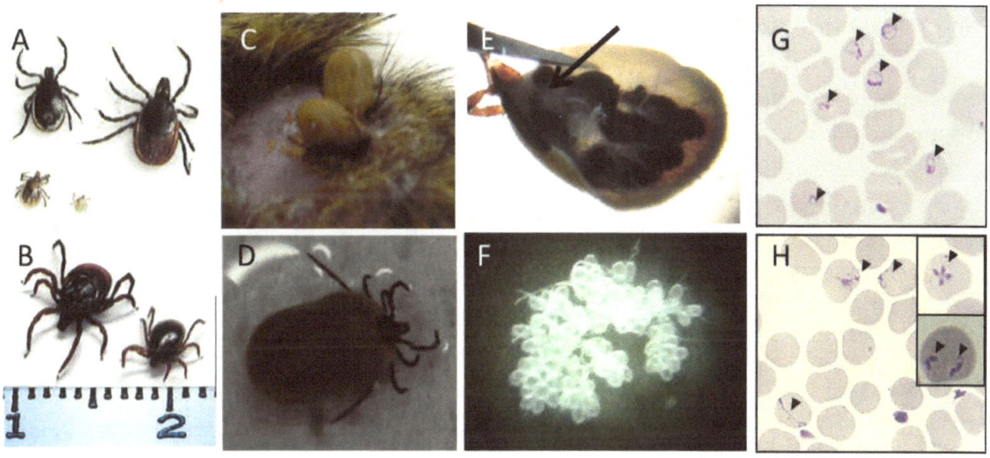

Figure 9: Ticks, salivary glands, and parasite isolation. (A) All stages of *Ixodes persulcatus* - adult male (upper left), adult female (upper right), nymph (bottom left) and larva (bottom right). (B) *Ixodes ovatus* adult female (left) and adult male (right). (C) Partially engorged *I. persulcatus* attached to gerbil at 4 days of feeding. (D) Partially engorged *I. persulcatus* removed from gerbil. (E) *I. persulcatus* salivary glands *in situ* in tick horizontally bisected. (F) Salivary glands dissected from *I. persulcatus*. (G) Giemsa-stained blood film of *Babesia microti* U.S. lineage isolated via hamster inoculation from *I. persulcatus* female collected in Hokkaido, Japan. (H) Giemsa-stained blood film of *B. microti* Hobetsu lineage isolated via hamster inoculation from *I. ovatus* female collected in Hokkaido, Japan.

results of our present epidemiological studies, however, indicate that the U.S. lineage is distributed more widely over the eastern Pacific coast than previously thought.

On Awaji Island, where the Kobe and Hobetsu lineages were isolated from *A. speciosus* rodents, *I. ovatus* and *H. flava* were predominantly collected at the same spots where the rodents were captured (Wei *et al.*, 2001). Of 180 *I. ovatus* examined, 11 pools were positive for *B. microti* group and classified to be exclusively of the Hobetsu lineage. No positive signal for *B.*

microti was found in *H. flava*. The 2 main tick species tested, *I. ovatus* and *H. flava*, were nega-tive for the Kobe lineage suggesting there is possibly another tick vector involved. *I. persulca-tus*, which is identified to be a vector of U.S. lineage above, does not occur in the western part of Japan including Awaji Island, or on Mikura Island and Shimane where parasites of Kobe lineage were isolated from rodents (Fujisawa *et al.*, 2011; Tabara *et al.*, 2007). Therefore *I. per-sulcatus* also should not be involved as a vector for Kobe lineage.

In summary, by collecting ticks in selected areas and performing specific PCR, we demonstrated that the U.S. and Hobetsu lineages were independently carried by *I. persulcatus* and *I. ovatus*, respectively, in nature. However, no tick vector was identified for the Kobe line-age in this study. The Kobe is possibly vectored by tick species other than *I. ovatus* and *I. per-sulcatus*.

2.3   Isolation of Parasites from Salivary Glands

PCR examination revealed that *I. persulcatus* and *I. ovatus* carried U.S. and Hobetsu lineages, respectively. The vector competency of ticks may be demonstrated experimentally by showing the presence of infectious parasites biologically active to a naïve host in the tick salivary glands. The isolation of the U.S. and Hobetsu lineages was performed by using a susceptible laboratory animal, the hamster (Figure 9). We collected both male and female adult *I. persulca-tus* and *I. ovatus* (Figure 9A and B) in highly endemic sites. The male ticks were used to derive an infection rate that was then used to estimate a rate for the females. Females collected at sites where males were found with high infection rates were then used for isolation in hamsters following the method shown in Figure 9 (Zamoto-Niikura *et al.*, 2012).

I. persulcatus (Figure 9A) or *I. ovatus* (Figure 9B) adult female ticks were fed on a gerbil for 3 or 4 days (Figure 9C) to activate the parasites in the salivary glands to the infectious state, then removed manually (Figure 9D). The salivary glands were dissected from the tick under light microscopy (Figure 9E and F) and homogenized in phosphate buffered saline. A portion of the homogenate was subjected to DNA extraction and PCR to check for the presence of *B. microti* group DNA. The remaining homogenate was injected intraperitoneally into a hamster. The hamster was monitored every 2 or 3 days for appearance of the parasite in erythrocytes by microscopic examination of stained blood smears.

Three U.S. strains and two Hobetsu strains, as identified by classification-specific PCR, from adult *I. persulcatus* and *I. ovatus*, respectively, were successfully isolated in hamsters (Figure 9G and H). Intraerythrocytic parasites were detected at a parasitemia of 0.05% 19 to 24 days after inoculation for both lineages. Sequencing of *CCT7* and *β-tubulin* genes of the ham-ster-isolated parasites showed that the U.S. and Hobetsu lineages originating from *I. persulca-tus* and *I. ovatus*, respectively, were genetically identical to the parasite sequences found in the reservoir hosts, *A. speciosus* (Figure 5). The results from these field survey and parasite isola-tion studies strongly suggest that the U.S. and Hobetsu lineage life cycles are maintained by various rodent species and specific vector ticks, *I. persulcatus* and *I. ovatus*, respectively.

3   Conclusions

We have shown that the U.S., Hobetsu and Kobe lineages in the *B. microti* group in Japan are vectored by different vector ticks, *I. persulcatus*, *I. ovatus*, and other as yet unidentified tick spe-cies, respectively. This was achieved by conducting a carefully designed survey and utilizing the classification specific PCR system for parasite identification. The significant biological finding strongly correlates with genetic and antigenic distinction, as well as geographical distribution to some extent, of the *B. microti* group (Wei *et al.*, 2001; Nakajima *et al.*, 2009; Tsuji *et al.*, 2001; Zamoto *et al.*, 2004a; Zamoto *et al.*, 2004b).

I. persulcatus is distributed in Russia and northeastern Asia, including the eastern half of Japan, where parasites of East Asia sub-lineage were detected (Figure 5), indicating *I. persulcatus* specifically carries parasites in this sub-lineage. Interestingly, Europe-central Asian, North American, and the East Asian sub-lineages are each mainly vectored by single tick species, *I. ricinus*, *I. scapularis* (*I. dammini*) and *I. persulcatus*, respectively, but are carried in various mammalian hosts (Figure 5). Genetically *I. ricinus*, *I. persulcatus* and *I. scapularis* are closely related, and are designated the *I. ricinus* species complex (Xu *et al.*, 2003). While ticks belonging to this complex are distributed over Holarctic and Arctic zones, each species has common distribution pattern. Because the geographical distributions of *I. ricinus*, *I. persulcatus* and *I. dammini* overlap those of *B. microti* parasites in Europe-central Asia, East Asia, and North America, respectively, it is speculated that ancestors of the U.S. lineage and *I. ricinus* complex were associated and recently co-evolved with geographical expansion over the northern hemisphere. Further studies should provide the population size of the gene pools for each lineage of the *B. microti* group, each of which may have different level of efficiency in transmission by vector ticks. Consequently, significance of the co-evolutionary scenario and parasite-vector interactions will be evaluated.

I. ovatus is distributed in the Far East Asia including throughout Japan. Geographically wide distribution of the Hobetsu lineage over the country appears to be attributable to the large population of its vector tick, *I. ovatus*. To date, this lineage has not been found outside of Japan. More extensive surveys in Far East Asia will elucidate whether the Hobetsu lineage is only endemic to Japan. Since inapparent infection in humans has been reported (Arai *et al.*, 2003), and *I. ovatus* as well as *I. persulcatus* feed on people, it is important to reveal endemic areas in order to estimate the risk of acquiring infection and bring this information to the attention of health workers.

In a previous report, we speculated that the observed low infection rate of U.S. lineage in *I. persulcatus* might be relevant to weak transmission competency of the tick as a vector and extremely narrow distribution of the lineage in Nemuro (Zamoto-Niikura *et al.*, 2012). However, in this study infection rates of the U.S. lineage in vector ticks were comparable to those of Hobetsu lineage which is distributed over the country. The exact reason why the U.S. lineage is confined to eastern Hokkaido is still unclear. One possible reason may be the lineage entered Hokkaido Island from the Eurasian Continent, which had been connected with Hokkaido until approximately ten thousand years ago, and has remained confined to the area. Another reason may be the lineage was imported to a location in eastern Hokkaido and expanded its distribution in that area. It will be interesting to monitor whether the lineage crosses the mountains and emerges into another region of Hokkaido. This seems likely to occur in the near future because wild Sika deer, the main host for adult *I. persulcatus*, have become overabundant. Although the deer does not serve as a reservoir for *B. microti*, its availability supports the tick population.

Authors

Aya Zamoto-Niikura
Division of Experimental Animal Diseases, National Institute of Infectious Diseases, Japan

Masayoshi Tsuji, Rui Nakajima, Haruyuki Hirata, Chiaki Ishihara
School of Veterinary Medicine, Rakuno-Gakuen University, Japan

Qiang Wei
Institute of Laboratory Animal Science, Chinese Academy of Medical Sciences & Peking Union Medical College, China

Shigeru Morikawa
Department of Veterinary Science, National Institute of Infectious Diseases, Japan

Patricia J. Holman
Department of Veterinary Pathobiology, College of Veterinary Medicine and Biomedical Sciences, Texas A&M University, U.S.A.

Acknowledgement

We acknowledge the late Professor Masayoshi Tsuji for his seminal contributions to this research. Dr. Tsuji, who departed on December 19, 2006, provided the guidance and advice for the demarcation of the *B. microti*-group and improvement of methodology. Financial support for this study was provided in part by Grants-in-Aid from the Ministry of Education, Science and Culture of Japan, by a Health Science Grants for Research in Emerging and Re-emerging Infectious Diseases from the Ministry of health, Labor and Welfare of Japan (H25-Shinko-Ippan-008 and H25-Shinko-Shitei-009) and by Research Program on Emerging and Re-emerging Infectious Diseases (40101906) . The authors report no conflicts of interest.

References

Arai, S., Tsuji, M., Kaiho, I., Murayama, H., Zamoto, A., Wei, Q., Okabe, N., Kamiyama, T., & Ishihara, C. (2003). *Retrospective seroepidemiological survey for human babesiosis in an area in Japan where a tick-borne disease is endemic. J Vet Med Sci, 65, 335-340*

Beattie, J. F., Michelson, M. L., & Holman, P. J. (2002). *Acute babesiosis caused by Babesia divergens in a resident of Kentucky. N Engl J Med, 347, 697-698*

Beck, R., Vojta, L., Curkovic, S., Mrljak, V., Margaletic, J., & Habrun, B. (2011). *Molecular survey of Babesia microti in wild rodents in central Croatia. Vector Borne Zoonotic Dis, 11, 81-83*

Centers for Disease Control and Prevention (CDC). (2012). *Babesiosis surveillance – 18 states, 2011. MMWR Morb Mortal Wkly Rep. 61:505–509*

Clark, K., Savick, K., & Butler, J. (2012). *Babesia microti in rodents and raccoons from northeast Florida. J Parasitol, 98, 1117-1121*

Duh, D., Petrovec, M., Trilar, T., & Avsic-Zupanc, T. (2003). *The molecular evidence of Babesia microti infection in small mammals collected in Slovenia. Parasitology, 126,* 113-117

Escalante, A. A. & Ayala, F. J. (1995). *Evolutionary origin of Plasmodium and other Apicomplexa based on rRNA genes. Proc Natl Acad Sci USA, 92,* 5793-5797

Foppa, I. M., Krause, P. J., Spielman, A., Goethert, H., Gern, L., Brand, B., & Telford, S. R., 3rd. (2002). *Entomologic and serologic evidence of zoonotic transmission of Babesia microti, eastern Switzerland. Emerg Infect Dis, 8,* 722-726

Fujisawa, K., Nakajima, R., Jinnai, M., Hirata, H., Zamoto-Niikura, A., Kawabuchi-Kurata, T., Arai, S., & Ishihara, C. (2011). *Intron sequences from the CCT7 gene exhibit diverse evolutionary histories among the four lineages within the Babesia microti-group, a genetically related species complex that includes human pathogens. Jpn J Infect Dis, 64,* 403-410

Goethert, H. K., Lubelcyzk, C., LaCombe, E., Holman, M., Rand, P., Smith, R. P., Jr., & Telford, S. R., 3rd. (2003). *Enzootic Babesia microti in Maine. J Parasitol, 89,* 1069-1071

Goethert, H. K., & Telford, S. R., 3rd. (2003). *What is Babesia microti? Parasitology, 127,* 301-309

Haselbarth, K., Tenter, A. M., Brade, V., Krieger, G., & Hunfeld, K. P. (2007). *First case of human babesiosis in Germany - Clinical presentation and molecular characterisation of the pathogen. Int J Med Microbiol, 297,* 197-204

Herwaldt, B., Persing, D. H., Precigout, E. A., Goff, W. L., Mathiesen, D. A., Taylor, P. W., Eberhard, M. L., & Gorenflot, A. F. (1996). *A fatal case of babesiosis in Missouri: identification of another piroplasm that infects humans. Ann Intern Med, 124,* 643-650

Herwaldt, B. L., Caccio, S., Gherlinzoni, F., Aspock, H., Slemenda, S. B., Piccaluga, P., Martinelli, G., Edelhofer, R., Hollenstein, U., Poletti, G., Pampiglione, S., Loschenberger, K., Tura, S., & Pieniazek, N. J. (2003). *Molecular characterization of a non-Babesia divergens organism causing zoonotic babesiosis in Europe. Emerg Infect Dis, 9,* 942-948

Herwaldt, B. L., de Bruyn, G., Pieniazek, N. J., Homer, M., Lofy, K. H., Slemenda, S. B., Fritsche, T. R., Persing, D. H., & Limaye, A. P. (2004). *Babesia divergens-like infection, Washington State. Emerg Infect Dis, 10,* 622-629

Hirata, H., Kawai, S., Maeda, M., Jinnai, M., Fujisawa, K., Katakai, Y., Hikosaka, K., Tanabe, K., Yasutomi, Y., & Ishihara, C. (2011). *Identification and phylogenetic analysis of Japanese Macaque Babesia-1 (JM-1) detected from a Japanese Macaque (Macaca fuscata fuscata). Am J Trop Med Hyg, 85,* 635-638

Hildebrandt, A., Hunfeld, K. P., Baier, M., Krumbholz, A., Sachse, S., Lorenzen, T., Kiehntopf, M., Fricke, H. J., & Straube, E. (2007). *First confirmed autochthonous case of human Babesia microti infection in Europe. Eur J Clin Microbiol Infect Dis, 26,* 595-601

Holler, J. G., Roser, D., Nielsen, H. V., Eickhardt, S., Chen, M., Lester, A., Bang, D., Frandsen, C., & David, K. P. (2013). *A case of human babesiosis in Denmark. Travel Med Infect Dis, 11,* 324-328

Hu, R.-J., & Hyland, K. E. (1997). *Human babesiosis in the United States: a review with emphasis on its tick vector. Sys Appl Acarol, 2,* 3-16

Hunfeld, K. P., Lambert, A., Kampen, H., Albert, S., Epe, C., Brade, V., & Tenter, A. M. (2002). *Seroprevalence of Babesia infections in humans exposed to ticks in midwestern Germany. J Clin Microbiol, 40,* 2431-2436

Kim, J. Y., Cho, S. H., Joo, H. N., Tsuji, M., Cho, S. R., Park, I. J., Chung, G. T., Ju, J. W., Cheun, H. I., Lee, H. W., Lee, Y. H., & Kim, T. S. (2007). *First case of human babesiosis in Korea: detection and characterization of a novel type of Babesia sp. (KO1) similar to ovine Babesia. J Clin Microbiol, 45,* 2084-2087

Main, A. J., Carey, A. B., Carey, M. G., & Goodwin, R. H. (1982). *Immature Ixodes dammini (acari: Ixodidae) on small animals in Connecticut, USA. J Med Entomol, 19,* 655-664

Meer-Scherrer, L., Adelson, M., Mordechai, E., Lottaz, B., & Tilton, R. (2004). *Babesia microti infection in Europe. Curr Microbiol, 48,* 435-437

Nakajima, R., Tsuji, M., Oda, K., Zamoto-Niikura, A., Wei, Q., Kawabuchi-Kurata, T., Nishida, A., & Ishihara, C. (2009). *Babesia microti-group parasites compared phylogenetically by complete sequencing of the CCTeta gene in 36 isolates. J Vet Med Sci, 71,* 55-68

Nguyen, H. D., Yoshihama, M., & Kenmochi, N. (2007). *The evolution of spliceosomal introns in alveolates. Mol Biol Evol, 24,* 1093-1096

Pancewicz, S., Moniuszko, A., Bieniarz, E., Pucilo, K., Grygorczuk, S., Zajkowska, J., Czupryna, P., Kondrusik, M., & Swierzbinska-Pijanowska, R. (2011). *Anti-Babesia microti antibodies in foresters highly exposed to tick bites in Poland. Scand J Infect Dis, 43,* 197-201

Persing, D. H., Herwaldt, B. L., Glaser, C., Lane, R. S., Thomford, J. W., Mathiesen, D., Krause, P. J., Phillip, D. F., & Conrad, P. A. (1995). Infection with a Babesia-like organism in northern California. N Engl J Med, 332, 298-303

Piesman, J., Mather, T. N., Dammin, G. J., Telford, S. R., 3rd, Lastavica, C. C., & Spielman, A. (1987). Seasonal variation of transmission risk of Lyme disease and human babesiosis. Am J Epidemiol, 126, 1187-1189

Piesman, J., & Spielman, A. (1980). Human babesiosis on Nantucket Island: prevalence of Babesia microti in ticks. Am J Trop Med Hyg, 29, 742-746

Piesman, J., & Spielman, A. (1982). Babesia microti: infectivity of parasites from ticks for hamsters and white-footed mice. Exp Parasitol, 53, 242-248

Poisnel, E., Ebbo, M., Berda-Haddad, Y., Faucher, B., Bernit, E., Carcy, B., Piarroux, R., Harle, J. R., & Schleinitz, N. (2013). Babesia microti: an unusual travel-related disease. BMC Infect Dis, 13, 99

Qi, C., Zhou, D., Liu, J., Cheng, Z., Zhang, L., Wang, L., Wang, Z., Yang, D., Wang, S., & Chai, T. (2011). Detection of Babesia divergens using molecular methods in anemic patients in Shandong Province, China. Parasitol Res, 109, 241-245

Quick, R. E., Herwaldt, B. L., Thomford, J. W., Garnett, M. E., Eberhard, M. L., Wilson, M., Spach, D. H., Dickerson, J. W., Telford, S. R., 3rd, Steingart, K. R., Pollock, R., Persing, D. H., Kobayashi, J. M., Juranek, D. D., & Conrad, P. A. (1993). Babesiosis in Washington State: a new species of Babesia? Ann Intern Med, 119, 284-290

Ramharter, M., Walochnik, J., Lagler, H., Winkler, S., Wernsdorfer, W. H., Stoiser, B., & Graninger, W. (2010). Clinical and molecular characterization of a near fatal case of human babesiosis in Austria. J Travel Med, 17, 416-418

Rar, V. A., Epikhina, T. I., Livanova, N. N., & Panov, V. V. (2011). Genetic diversity of Babesia in Ixodes persulcatus and small mammals from North Ural and West Siberia, Russia. Parasitology, 138, 175-182

Rios, L., Alvarez, G., & Blair, S. (2003). Serological and parasitological study and report of the first case of human babesiosis in Colombia. Rev Soc Bras Med Trop, 36, 493-498

Saito-Ito, A., Tsuji, M., Wei, Q., He, S., Matsui, T., Kohsaki, M., Arai, S., Kamiyama, T., Hioki, K., & Ishihara, C. (2000). Transfusion-acquired, autochthonous human babesiosis in Japan: isolation of Babesia microti-like parasites with hu-RBC-SCID mice. J Clin Microbiol, 38, 4511-4516

Saito-Ito, A., Takada, N., Ishiguro, F., Fujita, H., Yano, Y., Ma, X. H., & Chen, E. R. (2008). Detection of Kobe-type Babesia microti associated with Japanese human babesiosis in field rodents in central Taiwan and southeastern mainland China. Parasitology, 135, 691-699

Shih, C. M., Liu, L. P., Chung, W. C., Ong, S. J., & Wang, C. C. (1997). Human babesiosis in Taiwan: asymptomatic infection with a Babesia microti-like organism in a Taiwanese woman. J Clin Microbiol, 35, 450-454

Senanayake, S. N., Paparini, A., Latimer, M., Andriolo, K., Dasilva, A. J., Wilson, H., Xayavong, M. V., Collignon, P. J., Jeans, P., & Irwin, P. J. (2012). First report of human babesiosis in Australia. Med J Aust, 196, 350-352

Sinski, E., Bajer, A., Welc, R., Pawelczyk, A., Ogrzewalska, M., & Behnke, J. M. (2006). Babesia microti: Prevalence in wild rodents and Ixodes ricinus ticks from the Mazury Lakes District of north-eastern Poland. Int J Med Microbiol, 296, S1, 137-143

Spielman, A. (1976). Human babesiosis on Nantucket Island: transmission by nymphal Ixodes ticks. Am J Trop Med Hyg, 25, 784-787

Spielman, A., Etkind, P., Piesman, J., Ruebush, T. K., 2nd, Juranek, D. D., & Jacobs, M. S. (1981). Reservoir hosts of human babesiosis on Nantucket Island. Am J Trop Med Hyg, 30, 560-565

Tabara, K., Arai, S., Kawabuchi, T., Itagaki, A., Ishihara, C., Satoh, H., Okabe, N., & Tsuji, M. (2007). Molecular survey of Babesia microti, Ehrlichia species and Candidatus neoehrlichia mikurensis in wild rodents from Shimane Prefecture, Japan. Microbiol Immunol, 51, 359-367

Tsuji, M., Wei, Q., Zamoto, A., Morita, C., Arai, S., Shiota, T., Fujimagari, M., Itagaki, A., Fujita, H., & Ishihara, C. (2001). Human babesiosis in Japan: epizootiologic survey of rodent reservoir and isolation of new type of Babesia microti-like parasite. J Clin Microbiol, 39, 4316-4322

Tsuji, M., Zamoto, A., Kawabuchi, T., Kataoka, T., Nakajima, R., Asakawa, M., & Ishihara, C. (2006). Babesia microti-like parasites detected in Eurasian red squirrels (Sciurus vulgaris orientis) in Hokkaido, Japan. J Vet Med Sci, 68, 643-646

Vannier, E., & Krause, P. J. (2009). Update on babesiosis. Interdiscip Perspect Infect Dis, 2009, 984568

Vannier, E., & Krause, P. J. (2012). Human babesiosis. N Engl J Med, 366, 2397-2407

Wei, Q., Tsuji, M., Zamoto, A., Kohsaki, M., Matsui, T., Shiota, T., Telford, S. R., 3rd, & Ishihara, C. (2001). *Human babesiosis in Japan: isolation of Babesia microti-like parasites from an asymptomatic transfusion donor and from a rodent from an area where babesiosis is endemic. J Clin Microbiol, 39, 2178-2183*

Western, K. A., Benson, G. D., Gleason, N. N., Healy, G. R., & Schultz, M. G. (1970). *Babesiosis in a Massachusetts resident. N Engl J Med, 283, 854-856*

Xu, G., Fang, Q. Q., Keirans, J. E., & Durden, L. A. (2003). *Molecular phylogenetic analyses indicate that the Ixodes ricinus complex is a paraphyletic group. J Parasitol, 89, 452-457*

Yao, L. N., Ruan, W., Zeng, C. Y., Li, Z. H., Zhang, X., Lei, Y. L., Lu, Q. Y., & Che, H. L. (2012). *[Pathogen identification and clinical diagnosis for one case infected with Babesia]. Zhongguo Ji Sheng Chong Xue Yu Ji Sheng Chong Bing Za Zhi, 30, 118-121*

Zamoto-Niikura, A., Tsuji, M., Qiang, W., Nakao, M., Hirata, H., & Ishihara, C. (2012). *Detection of two zoonotic Babesia microti lineages, the Hobetsu and U.S. lineages, in two sympatric tick species, Ixodes ovatus and Ixodes persulcatus, respectively, in Japan. Appl Environ Microbiol, 78, 3424-3430*

Zamoto, A., Tsuji, M., Kawabuchi, T., Wei, Q., Asakawa, M., & Ishihara, C. (2004a). *U.S.-type Babesia microti isolated from small wild mammals in Eastern Hokkaido, Japan. J Vet Med Sci, 66, 919-926*

Zamoto, A., Tsuji, M., Wei, Q., Cho, S. H., Shin, E. H., Kim, T. S., Leonova, G. N., Hagiwara, K., Asakawa, M., Kariwa, H., Takashima, I., & Ishihara, C. (2004b). *Epizootiologic survey for Babesia microti among small wild mammals in northeastern Eurasia and a geographic diversity in the beta-tubulin gene sequences. J Vet Med Sci, 66, 785-792*

.

Community-Centred Eco-Bio-Social Approach to Control Dengue Vectors: An Intervention Study from Myanmar

KhinThet Wai, Pe Than Htun, Tin Oo, Axel Kroeger, Max Petzold

1   Introduction

Worldwide, there are over 100 million cases of dengue annually. In South East Asia, dengue is reemerging and the leading cause of paediatric hospitalization and death. In Myanmar, dengue has been occurring since the 1970s with epidemics reported in three to four years cycles (Aung Than Batu, 2003). There is a simultaneous circulation of the four serotypes which are closely related viruses (DEN 1, DEN 2, DEN 3 and DEN 4) and transmitted to humans by the bite of an infected *Aedes aegypti* mosquito. These mosquitoes mostly breed in clean water containers inside or around houses. Climatic variation, socio-cultural norms, life style and vulnerable conditions linking to quality of breeding sites and household container management practices are associated with high vector densities. In Myanmar, there is a lack of model for sustainable vector control and weaknesses in entomological surveillance. As there is no vaccine available at present and no specific antiviral drug for the treatment of dengue (WHO, 2009), vector control remains essential for the reduction of vector density below threshold values. The Vector Borne Disease Control (VBDC) program from the Department of Health, Myanmar is responsible for establishing effective disease and vector surveillance systems and to undertake disease prevention through selective, stratified and integrated vector control and to increase community awareness and collaboration. Pupal surveys able to target the most productive container types (Tun Lin *et al.*, 1995) are not included in their routine activities and other novel approaches of integrated vector management (WHO, 2009) are not recognized.

Continuous community efforts for integrated vector control together with environmental management can be expensive and without the support of key stakeholders, sustainability is questionable (Kroeger *et al.*, 2006; Arunachalem *et al.*, 2010). A strategy of targeted source reduction was proposed (Tun Lin *et al.*, 1995) directed solely against highly productive containers that may be sufficient to control dengue vectors; the cost-effectiveness of such an approach was confirmed later in a multi-country study (Tun Lin *et al.*, 2009). Present vertical programs are inefficient and educational messages are often unclear; staffing levels, capacity building, management and organization, funding and community engagement tend to be insufficient (Horstick *et al.*, 2010). There is a need to attempt for community capacity building giving priority to vulnerable sites. This may further lead to community development which means that a community itself engages in a process aimed at improving the social, economic and environmental situation of the community. The very first step is the critical analysis for health disparities through identification of the underlying social, economic, and environmental forces that create health and social inequities (Lavery *et al.*, 2005). The community action model as proposed by Paulo Freire, a Brazilian educationalist in 2004 included 5-step, community-driven model designed to build communities' capacity to address health disparities through mobilization. The diagnosis or action research component is one of the central facet of that particular community action model (Ledwith, 2011).

As early as 1958, Sanders argued community development as a process moving from stage to stage; a method of working towards a goal; a program of procedures and as a movement sweeping people up in emotion and belief. Later, it has been widely recognized that the community development approach encompasses health as a human condition and participation as the planning and managing of health activities by the community using professionals as resources and facilitators (Rifkin and Pridmore, 2001). However, there is an ongoing challenge to assess the sustainable community participation and to evaluate its impact on desired program outcomes and broader health improvements. Draper *et al.* (2010) highlighted the indicators to enable the analysis of the different ways of community participation in the intervention delivery of health and health related programmes.

This present study is focused to conduct as part of a comprehensive research programme in six Asian countries which aimed at elucidating contextual factors of dengue vector abundance in a comprehensive way and then to design and implement the site-specific interventions. The programme was guided by a conceptual framework which included ecological (eco), biological (entomological) and social ("eco-bio-social") determinants of vector density as key factors for dengue transmission (see details of the comparative situation analysis in Arunachalam *et al.* 2010 and Tana *et al.*, 2012). During the baseline studies of this research programme (Arunachalem *et al.*, 2010) in Yangon City, the most productive water container types for *Aedes* pupae as a proxy measure for vector density in households were identified (see resultssection). These were metal drums, cement tanks, ceramic jars and ceramic bowls which contributed over 85% of total pupae count and could be specifically targeted for vector control interventions.

The ecosystem approach based upon transdisciplinarity, multi-stakeholder partnership and participatory actions is desirable to formulate locally relevant and appropriate health interventions. The scope of research is beyond exposure assessment and epidemiological studies (Boischio *et al.*, 2009). This will promote sustainable dengue vector control by means of intersectoral collaboration and coordination. It was decided to conduct an intervention study with the objectives to build up and analyze the feasibility, process and effectiveness of a partnership driven ecosystem management intervention in reducing vector densities and constructing sustainable partnerships among multiple stakeholders. Therefore, the interconnected links between epidemiological surveillance of dengue vector breeding, extensive evidence-based research findings and concerted community efforts for integrated vector management within the context of multiple stakeholder environment have been critically analyzed and presented in this book chapter.

2   Research Methods

2.1   Study Design, Timeline and Study Site

A community-based intervention study using a cluster randomized balanced design was carried out fromMay2009 to January 2010 in Yangon City (96° 09′ longitude and 16° 48′ latitude).

The total population as of 2008-09 in the City was around 6.8 million and the population density was 666 persons per square kilometer. Two peri-urban eco-settings in Yangon Region were selected purposively and stratified on the basis of reported dengue incidence for three years: North Dagon (zone 1inthenorth-eastern part) with low to moderate dengue transmission and Insein (zone 2 in the north-western part) with moderate to high dengue transmission. The study neighborhoods were overall reasonably well developed urban areas with electricity and many (75%) with paved streets; water was mainly drawn by hand pumps (79.1% of households); most toilets (83.1%) were in the patio - half of them latrines, half septic tanks. Waste collection was at least once per week in all study neighborhoods. Three quarter of neighborhoods were mainly residential, the remainder mixed commercial/residential areas. In the majority the poorer social strata were included in the study, but the housing conditions, mainly one story buildings, were generally satisfactory to good. One third had patios/ gardens and some of these trees and/or bushes. Green areas were frequent but rarely for leisure activities. There were no neighborhoods with cemeteries, half of them with schools and almost half of them with small market places. Many study clusters had visible garbage dumps or open water pools and about one third had tire capping facilities (Wai *et al.,* 2012).

2.2   Weather Variables

Temperature, rainfall and relative humidity throughout the period of the intervention were collected by the Kabar Aye weather station in Yangon, approximately 10 kilometers away from zone 1 and 8 kilometers away from zone 2.This station was under the Department of Meteorology and Hydrology, Nay Pyi Taw.

2.3   Sampling of Study Neighborhoods

During phase 1, a map of each study site was taken using Google Earth software (Google Inc., Mountain View, CA, United States of America). A grid with 200 squares was placed upon it. The squares were numbered and 20 squares were randomly selected using simple random numbers. In order to ensure a good representation of high and low dengue transmission areas, the study universe was further stratified into high and low transmission strata according to reported annual dengue case incidence for the preceding two to six years. Half of the squares were thus located in high and half in low transmission areas. In the baseline survey in phase 1,20 urban neighborhoods or "clusters" were randomly selected and analyzed (Arunachalem *et al.,* 2010). Ten clusters from each site (100 households per cluster) were included by means of geographical grid sampling. However, in phase 2, the cluster background information was used to stratify six high risk clusters and six low risk clusters out of 20 clusters. Cluster background characteristics covered 33 items: approximate total surface area, socioeconomic characteristics, housing condition, residential function, type of majority of house, approximate mean distance between houses, presence of gardens and outdoor space, presence of green areas, defined public spaces for leisure activities, presence of small pools of water, visible garbage dumps, piped water supply, availability of electricity, types of roads and pavements, presence of tire capping facilities, frequency of solid waste disposal from the area, presence of school premises, presence of religious sites, presence of market, presence of railway/bus station, presence of cemetery, presence of ferry/jetty, presence of health facility and presence of cinema/theater hall, commercial mall, motorcar service station, any vector control intervention within past 6 months, any kind of community work, any community meeting during last 6 months, presence of a lake/puddle, presence of vegetative land cover, presence of tire capping facility, and presence of any garbage dumping area. These selected clusters were randomly allocated to intervention and routine services areas respectively. To have a balanced design in each area, 3 high risk and 3 low risk clusters were selected at random. Each cluster included roughly, 100 households. Considering the flight range of mosquitoes, a buffer zone of at least 100 meters around the intervention and routine services areas was taken into account.

2.3.1   Definition of Clusters within Squares

In each of the selected squares, the left lower corner was identified on the map and the exact location was determined by GPS methods. Then, this point was physically located in the real city. Starting from this point, the closest crossing of two streets was identified, one street representing the vertical line of the square in the map, and the other the horizontal line of the square. Then, the researcher went roughly 100 meters on the horizontal line or street, turned left and looked into the "vertical" direction and identified a street which was parallel to the first vertical street. Now, a U shaped form was obtained. In order to close the U to a cluster area, the researcher looked for 100 households (houses, flats, small business units) within the U shaped area. After completion of them, the U was closed and bordered the cluster. A simple map was drawn for orientation. If the square fell over a football ground or large park or any open public space, then the next corner of two crossing streets and U was constructed. All houses as well as public and private open spaces were included in the cluster analysis (Arunachalem *et al.*, 2010; Wai *et al.*, 2012).

2.4   Sample Size

For phase 1, the mean number of pupae per person in households in high transmission areas was assumed as being 3 and in low transmission areas being 0.3 considering negative binomial distribution with a dispersion factor of 0.02 (field data in Venezuela). At significance level of 5% and power of 80%, and intra cluster coefficient (ICC) of 0.05, the needed numbers of clusters per area was found to be 8.9 suggested of a random selection of 10 clusters per area (Lwanga and Lemeshow, 1991) with approximately 1000 (10 x 100) households were included. For the post-intervention cross-sectional analysis of intervention clusters *versus* routine services clusters, the following sample sizes were needed for a significance level of 5% and a power of 80%. As for PPI (pupae per person index), by anticipating a mean level of 0.3 in routine services clusters and 0.1 in intervention clusters with a standard deviation of 0.1, the needed number of cluster per arm was 4 to 6. As for BI (Breteau Index), by anticipating a mean level of 40 in control clusters and 10 in intervention clusters with a standard deviation of 20, the needed number of cluster per arm was 7. Thus considering for both PPI and BI values, 6 clusters per arm were selected, three each in *high and low transmission clusters* regardless of Zones and randomized to introduce intervention measures.

Ten focus group discussions (FGD) comprised either heads of the households or assigned persons and 6 FGDs with dengue volunteer groups were organized in intervention clusters, which were facilitated by the research team. Each FGD had 10 to 12 participants. The core topic was satisfaction with and opinions about the intervention which had been done in their homes. Furthermore, 10 in-depth interviews (IDIs) were conducted with eco-health friendly groups (EFGs), Health Department and Municipal services on feasibility and sustainability of the intervention programme. Additionally, one multi-stakeholder discussion with 20 participants from different social sectors focusing the importance and sustainability issues was conducted in the intervention neighborhoods. All FGDs and IDIs were audio-taped after a written informed consent. The analysis was facilitated by using SAS[2] methods (Chevalier & Buckles, 2010) for "priority options" and "feasibility". Themes and sub themes were analyzed manually and triangulated with quantitative data.

2.5   Household Surveys

A formal household survey for the acceptance of intervention tools was done in 6 intervention clusters at the end of phase 2 by using the pre-tested interview forms. Altogether 555 house-holders were interviewed. The safety of the intervention was measured by regular monitoring and recording side effects of chemical larvicides by volunteers.

2.6   Intervention Methods

2.6.1   Rationale for the Intervention Package

Phase 1 findings inclusive of varying causes of dengue vector breeding, most productive container types, current vector control measures, limited mobilization of health and health related networks, weaknesses in supervision of volunteers and their capacity pointed out to the need of changing the strategy and developing a new vector control model for effective source reduction at low cost either chemical alone or in combination with non-chemical and biological measures as an integrated approach. This is in line with research findings from the remaining 5 countries in Asia and the Pacific applying eco-bio-social principles (Tana *et al.,* 2012). It was also felt that the vertical control strategy should be replaced by a community-based model for larval control operations leaded by a multi-stakeholder partner group with the Township Health Department (THD) being the focal point. The community-based model covered interested stakeholder partner groups and volunteers together with highly motivated householders to augment the routine vector control activities by the Township Health Department.

2.6.2   Selection and Capacity Building of Partners

a)   Eco-health Friendly partner Groups (EFG) *(Thingaha)* were formed, one in each selected intervention cluster by recruitment of existing viable groups led by ward authorities jointly with midwives, members of Maternal and Child Welfare Association (MCWA), credible and trusted persons and school teachers. Each group comprised one leader and four core members. They were trained for information dissemination and how to manage vector control tools. Their functions included to set local targets for household coverage, to liaise between Township Dengue Control Committee (TDCC) and householders, to organize/mobilize householders to accept interventions and environmental management, supervision of volunteers, and deployment of intervention tools. *Thingaha* groups distributed pictorial booklets and pamphlets regarding dengue already in use by MCWA members.

b)   Local manufacturers were explained to produce tightly fitted lid covers at low cost which should serve as a model to be replicated by community members.

c)   Ward-based volunteers were selected by EFG, 10 in each cluster to participate actively in controlling dengue vectors. Each volunteer was responsible for local target setting of households to be visited, to provide information and to assist in the inspection and removal of larvae. Each volunteer was provided with a record book to note the vector control tool preference of each household and any problems if encountered in each visit. Their activities were monitored weekly by EFG. Two days training on communication of dengue issues and the use of cotton-net sweepers and a half day of field demonstration was done by the research team jointly with TDCC.

d) An intensive awareness-raising for the local communities was done through group discussions. Interpersonal communication reinforced by information leaflets and booklets distributed in house to house visits were carried out explaining three sets of intervention tools for targeted containers (chemical or non-chemical measures or both). The TDCC scheduled household monitoring visits weekly either on Wednesday or Saturday accompanied by EFG. Monthly meetings and feedback regarding constraints and solutions were carried out in the Township Health Department throughout the intervention for three times.

2.6.3   Vector Control Tools

The selective mechanical, chemical and biological vector control measures were applied in intervention clusters. Among 10 different types of containers, 4 of them produced more than 80% of all pupae as proxies for adult mosquitoes: drum (200 L), cement tank (100-950 L), ceramic jar (50-100 L) and spiritual bowl (1-2 L) were regarded as most productive containers. Four intervention tools were applied according to the type of container and peoples' preferences (see below). Pyriproxyfen sand granules and *Bacillus ThurigiensisIsraelensis (Bti)* as chemical control, lid covers and cotton-net sweepers as mechanical control, dragon fly nymphs as biological control and waste-collection bags for water retaining discarded small containers in households were used for environmental management covering the period of six months. In control clusters, only routine control measures were carried out. The following vector control options were offered to heads of households being asked to choose the most appropriate one for them.

- For metal drums and ceramic jars, available choices were (a) Pyriproxyfen sand granules or (b) lid covers and cotton-net sweepers. Pyriproxyfen, a non-toxic insect growth inhibitor does not even in high concentrations- inhibit ovi-position and treated water does not taste tainted and can retain efficacy for six months (Kroeger *et al.*, 2006). Households choosing tightly fitted metal/zinc sheet covers were visited bi-weekly by volunteers for removal of immature stages of mosquitoes if any by cotton-net sweepers (Tun Lin *et al.*, 1994). Pyriproxyfen sand granules were applied at the rate of 2 mg/liter to obtain 0.01mg/liter every two months.

- For cement tanks which cannot be covered or emptied regularly, available choices were (a) Pyriproxyfen sand granules or (b) dragonfly nymphs. These were offered after thorough explanation of their predator potential. Two to four dragon fly nymphs *B. geminator* (Rambur) were seeded into cement tanks. They were culturally accepted because clean water was clearly observed in cement tanks and cement drums where there were dragon fly nymphs.

- For culture specific ceramic bowls to worship spirits, available choices were (a) *Bti* in a slow release formulation) granules to be applied by householders themselves under observation of volunteers or (b) weekly regular cleaning by themselves.

- As an additional measure, waste collection bags made of durable material of low cost were distributed to collect water retaining discarded small containers linking to ward organized collection and recycling scheme on bi-weekly basis.

The list of options for each container type was shown to heads of the household or the assigned person. They had to choose, decide and sign the form which was plastic coated and hung on the entrance of the premises so that the entomological team could apply the desired intervention at specific times.

2.6.4   Entomological Surveys and the Intended Measurement of Effectiveness

Larval/pupal surveys conducted during the dry and the wet season followed standard operating procedures (TDR-WHO, 2011). The teams trained six research assistants for the procedures and use of the common data collection instrument. The trained staff inspected household areas including spaces in and around the households in each cluster. They classified containers according to type, source of water, volume, location, presence of vegetation, presence of larval control measures, and the presence of a proper/suitable cover. The trained staff examined containers with water ("wet containers") only. The surveyor determined the presence or absence of *Aedes* larvae in each container. For pupae, the surveyor counted all the pupae present in each container. For large water containers, the surveyors employed the sweeping method. The teams examined the sample of pupae from different container types in the laboratory and left to develop into adults. The adults were then identified by species and sex (KhinThet Wai *et al.*, 2012). The effectiveness of integrated vector management that covered the use of combined chemical and non-chemical methods and environmental management through social mobilization efforts was measured by comparison of pupa and larva indices between intervention and routine services clusters during three rounds of evaluation surveys. The PPI (total number of *Ae. aegypti*pupae by number of inhabitants) was used as a proxy indicator for adult density. The pupae per container index (PCI) was used as an indicator for the infestation levels of different container types. As secondary measures, the larval indices were used: BreteauIndex (BI), House Index (HI) and Container index (CI). Assuming the sero-prevalence rate as 33%, the estimated threshold level of PPI of 0.19 at the average temperature of 30ºC at the given period was kept in mind (Arunachalem *et al.*, 2010). Before the start of the intervention study, cyclone Nargis struck the city in May 2008 so that all research activities had to be postponed. The public response included massive larviciding of all water containers by the control programme. For saving resources, the intervention areas were covered by the project staff and the control clusters by personnel from Ministry of Health using temephos treatment of water containers which was donated by foreign aid for the relief operations. This situation limited the possibilities of determining the effectiveness of our intervention package against purely untreated control group.

2.6.5   Performance Measurement

The quality of the delivery of the intervention package was assessed by observing program performance and analyzing whether targets were reached. Furthermore, the adequate program performance in terms of timeliness, rational use of resources, competencies, relations between volunteers and householders, level of community satisfaction and coordination between volunteers and eco-health friendly partner groups was assessed in a qualitative way.

2.7   Data Management and Analysis

Field supervisors checked all data for errors prior to entry. Then, double entry was done by trained data entry personnel for quality assurance. All data files were checked and cleaned by data entry supervisors. For data entry, Epi Data 3.0 (http://www.epidata.dk) was used since it is equipped with range check and skip check and also data export facilities. The data files were re-checked in the data management centre of Gothenburg, Sweden and analyzed by SPSS version 17.0. The unit of analysis is a cluster. Analyses regarding factors associated with pupal production were performed for different units of analysis; container (pupae counts, pupae/larvae positive), household (pupae counts) and study cluster (pupae per person, house index, and Breteau index).

2.8   Ethical Considerations

The study was approved by the Ethics Review Committee, Department of Medical Research (Lower Myanmar) and from the Ethical Review committee (ERC), WHO, Geneva. The informed consent was obtained from householders during entomological and feasibility surveys, focus group and stake-holder group discussants and in-depth interviewees. Privacy, anonymity and confidentiality issues were ensured.

3   Results

3.1   Situation Analysis

Yangon City has a tropical monsoon climate and vector *Aedesaegypti* has been responsible for dengue transmission. The most productive man-made containers such as metal drums, cement drums, cement tanks and culture-specific ceramic bowls for spirit worship were identified in the peri-urban neighborhoods during wet and dry season entomological surveys and this led to the formulation of locally appropriate and acceptable vector control measures (Arunachalem *et al.*, 2010). The most frequently infested container types by Aedes immature stages in the dry and wet season were completely different. The second striking observation was that the container types most frequently infested by immature stages differed from the productive container types (i.e. those which produce together more than 70% of all pupae). In the dry season, two out of three productive container types (for Aedes pupae and adults) would be missed by larval surveys. Phase 1 findings underlined the importance of determining "productive container types" being responsible for the development of the majority of dengue vectors to its adult stage, as these were clearly different from containers infested with Aedes larvae/ pupae, represented by the classical stegomyia indices such as the house index, container index and Breteau Index (Wai *et al.*, 2012).

During household surveys in phase 1, all respondents (n = 2,000) in 20 clusters resided by 10,488 dwellers had heard of dengue haemorrhagic fever. The majority perceived dengue illness as serious and being lethal also noted during focus group discussions and semi-structured interviews. Over 75% knew that dengue was due to mosquito bite and 93% knew that dengue can be prevented. It was a good indicator to note that over 80% had ever seen larvae in water (Arunachalem *et al.*, 2010) and nearly 100% expressed their attitude that it mattered when larvae were present in water containers at home. Water storage was universal in study households. The percentage of storing water for drinking purpose was lower than for other purposes (79% *vs.* 64%). Householders reported that they had never emptied large containers of over 200 liters capacity (52.2%). Results indicated the presence of barriers for emptying practices due to size of containers, not paying attention much for that specific action and busy urban life style also reported during FGDs and stakeholder consultations. Gender specific needs on water use, and gender roles in cleaning water storage containers and waste disposal did not differ across all clusters. Three common practices recommended by cluster dwellers included cleaning rubbish (32%), using mosquito coils and other chemicals (30%) and to cover water containers (16%). Very few recommended to put fish in water (5%; Arunachalem *et al.*, 2010).

3.2   Characteristics of the Study Population in Post Intervention

The majority of householders from the 6 intervention clusters participated in structured interviews (555/600, 92.5%). The total number of dwellers was 3,054 with an average of 5.5 individuals per household. Only 10.3% of household heads were unemployed and 15% to 24% were children under 15 years. In terms of distribution by age group, 1.5% (47/3054) were 0-1 years age group, 2.8% (87/3054) were 2-4 years age group and 13.2% (402/3054) were 5-14 years age group. Most of the inhabitants were Buddhists except in one cluster in which equal proportions of Buddhists and Christians were found. Those characteristics confirmed what had been found in the whole study population in phase 1 (Arunachalem *et al.*, 2010).

3.3   Productive Containers to be Targeted by the Intervention

During the intervention period, percent filled with piped water increased in both intervention and routine services areas compared to base-line studies in wet season (Arunachalem *et al.*, 2010). Cement based containers tended to harbor dragon fly nymphs naturally due to thin growth of algae at the wall and it provided alternate food for the nymphs. All productive containers were man-made and mostly situated in and around the households. Most frequent container types in intervention area were flower vases over 48% and cement tanks and drums/barrels around 30%. Likewise, in routine services area, flower vases contributed over 50% and cement tanks and drums/barrels were approximately 25%.The most productive water container types for *Aedes*pupae at baseline were man-made spiritual worshipped bowls, cement tanks and flower vases. In the subsequent surveys, metal or cement drums replaced the flower vases (Table 1). The most infested container types by *Aedes* larvae were rarely the most productive ones for adult mosquitoes. Total number of pupae in all containers reduced to 18.6% in evaluation 2 and 44.1% in evaluation 3 in intervention area. However, in routine services area, more reduction was observed. Types of productive containers in both areas such as flower vases, spiritual bowls, cement tanks, drums/barrels were more or less the same with slight variations. At baseline, less than 20% of water containers were properly covered in intervention clusters and less than 5% in clusters of the routine services area (Table 1). Householders' confidence and trust in community groups improved and their misperceptions and negative attitudes towards dengue vector control activities disappeared or was rarely mentioned in group discussions after interventions.

Characteristic	Intervention area (I) (n =6) 6				Routine services area (R)(n =6) 6		
	Baseline (Wet)*	Eval 1 (Wet)	Eval 2 (Semi-wet)	Eval 3 (Dry)	Eval 1 (Wet)	Eval 2 (Semi-wet)	Eval 3 (Dry)
Number of households	2,000	593	592	592	600	599	600
Total number of water containers	18,510	4802	4857	4460	5110	5135	4697
% Indoor containers	37.5	60.3	61.4	60.9	61.9	63.6	64.7
%Tap water filled	81.6	91.5	95.4	99.3	82.3	96.2	98.6
%Containers fully covered	14.5	16.5	16.0	15.7	4.4	3.8	3.4
Most frequent container types (% of all container types)	Flower vase (48.7%)	Flower vase (47.9%)	Flowervase (50.5%)	Flowervase (49.8%)	Flower vase (51.8%)	Flower vase (53.8%)	Flower vase (56.8%)
	Cement tank† (14.3%)	Cement tank(16.5%)	Cement tank (16.0%)	Cement tank (16.8%)	Cement tank(14.2%)	Cement tank(14.2%)	Cement tank (14.7%)
	Drum/ barrel (12.4%)	Drum/ barrel (14.6%)	Drum/ barrel (14.0%)	Drum/ barrel (14.6%)	Drum/ barrel (11.3%)	Drum/ barrel (10.9%)	Drum/ barrel (10.6%)
Total number of pupae in all containers	2155	295	240	165	1117	874	493
% reduction of pupae	-	-	18.64	44.06	-	21.75	55.86
Most productive container types (% of all pupae)	Spiritual bowl (51.7%)	Drum /barrel (34.1%)	Drum/ barrel (38.2%)	Cement tank (31.0%)	Cement tank (38.9%)	Drum/ barrel (41.4%)	Cement tank (41.0%)
	Cement tank† (19.5)	Ceramic jar (19.0%)	Flower vase (19.7%)	Bucket (26.8%)	Ceramic jar (26.1%)	Cement tank(16.8%)	Drum/ barrel (27.6%)
	Flower vases (7.2%)	Cement tank (16.3%)	Ceramic jar (17.2%)	Drum/ barrel (24.7%)	Drum/ barrel (17.2%)	Ceramic jar (16.4%)	Spiritual bowl (21.9%)

Notes: *Source: Arunachalam *et al.,* 2010, p. 179.
†Cement tanks included cement drums in baseline studies.

Table 1: Vector breeding places and productivity in clusters at baseline and three rounds of evaluation.

3.4   Preferred Choices and Strategies of Interventions

At baseline, there was little collaboration and partnership among stakeholders in dengue vector control and the community was a passive recipient of public health interventions. The intervention package mainly delivered by EFG improved the understanding and shared responsibility among local authorities and the community. Distributing pamphlets and booklets and assisting people in the application of targeted container interventions strengthened the leadership of EFG and the development of sense of ownership by community members. Managerial skills, leadership roles and the participation of EFG and volunteers in activities to reduce dengue vectors were strengthened. A practical 'matrix-based decision-making tool' illustrating vector control options to facilitate the decision by heads of household was well accepted. According to Table 2, combined measures were most frequently favored (44.8% of cluster dwellers) while chemical measures were the second choice (34.2% of cluster dwellers) and mechanical measures the third choice (16.5% of cluster dwellers). Biological measures were preferred in a combined package but rarely alone.

Initial choice expressed by cluster dwellers (n = 6)	Average	Percent
Combined (chemical, mechanical and biological measures)	45	44.8
Chemical measures (pyriproxyfen&Bti) only	34	34.2
Mechanical measures (lid covers and cotton net sweepers) only	17	16.5
Biological measures (dragon fly nymphs) only	1	0.7
Refusal	4	3.8

Table 2: Initial choice of intervention measures in six clusters in relation to type of water container

3.5   Stakeholder Processes

Sixmulti-stakeholder groups involved in dengue prevention and control activities existed at baseline in form of "Dengue Control Committees" in the Townships of Yangon Region (TDCC) since 2003-2004. Dengue control in a collective way involving actively local communities was meant to be carried out at that time but was felt to be inadequate. Therefore, in the first phase of this research programme, power, legitimacy, interests and interactions towards controlling dengue vectors in each stakeholder group were thoroughly discussed and analyzed. In phase 2, the importance as well as favorable and unfavorable conditions related to the 6 strategic options to reduce dengue vector breeding was discussed and scores were given to ascertain the feasibility and sustainability of each option. These strategic options included: formation of EFG, recruitment of ward-based volunteers, informed choices of vector control tools for most productive containers, targeted container approach for implementation of chemical measures, inspection and removal of larvae and pupae, keeping separate waste collection bags for water retaining discarded materials and integrated use of mechanical and biological measures. The preferred options were a) to train volunteers, b) to target and manage productive container sandc) to use waste collection bags. Discussants realized also the importance of forming multi-stake holder groups at ward level which was feasible and necessary for extended ownership of the programme.

3.6   Intervention Effect on People's Knowledge, Attitudes and Practices

At baseline, the overall knowledge of 2,000 respondents on dengue related issues was high (Arunachalem *et al.*, 2010) but their container management practices were inadequate especially for productive large size containers. Qualitative evaluations after the intervention captured that people`s awareness of appropriate vector control options for specific containers was highly improved as well as positive attitudes towards joint actions. At the end of the intervention period (see Table 3), nearly 45% of cluster dwellers accepted pyriproxyfen alone or in combination with other measures.

Cluster dwellers who accepted †	Average ofclusters	% acceptance
Pyriproxyfen		
Very desirable/extremely beneficial	5.17	44.6
Definitely feasible in households	5.17	43.9
Very important	4.67	39.4
Confident	72	59.3
Bti		
Very desirable/extremely beneficial	6	28.0
Definitely feasible in households	6	32.5
Very important	6	28.2
Confident	10	49.2
Lid covers		
Very desirable/extremely beneficial	27	51.6
Definitely feasible in households	26	50.5
Very important	24	46.1
Confident	31	60.5
Cotton-net sweepers		
Very desirable/extremely beneficial	15	32.7
Definitely feasible in households	14	31.2
Very important	14	30.3
Confident	14	30.3
Dragon fly nymphs		
Very desirable/extremely beneficial	7	57.4
Definitely feasible in households	7	59.4
Very important	7	58.0
Confident	8	64.3
Waste collection bags		
Very desirable/extremely beneficial	31	41.9
Definitely feasible in households	29	38.1
Very important	31	41.5
Confident	39	53.0

† Multiple responses; Totals do not add up to 100

Table 3: Acceptability of six intervention tools in intervention clusters (n = 6).

They perceived the chemical as being extremely beneficial and nearly 60% had full confidence in it. Of cluster dwellers using *Bti* for their ceramic bowls, only 28% perceived it to be extremely beneficial. Lid covers were accepted by 52 households per cluster and 60% of cluster dwellers were fully confident to use them continuously which was important for vector control in the intervention clusters. Dragon fly nymphs were found in 12 households per cluster but nearly 60% of cluster dwellers found those nymphs as being extremely beneficial and perceived them as being important in removal of larvae and pupae from their water containers. Nearly 42% of cluster dwellers perceived waste collection bags as extremely beneficial for them and 52% was fully confident for continuity in use. There were no differences between high and low risk clusters. The results indicated that people were less enthusiastic about *Bti*- and cotton net sweepers. In the FGDs and observations following the intervention, it became clear that householders' responsibility in managing dengue vector breeding sites was enhanced. They became interested in the inspection and removal of larvae in their homes; they used lid covers and cotton net sweepers and scrubbed the containers and changed the water regularly in contrast to responses at baseline when household members did not regularly scrubbing and changing water especially of the large containers. It became also clear that cultural barriers persisted in the management of spiritual bowls and that, against original expectations, the use of dragon fly nymphs for cement tanks still needs promotion.

3.7   Reduction of Dengue Vector Density

After the entomological baseline survey during the wet season of 2007 in Phase 1, three entomological evaluations were conducted, the first during the wet season, the second during the semi-wet season and the third during the dry season (Figure 1). As mentioned before, after the baseline survey, cyclone Nargis struck the city and as a response by the vector control services a massive larviciding programme with temephos (Abate) was launched. The overall decrease in all entomological indices was detected at intervention clusters. The Pupae per Person Index (PPI) (decreased from 0.34 at the first evaluation to 0.23 at the last evaluation. Similarly, from 27.7 to 19.4 for Container Index (CI = % of all water holding containers infested by Aedes larvae or pupae), from 49.7 to 27.9 for Breteau Index(BI= number of containers infested by 100 houses) and from 6.3 to 3.7 for House Index (HI= % of houses with one or more infested containers) reduction were detected respectively. However, similar reduction in vector density was also detected at control clusters. The stratified data analysis for low risk and high risk intervention clusters indicated that pupae per person index (PPI) decreased at the last evaluation by 5.7% (0.35 to 0.33) in high risk clusters but in low risk clusters, PPI remarkably decreased by 63.6 % (0.33 to 0.12) (Figure 2). Regarding the BI, 38.8 % reduction was achieved at the high risk clusters and 48.0 % was achieved at low risk clusters. Reduction at control areas were also detected for BI. Routine vector control activities were significantly approved due to the availability and application of temephos which was complemented in the system after Cyclone Nargis.

Our community-centered multiple stakeholder intervention programme was as good in reducing vector densities (using as the PPI as the main outcome measure) as the massive intervention with temephos in the routine services areas (Figure 2). The Pupae per Person Index (PPI) decreased from 0.34 at the first evaluation to 0.23 at the last evaluation (32% reduction) in intervention clusters and from 0.33 to 0.15 (54.5% reduction) in routine services clusters. The PPI decreased in the last evaluation by 5.7% (0.35 to 0.33) in high risk clusters but much more in low risk clusters (63.6 % reduction, 0.33 to 0.12). Similarly, the Stegomyia indices decreased: Container Index from 27.7 to 19.4, BI from 49.7 to 27.9 and House Index from 6.3 to 3.7. The same level of reduction was detected in the clusters where routine larviciding activities with

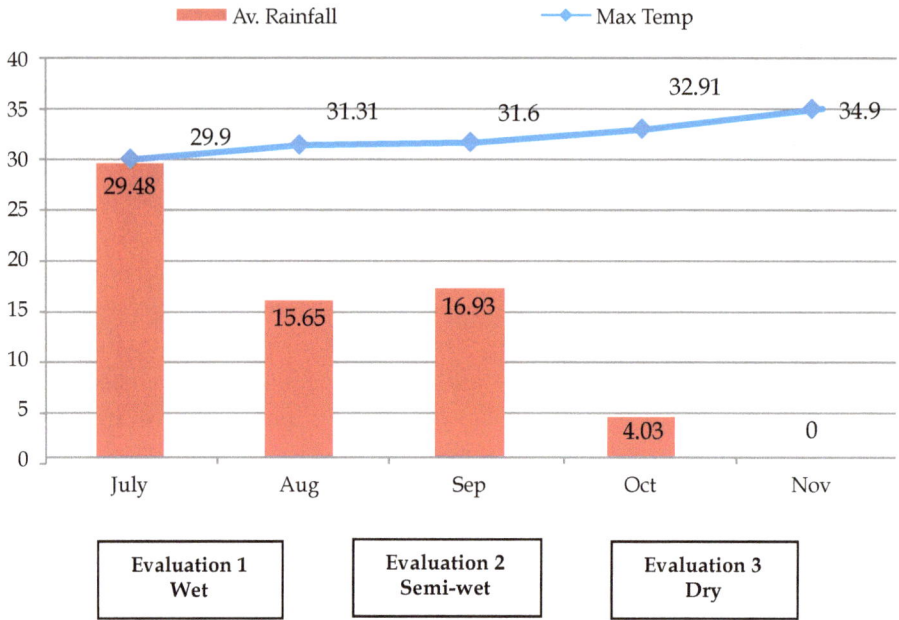

Figure 1: Distribution of average monthly rainfall, maximum daytime temperature and three rounds of entomological evaluation.

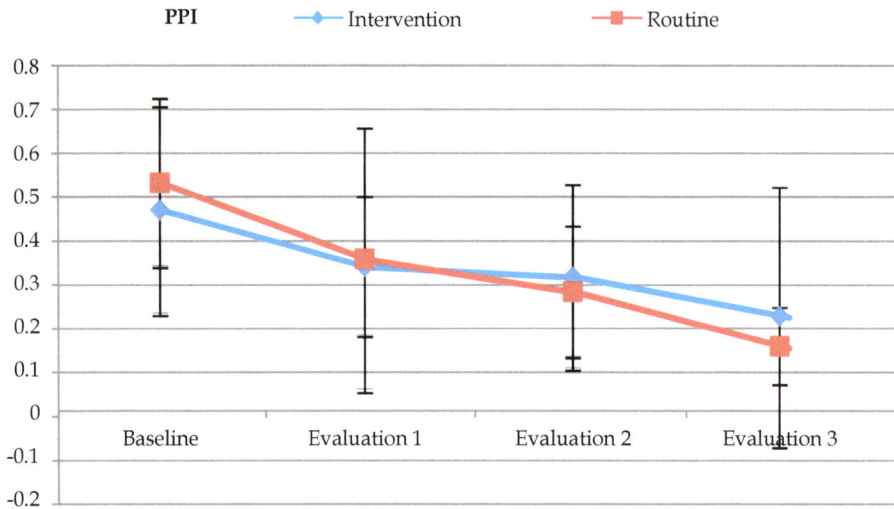

Figure 2: Mean pupae per person Index (PPI) and 95% confidence intervals at baseline and in three rounds of evaluation surveys in clusters of the community centered intervention (n = 6) and the areas with routine larviciding (n = 6).

Temephos were carried out especially during 2008 (the year of cyclone Nargis) and continued in 2009.

4   Discussion

4.1   Multi-stakeholder Partnerships in Urban Eco-health Interventions and Sustainability

It became clear during our study period that purely vertical interventions in dengue vector control are not sustainable particularly if they are built upon "crisis management" as in our case the response to the dengue threat after cyclone Nargis. This involved massive external emergency relief funds that included five metric tons of larvicides (temephos 1% sand granules) initially (WHO, 2008). Therefore, continued supply of temephos was available through the year 2009, which coincided with our intervention year, and still in 2010 when the stocks were emptied. Over 10 years prior to 2008, the routine services could not include temephos for larviciding due to limited resources and they will probably not be able to do it in the near future. Community participation in dengue vector control is desirable as it has prospects of better programme sustainability even if external funds are not anymore available. Equally important in our study was the multi-partnership approach: the EFG acted as the liaison between the community and the THD. They established close relationships among different partners and helped to build and maintain the sense of ownership. The eco-health component was particularly evident in the recognition of the vector ecology in particular in the identification and management of productive breeding places (Arunachalem *et al.*, 2010). This led to the development of a matrix illustrating vector control options according to productive water container types and was used for strengthening household decision-making on the specific intervention they preferred. It took only 1-2 days for volunteers to identify in 600 households, people`s preference of vector control options. Community acceptance was high throughout the 6 months of intervention for targeted containers. The disposition of providing active contributions, time and space for removal of larvae/or pupae was enhanced and not solely depended upon Basic Health Staff who had time constraints and excessive work load. Targeting productive container types was as effective in reducing the PPI as targeting all types in routine services areas but had lower implementation costs (Tun Lin *et al.*, 2009).

Community development improves the ability of communities to collectively make better decisions about the use of resources such as infrastructure, labor and knowledge (Lavery *et al.*, 2005). Active involvement of the community in project design and implementation influenced the sustainability of health interventions in Cuba (Toledo *et al.*, 2008). Sustainability of the current intervention package depends upon a) political commitment and continuing support by the local governance, b) the extent of interest of the community, acceptance and their active participation including the development of a sense of responsibility in using appropriate mechanical control tools (such as lid covers and cotton net sweepers) and c) on additional programme costs. These conditions were largely fulfilled in our study area. The leadership of EFGs was successful as they achieved that ward authorities developed a strong commitment in problem identification at base line and in scheduling, motivating people and distributing intervention materials and later on in monitoring the implementation and results. This is the positive outcome of this study contributing towards community engagement principles in real practice while outlining the impact of interventions on epidemiological indices reflecting active dengue transmission in the area. Suwanbumrang (2010) also pointed out that leadership of local group was essential for the process of social mobilization and human resource development in dengue prevention program. However, the attrition of EFG members and volunteers required not only continuous motivation through good leadership by the Township Health Department but also a system of replacement. Contemporary scenarios in India and Thailand using innovative approaches in controlling dengue vectors by cluster randomization through community participation also reported as successful in capacity building (Sommerfeld & Kroeger, 2012).

Local municipal authorities assisted in ward-based waste collection but challenges were sometimes inadequate manpower and vehicles. The recycling of water retaining discarded materials required private sector involvement. For maintaining community interest in managing mechanical control tools, the continuing support by EFGs for households was essential particularly by working with local manufacturers for any demand to replace or to purchase new water container lids and other tools at affordable costs. Continuing use of pyriproxyfen (approximately 50 USD per kilogram) will mean additional program costs but these can be obtained through the coordination between Regional Health Department and City Development Committee for the purchase of pyriproxyfen at lower cost by subsidization compared to temephos which was actually cheaper that is approximately 30 USD per kilogram. Moreover, the high acceptability of pyriproxiphen by users due to lack of smell may facilitate the program demand and sustainability. The PPI decreased higher in low risk compared to high risk dengue areas. In high risk clusters, the distance between each household and also to adjacent control clusters was closer than in low risk clusters according to cluster background information at baseline (Arunachalem *et al.,* 2010) so that *Aedes*mosquitoes in high risk areas could fly from control clusters into intervention clusters ("spill over effect" which increases the vector density in intervention clusters); this was much less the case in low transmission clusters.

4.2   Other Challenges in Controlling Dengue Virus Transmission

The PPI in three rounds of entomological surveys was reduced but not below the theoretical threshold limits for epidemic transmission of 0.19 (Figure 2) (Focks, 2004) indicating a persistent transmission risk. The exact correlation was unknown but the increase of vectors in the wet season coincided with the increase of dengue cases (Dengue season).The phase 2 study also underlined the importance of determining "productive container types" as in phase1 being responsible for the development of the majority of dengue vectors to its adult stage, as these were clearly different from containers infested with Aedes larvae/ pupae, represented by the classical stegomyia indices such as the house index, container index and Breteau Index. Doing the survey during the dry season would miss a number of productive containers during the wet season, but not the other way round. Pupal productivity surveys during the wet season will identify almost all productive container types relevant in the dry and wet season (Wai *et al.,* 2012).

Another challenge is the need for high coverage and repeated larviciding as shown in northern Argentina (Garelli *et al.,* 2009). Mass larviciding was however successful in Cambodia (Cheng *et al.,* 2008). Water storage practices, still existing despite improvement in municipal water supply, and population growth are other factors favoring dengue spread. Further improvement in feasible water resources and environmental management is essential in study sites so as to improve the situation of water scarcity, and water storage practices linking to pupae productivity. Caprara *et al.* (2009) underscored the chance of irregular water supply associated to more possible breeding sites and favorable conditions for *Aedesaegypti* survival. However, the relationship between domestic water supply, household water use and pupal production is complex (Phuanukoonnon *et al.,* 2005; Arunachalem *et al.,* 2010).

Demographic growth was noted in the study areas during five years (2005- 2009). There was a population increase of 9.7% from 49,922 to 54,777 in 6 wards where there were intervention clusters but less increase of 1.5% from 49,340 to 50,022 in 6 wards where there were control clusters. Congested areas and housing density may favor dengue transmission. Infrastructure changes especially piped water supply coverage was noted in both intervention and control clusters during the same period. But owing to cautiousness and social reasons, water storage practices in large containers still existed despite improvement in situation of water scarcity. The targeted container approach by integrated vector control options were acceptable which were based upon informed choices for most productive containers and provision of waste collection bags for storing water retaining discarded materials. The corresponding *Thingaha* groups could successfully manage for regular disposal of water retaining discarded materials from each cluster by connection to Municipal waste collection system.

The coverage in dimensions of activity, time and space for removal of larvae/ or pupae was improved by not solely depended upon Basic Health Staff (BHS) who had time constraints and excess work load. The collaboration of BHS in current implementation strategy was high and appreciated targeted container approach which seemed to be less time consuming for them. As proved by Tun-Lin *et al.,* (2010), targeting roughly half of all water holding container types was as effective as lowering the PPI as targeting all types in routine services areas at lower implementation costs. The role of pyirproxyfen in most productive containers was also found as an ease of handling, application and high level of acceptability similar to Cambodian study (Cheng *et al.,* 2008). Thus, complex public health response is imperative for effective reduction in the long run as noted in this project by incorporating integrated vector management principles (WHO, 2009) rather than focusing on larviciding only as in vertical programs.

5   Conclusion

The importance of community capacity building for prevention of dengue transmission by knowledge translation of evidence-based findings during phase 1 through multiple stakeholder groups, community volunteers, and householders was underscored. The efficacy of the community and multi-partnership based intervention was equivalent to the massive vertical larviciding organized as a vertical programme in the aftermath of cyclone Nargis. However, in terms of sustainability and empowerment of communities and other stakeholders, the partnership approach with targeted container interventions was found to be superior to the vertical approach. The policy implications are: partnerships between community and municipal services are to be strengthened further in terms of waste segregation, adequate and continuous water supply, and improved water management. Vector control efforts are required to focus on the most productive water container types and environmental sanitation activities dealing with solid waste disposal focused at integrated vector management. Further research is required on establishing the long term sustainability of the intervention package and its delivery in high risk transmission areas. This will promote better understanding related to applicability of epidemiological-biological indicators in real practice for prevention of dengue transmission at vulnerable sites.

Authors

KhinThet Wai, Pe Than Htun, Tin Oo
Department of Medical Research, Ministry of Health, Myanmar

Axel Kroeger
Liverpool School of Tropical Medicine, United Kingdom

Max Petzold
Health Metrics at Sahlgrenska Academy, University of Gothenburg, Sweden
School of Public Health, Faculty of Health Sciences, University of the Witwatersrand, Johannesburg, South Africa.

References

Arunachalem N, Tana S, Espino FE, Kittayapong P, Abeyewickereme W, Wai KT et al. (2010). *Eco-bio-social determinants of dengue vector breeding: a multicountry study in urban and periurban Asia. Bull World Health Org, 88, 173-184.*

Aung Than Batu (2003).*The growth and development of medical research in Myanmar (1886 to 1986).Myanmar Academy of Medical Science.*

Boischio A, Sanchez A, Orosz Z &Charron D (2009). *Health and sustainable development: challenges and opportunities of eco-system approaches in the prevention and control of dengue and Chagas. Cadernos de SaudePublica.25 (Suppl, 1), S149-154.*

CapraraA,Lima JWD, Marinho ACP, Calvasina PG, Landim LP &Sommerfeld J, (2009). *Irregular water supply, household usage and dengue: a biosocial study in the Brazilian Northeast. Cad. SaúdePública, Rio de Janeiro, 25 Suppl:S125-136.*

Cheng MS, Setha T, Nealon J, Socheat D & Nathan MB (2008). *Six months of Aedes aegypti control with a novel controlled release formulation of pyriproxyfen in domestic water storage containers in Cambodia. Southeast Asian J Trop Med Public Health, 39, 5-12.*

Chevalier J & Buckles D. (2010). *Guide to SAS²: Concepts and tools for collaborative inquiry and social innovation. Available at http://www.sas2.net*

Draper AK, Hewitt G & Rifkin S. (2010). *Chasing the dragon: Developing indicators for the assessment of community participation in health programmes. Social Science and Medicine 71, 1102-1109.*

Focks DA (2004). *A review of entomological sampling methods and indicators for dengue vectors Geneva: World Health Organization, (TDR/IDE/Den/03.1).*

Garelli FM, Espinosa MO, Weinberg D et al. (2009). *Patterns of Aedesaegypti (Diptera: Culicidae) Infestation and Container Productivity Measured Using Pupal and Stegomyia Indices in northern Argentina. J. Med. Entomol., 46 (5), 1176 - 1186.*

Horstick O, Runge-Ranzinger S, Nathan MB, &Kroeger A (2010). *Dengue vector-control services: how do they work? A systematic literature review and country case studies. Trans R Soc Trop Med Hyg.104 (6), 379-386.*

Kroeger A, Lenhart A, Ochoa M, Villegas E, Levy M, Alexander N & McCall PJ. (2006). *Effective control of dengue vectors with curtains and water container covers treated with insecticide in Mexico and Venezuela: cluster randomisedtrials.BMJ. 3-6. BMJ Online first. http://www.bmj.com*

Kroeger A, Lenhart A, Ochoa M, Villegas E, Levy M, Alexander N, &Mc Call PJ (2006). *Effective control of dengue vectors with curtains and water container covers treated with insecticide in Mexico and Venezuela: Cluster randomised trials. British Medical Journal, 332, 1247-1252.*

Lavery SH, Smith ML, Esparza AA, Hrushow A, Moore M, & Reed DF. (2005). *The Community Action Model: A Community-Driven Model Designed to Address Disparities in Health.American Journal of Public Health, 95 (4), 611-616.*

Ledwith M (2011). *Community development: a critical approach. The Policy Press, University of Bristol, UK. Second Edition. 53-73.*

Lwanga SK &Lemeshow S (1991).*Sample size determination in health studies: a practical manual. Geneva: World Health Organization.*

Phuanukoonnon S, Mueller I & Bryan JH (2005). *Effective dengue control practices in water containers in Northeast Thailand. Trop. Med. Int. Health. 10 (8), 755-63.*

Rifkin SB & Pridmore P (2001). *Partners in planning, information, participation and empowerment. London: Macmillan Eduaction Ltd.*

Sanders, I.T.(1958)*Theories of Community Development.Rural Sociology 23(1), 1-12.*

Sommerfeld,J.& Kroeger A (2012).*Eco-Bio-Social research on dengue in Asia:a multicountry study on ecosystem and community-based approaches for the control of denguevectors in urban and peri-urban Asia. Pathogens and Global Health, 106(8): 428-435.*

Suwanbamrung C (2010). *Community capacity for sustainable community-based dengue prevention and control:domain, assessment tool and capacity building model. Asia Pacific Journal of Tropical Medicine, 499-504.*

Tana S, Abeyewickreme W, Arunachalem N, Espino F, Kittayapong P, Wai KT, Horstick O & Sommerfeld J (2012). *Eco-bio-social research on dengue in Asia: General Principles and a case study from Indonesia. In: D.F. Charron (ed.), Ecohealth Research in Practice: Innovative Applications of an Ecosystem Approach to Health, Insight and Innovation in International Development 1, DOI 10.1007/978-1-4614-0517-7_16, © International Development Research Centre. 173-184.*

TDR-WHO (2011).*Operational guide for assessing the productivity of Aedesaegypti breeding sites. Web version. World Health Organization, Geneva.www.who.int/entity/tdr/publications/documents/sop-pupal-surveys.pdf*

Toledo ME, Baly A, Vanlerbergh V, Rodrı´guez M, Benitez JR, Duvergel J & Van der Stuyft P (2008). *The unbearable lightness of technocratic efforts at dengue control. Tropical Medicine and International Health, 13 (5), 728-736.*

Tun Lin W, Lenhart A, Nam VS, Rebollar-Téllez E, Morrison AC,Barbazan P, Cotev M,Midega J,Sanchez F, Manrique-Said P, Kroeger A, Nathan MB, Meheus F, &Petzold M (2009). *Reducing costs and operational constraints of dengue vector control by targeting productive breeding places: a multi-country non-inferiority cluster randomized trial. Trop. Med. Int. Health, 14 (9), 1143-1153.*

Tun-Lin W, Kay BH & Barnes A (1995).*Understanding productivity, a key to Aedesaegypti surveillance. Am. J. Trop. Med. Hyg. 53, 595 - 598.*

Wai KT, Arunachalam N, Tana S, Espino FE, Kittayapong P, Abeyewickreme W,Hapangama D,Tyagi BK, Htun PT, Koyadun S,Kroeger A,Sommerfeld J &Petzold M (2012). *Estimating dengue vector abundance in the wet and dry season: implications for targeted vector control in urban and peri-urban Asia. Pathogens and Global Health.*

WHO (2008). *Action Plan. Scaling up dengue prevention and control for the cyclone Nargis affected populations.June to September.Office of World Health Organization, Yangon, Myanmar. Unpublished document.*

WHO (2009).*Integrated Vector Management. Working Group Meeting Reports. World Health Organization. WHO/HTM/NTD/VEM/2009.2*

Molecular and Cell Culture Methods for Evaluate Viral Contamination in Environmental Samples using Human Adenoviruses as Model

Gislaine Fongaro, Vanessa Moresco, Lucas Ariel Totaro Garcia
Elmahdy Mohamed Elmahdy, Doris Sobral Marques Souza,
Mariana de Almeida do Nascimento, Mariana Rangel Pilotto, Célia Regina Monte Barardi

1   Background

Gastroenteritis, diarrhea, and other diseases can be caused by enteric viruses transmitted by fecal-oral route. These viruses are usually introduced into aquatic environments by human, industrial, or agricultural activities and are widely distributed around the world. They have the common characteristics to be structurally stable and can also absorb to solid particles, thereby protecting themselves from inactivating factors. However, among the enteric viruses, Human Adenoviruses (HAdV) are one of the most resistant pathogen to water and sewage treatments since they are related to occur very frequently in public water systems and have the potential to cause gastroenteritis and other diseases such as otitis, respiratory diseases, cystitis therefore being indicated as a model of enteric viruses in environmental samples. Molecular techniques, such as PCR-based methods, are commonly used to detect and identify viral contamination in water, particularly those viruses that do not multiply easily in cell culture. Although molecular methods have the highest degree of sensitivity and specificity, the concentration of PCR inhibitors in environmental samples and the ability of such techniques to detect free viral genomes may represent a limitation for their use. In addition, PCR alone does not allow the discrimination between infectious and non-infectious viral particles. A combination of cell culture and PCR has allowed detection of infectious viruses that grow slowly or fail to produce cytopathic effects (CPE) in cell culture. Integrated cell culture PCR (ICC-PCR) has the benefits of cell culture coupled to PCR and attempts to compensate for several cell culture disadvantages, such as time-consuming and limited detection sensitivity. Therefore, other strategies are required to confirm infectious viruses by assaying infection of the permissive cells. This can be based on the use of viral mRNA transcribed into infected cells by using RT-PCR templates (ICC-RT-qPCR). Thus, the detection of viral mRNA in cell culture indicates the presence of infectious viral particles. Plaque assay is another method that can be used to infer the ability of viruses to infect and cause lysis in a cell monolayer. Enzymatic assays can also be used to check the integrity of the viral capsid by using nucleases and genetic material that is not protected by a viral capsid will be degraded by these nucleases. All of the mentioned characteristics have encouraged studies to indicate not only HAdV as a viral bioindicator, but also the use of molecular techniques coupled to cell culture to safely evaluate the viral disinfection in environmental matrices.

1.1   Human Enteric Virus: Adenoviruses as a Model

Enteric viruses presence in the aquatic environment may be extremely hard to detect and causing a broad range of diseases. Waterborne viral infections are among important causes of human morbidity, and related diseases continue to pose public health threat and socioeconomic implications worldwide. According to existing reports in the literature, there are hundreds of different types of human viruses present in human sewage, which can become a source of contamination of drinking and recreational water. In many countries, water quality is evaluated according to bacteriological standards, even though bacterial contamination is not correlated with the presence of human enteric viruses and other pathogens (Fong, Griffin & Lipp, 2005).

Food and waterborne diseases, as gastroenteritis and enteric hepatitis, can be caused by enteric viruses (human and zoonotic), such Adenovirus (HAdV), Rotavirus A and C (RVA and RVC), Enterovirus, Sapovirus (SAV), Norovirus (HNoV), Hepatitis A virus (HAV) and Hepatitis E virus (HEV). These viruses replicate in the gastrointestinal tract and are excreted in high concentrations in the feces of infected humans and animal (10^8–10^{11} particles/g of feces) (Bosch *et al.*, 2008).

Most of waterborne diseases are due to unsafe water supplies and inadequate sanitation. Drinking and recreational water are the main ways of human viral contamination, which can be responsible for multiple diseases. Water-related human pathogenic viruses include HAdV, polyomaviruses, enteroviruses, HNoV, rotaviruses, astroviruses, HAV and HEV (Bofill-Mas *et al.*, 2013). HNoV and HAV are the most prevalent viruses in United States outbreaks related to drinking water between 1971 and 2006 (Craun *et al.*, 2010). Polyomaviruses and HAdV are widely detected in surface water and sewage worldwide (Bofill-Mas *et al.*, 2013). Drinking and recreational waters, such swimming pool and seawater are also contaminated and outbreaks of HAdV infection described in day care centers, hospitals and swimming pools (Mena & Gerba; Jiang, 2006). Genomic methods target the unique and conservative gene sequences in the HAdV genome are commonly employed, however do not detect viable virus. Most of human adenovirus can be cultured in cells, but some HAdV serotypes, such enteric HAdV serotypes 40 and 41 are fastidious and produce little or no cytopathic effect (CPE) (Jiang, 2006).

The food contamination may happen in different steps of the production process; in primary production or during further processing. Among the food matrices that may be involved in foodborne outbreaks, shellfish (oysters, clams and mussels) and fresh produce (fruits and vegetables, including leafy vegetables) are important vehicles of human pathogens, including viruses. Foodborne diseases are responsible for approximately 48 million illnesses each year in the United States. During 1998–2008, CDC received 7,998 outbreaks reports with a known etiology. Among them, 3,633 (45%) were caused by viruses (CDC, 2013). DiCaprio *et al.*, (2012) showed that norovirus may be internalized by lettuce impairing its removal. This genus is recognized as the main agent of viral epidemics gastroenteritis in the world (Glass, Parashar & Estes, 2009). Bivalve shellfish, principally oysters, are commonly associated with norovirus infection (Guillois-Bécel *et al.*, 2009; Doré *et al.*, 2010; Mesquita *et al.*, 2011) because they are filter-feeding and due to their raw or lightly cooked consumption. Some norovirus may remain adsorbed in oysters cells hindering their removal during the purification procedures (Mcleod *et al.*, 2009). They may bind to the oyster tissues carbohydrates, which are similar to the human histo-blood antigens (HBGAs). These HBGAs, presents in some human cells as red blood cells and others, are required for start the HNoV infection (Maalouf *et al.*, 2011, Le Guyader *et al.*, 2006). HAV is also frequently associated in food outbreaks (Broman *et al.*, 2010), including oysters. Some authors showed that HAV may remain in basal cells of stomach epithelium in some oyster species (Romalde *et al.*, 1994) and it can persist into their tissues during 3 weeks, after the initial contamination (Romalde *et al.*, 1994; Kingsley & Richards, 2003). Beyond HNoV and HAV, other viral pathogens may be associated with oysters' consumption, as hepatitis E viruses (HEV), sapovirus (SAV), astrovirus (HAstVs), RVA and RVC, Aichi virus (AiV), HAdV, poliovirus (PV) and other enteric viruses (Richards, McLeod & Le Guyader, 2010). The shellfish growing areas are worldwide classified as A, B, C or improper based only in bacterial levels (*Escherichia coli* or coliforms monitoring), and since the enteric viruses are more resistant to be inactivated by environmental stressors than bacteria, their correlation is not well accepted by the scientific community (Noble, Lee & Schiff, 2004; Moresco *et al.*, 2012; Souza *et al.*, 2012). Viral investigation in food matrices is not an easy task, because of the many kind of inhibitors that can interfere on the enzymatic reactions, the low concentration of viruses in some samples (the infectious dose for HNoV and HAV is about 10-100 infectious particles) and the cytotoxicity of some food extracts when cell culture assays are applied to access viral infectivity. The choice of virus concentration as well as the kind of analysis employed for food contamination purposes is dependent on the food matrix involved (Bosch *et al.*, 2011).

The direct approach to detect pathogenic enteric viruses involves the use of molecular biology based techniques associated or not with cell culture. Cell culture techniques has some shortcomings; detects only infectious viral particles, but is not useful for uncultivable viruses or wild types viral strains isolated from environmental matrices (e.g. HNoV, HEV, HAV, Rotavirus, etc) and is time consuming, it takes up to 3 days from inoculating virus to the time when cytophatic effects (CPE) become visible by light microscopy. Molecular-based methods, when employed alone, although very powerful (due to sensitivity, specificity and rapidness), do not give any information about the infectious state of the detected virus. However, the presence of viral nucleic acid does not necessarily represent an infectious virus, which has important implications for water and food safety, particularly when microbial inactivation treatments are employed (Sobsey *et al.*, 1988).

Therefore, it is important to determine at least the potential of infectivity of the waterborne virus by nuclease treatment, because this can reduce free nucleic acid, in order to check the integrity of the virus particles when the use of permissive cells for infection, is not possible. Sometimes, viral inactivation data (reduction in the number of infectious units) can result in false negatives not because of viral inactivation itself but due to viral adhesion-aggregation (Gassilloud & Gantzer, 2005). The viral adhesion-aggregation processes are reversible and depend on: (a) viral serotype and the viral surface charge (Floyd & Sharp, 1979), (b) chemical properties of the medium such as pH, ionic strength, and the nature of the ions present (Totsuka, Ohtaki & Tagaya, 1978) and (c) the nature of the adsorbing surface which in turn is described in terms of surface charge and hydrophobicity (Voorthuizen, Ashbolt & Schäfer, 2001). Thus, the quantification of infectious virus without taking into account the adhesion-aggregation effect can produce a measurement bias (Gassilloud & Gantzer, 2005). These drawbacks are overcome by the ability to detect infectious virus, which can provide more reliable information for microbial risk assessment studies.

Human adenoviruses (HAdV) belong to the Adenoviridae family, and the serotypes that infect humans are classified in the *Mastadenovirus* genus. The HAdV virion particle consists of an icosahedral, non-enveloped capsid with a diameter ranging between 70 to 100 nm, and a double-stranded DNA genome of approximately 26 to 45 kb (Berk, 2007). Their structural characteristics make them quite stable in a variety of conditions (including variations in temperature, pH as well as some physical and chemical treatments). The adenoviruses are considered to be one of the most persistent enteric viruses in the environment (Thurston-Enriquez *et al.*, 2003). There are more than 52 known human serotypes, and they are distributed into six species, A- F (Wold & Horwitz, 2007). Of these, serotypes 40 and 41 (species F) are responsible for the majority of gastroenteritis outbreaks, affecting mainly young children. The other serotypes are responsible for asymptomatic (species A and D) or symptomatic (B and E) infections, and the viruses can be excreted in the feces for a long time after the infection, whether or not it is accompanied by diarrhea. They can be transmitted by both the respiratory and fecal-oral routes, causing infections in the upper and lower respiratory tract, conjunctivitis and gastroenteritis (Mena & Gerba, 2008; Rigotto *et al.*, 2010).

To evaluate the level of fecal contamination, classic microbiological indicators such as fecal coliforms (Bofill-Mas *et al.*, 2013). However, there is not a clear relationship between bacteria presence and virus detection in environmental samples, which turn the methods solely based on bacterial contamination unreliable and incomplete (Jiang, 2006).

HAdV have been indicated as potential markers of viral contamination in water (Wyer *et al.*, 2012; Bosch *et al.*, 2011; Wyn-Jones *et al.*, 2011; Calgua *et al.*, 2008; Fong, Griffin and Lipp, 2005; Hundesa *et al.*, 2006), since they are DNA viruses, which promotes more resistance to environmental degradation, such as UV radiation, temperature, chlorine treatment and pH extremes, including sewage treatment procedures (Carter, 2005; Fong and Lipp, 2005; LeChevallier & Au, 2004; Pina *et al.*, 1998). In addition, the genetic variation of DNA viruses is less prevalent than RNA viruses (Hijnen *et al.*, 2006; Thurston-Enriquez *et al.*, 2003; Enriquez *et al.*, 1995). Furthermore, HAdV have already been described as the most prevalent contaminant in drinking water (Fong, Griffin & Lipp, 2005; Garcia *et al.*, 2012; Rigotto *et al.*, 2010), recreational waters (Miagostovich *et al.*, 2008; Sinclair *et al.*, 2009; Fongaro *et al.*, 2012), associated with disease outbreaks in swimming pools (Papapetropolou and Vantarakis, 1995; Harley *et al.*, 2001), and in polluted fresh and ocean waters (Pina *et al.*, 1998; Laverick *et al.*, 2004; Lee *et al.*, 2004; Miagostovich *et al.*, 2008; Wong *et al.*, 2009; Rigotto *et al.*, 2010; Moresco *et al.*, 2012; Wong *et al.*, 2009; Wyn-Jones *et al.*, 2011; Garcia *et al.*, 2012, Fongaro *et al.*, 2012).

A current list of microorganisms candidate markers of contamination of the aquatic environment (CCL3) prepared by the Environmental Protection Agency from United States (USEPA) lists the contaminants that are not currently subject to any regulations which are expected to occur in public systems water, requiring that legislation of laws in ensuring the quality of drinking water. Among other viruses, adenovirus is considered a high priority emerging contaminant present in drinking water, candidate parameter for contamination of the aquatic environment (USEPA, 2009).

2   Methods for Environmental Viral Investigation

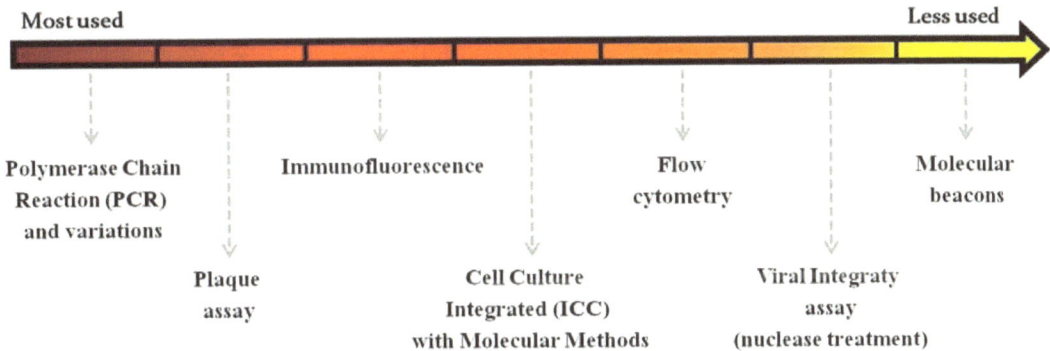

Figure 1: Molecular and cell culture main methods used to detect human enteric viruses, using human adenovirus as model. These methods are presented in this review.

2.1   Genome based Detection

2.1.1   Polymerase Chain Reaction (PCR) and Variations

The polymerase chain reaction (PCR) technique and their variations are widely used to amplify sequences of microorganisms present in environmental samples as contaminants (Abbaszadegan, Stewart & LeChevallier, 1999; Carducci *et al.*, 2003), in addition to rapidity and sensitivity, assay specificity is another advantage of PCR. Despite PCR, do not indicate the presence of infectious viral particles, is still considered as a gold technique for monitoring viral contamination in environmental samples, because it is rapid, practical and very sensitive (Abbaszadegan, Stewart & LeChevallier, 1999; Gofti-Laroche *et al.*, 2001; Carducci *et al.*, 2003, Domingo *et al.*, 2012). Due to the abundant occurrence of enteric virus in many water and food sources, this is considered a major health threat concern worldwide in recent years. Some studies focused on the detection of these viruses in water sources and foodstuff have been performed (Papapetropoulou & Vantarakis, 1995; Sinclair, Jones & Gerba, 2009)

PCR can be used to determine DNA integrity, but its effectiveness will depend on the length of the amplicon that is analyzed (Rodríguez, Bounty & Linden, 2013). Long-target (LT) PCR is able to detect undamaged viral DNA, once the generated amplicon is very large (up to

10 kb). Although DNA integrity confirmation, LT-PCR also cannot infer about viral infectivity. This technique is rarely employed to detect virus in environmental matrices (Rodríguez, Pepper & Yerba 2009; Rodríguez, Bounty & Linden, 2013).

The advent of quantitative real-time PCR (qPCR) allowed that the viral genome copies present in environmental samples could be precisely quantified. The qPCR uses fluorescent probes or fluorescent DNA-binding dyes and primers to detect and quantify products generated on each amplification cycle (Sugden & Winter, 2008). Among the advantages of qPCR use are the high yield, high sensitivity (up to 10 copies), and accuracy. It also avoids PCR product manipulation, lowering contamination risk (Sugden & Winter, 2008).

There are many ways to quantify viral genome copies by qPCR, but, in environmental studies, SYBR® Green DNA-binding dye and fluorogenic TaqMan probes are the two approaches most commonly used (Goyer & Dandie, 2012).

Viral genome quantification in the environment by SYBR® Green is unusual, but may be performed (Scipioni *et al.*, 2008; Haramoto *et al.*, 2009; Dong, Kim & Lewis, 2010; He *et al.*, 2011; Ye *et al.*, 2012). SYBR® not require the use of specific probes, it is a cheaper technique and as sensitive as the former one (Sugden & Winter, 2008). As disadvantages, this dye binds to all double-stranded formed, including nonspecific products and primer dimers when formed. To assess the efficiency of amplification with the use of SYBR® Green is necessary to construct a melting curve. The configuration of only one denaturation peak means the absence of nonspecific binding or primer dimers formation (Sugden & Winter, 2008; Goyer & Dandie, 2012). TaqMan probe is widely used for virus detection in environmental matrices (Fong, *et al.*, 2010; Wong & Xagoraraki, 2011; Hamza *et al.*, 2011; Calgua *et al.*, 2011; Wyn-Jones *et al.*, 2011; Fongaro *et al.*, 2012; Garcia *et al.*, 2012). This probe is a fluorogenic oligonucleotide that binds in the DNA in a region between the primers. When hydrolysis of probe occurs by exonuclease 5´-3´ activity of the DNA polymerase there is a fluorescence emission. The requirement of a specific probe turns the assay more specific, avoiding the primer dimers and nonspecific products. However the synthesis of this fluorogenic oligonucleotide is more expensive. Furthermore, the use of specific probes with different fluorophores enables detection and quantification of multiple PCR products, also known as multiplex (Sugden & Winter, 2008; Goyer & Dandie, 2012).

Quantification by qPCR may be relative, using a reference gene or DNA sequence, or absolute, which uses a standard (Sugden & Winter, 2008). For detection of viruses in samples usually is used absolute quantification. For this, is necessary to make a standard that contains known amounts of genome copies. Usually it is used target viral genes cloned in plasmids or viral purified genome dilutions. It is extremely important to be very careful when prepare and handle with standards, since they generate large amounts of amplicons that can easily contaminate the assay and the lab environment (Goyer & Dandie, 2012).

The qPCR reaction efficiency is directly linked to the primers quality, amplicon size, genome copies (GC) and sample impurities. These factors may affect the primer binding, target sequence melting point and the Taq polymerase efficiency (Sugden & Winter, 2008). Environmental samples such as water, sediment, sewage and shellfish can contain inhibitors (i.e. humic and fulvic acids, ions and heavy metals) that can be co-extracted with the target nucleic acid. These contaminants can input on the reaction, a large amount and types of impurities and inhibitors (Le Guyader *et al.*, 2009; Baar *et al.*, 2011; Goyer & Dandie, 2012; Bustin, Zaccara & Nolan, 2012). Also, different techniques of viral concentration/elution, such as beef extract, and genome extraction methods may have PCR inhibitors, with may generate false-negative results (Sugden & Winter, 2008). To avoid this, it is necessary to evaluate different sample dilutions to avoid inhibitors interference.

2.1.2   Enzymatic test

Enzymatic assays can be used to check the integrity of the viral capsid by using DNase or RNase nucleases. Genetic material that is not protected by the viral capsid will be degraded by these nucleases (Nuanualsuwan & Cliver, 2002). Studies have proposed the pre-treatment of the samples using nucleases in order to differentiate an undamaged virus (potentially infectious) from a damaged (inactivated) virus (Girones *et al.*, 2010). For this assay, the environmental samples are treated with nuclease (DNase or RNase) and the enzymatic reaction occurs at room temperature (nuclease should be inactivated). Later the nucleic acids should be extracted and reverse transcription reaction and qPCR or PCR is performed (Nuanualsuwan & Cliver, 2002; Fongaro *et al.*, 2012).

Viral infectivity studies often include experiments to demonstrate a cytopathic effect in cell culture. Such experiments are laborious, and many viruses do not produce cytopathic effects (Rodríguez, Pepper & Yerba, 2009). Factors such as temperature, pH and UV radiation are known to cause moderate conformational changes in the viral capsid, resulting in loss of infectivity, but not of integrity (Thurston-Enriquez *et al.*, 2003; Fong & Lipp, 2005).

For undamaged HAdV investigation, the samples should be treated with DNAse I in order to infer the presence of intact and potentially infectious virus particles (Nuanualsuwan & Cliver, 2002). After the reaction, the nucleic acids should be extracted and the qPCR or PCR should be performed in order to evaluate the number of undamaged virus (Bofill-Mas *et al.*, 2006; Fongaro *et al.*, 2013).

Bofill-Mas *et al.*, (2006) treated sewage samples with DNAse, and did not observe notable differences in the number of HAdV and JC-Polyomavirus detected in treated and untreated samples. However, this methodology was used by other authors in environmental samples and they observed notable differences in the number of HAdV on treated and untreated samples, confirming the applicability of this technique (Fongaro *et al.*, 2012).

2.2   Cell Culture based: Infectious Virus Detection

2.2.1   Plaque Assay

Plaque assay is a cell culture technique that relies on the ability of the virus to produce cytopathic effect (CPE) in *in vitro* cell culture. After infecting the host cells with the virus, a semi-solid medium is added, such as agar or carboxymethyl cellulose, which restricts the spread of the viral progeny only to neighboring cells. The infected cells will lyse, only adjacent cells will be infected, and a circular empty area of lysed infected cells will be produced. This area is called plaque.

The technique was first described by Dulbecco (1952), based on the methodology used to detect and calculate the titer of bacteriophages stocks. Nowadays, plaque assays are one of the standard procedures not only to detect infectious virus in environmental samples, but also to titer virus stocks.

The plaque assay has the same drawbacks that any other cell culture technique: it is laborious, expensive and depends on the capacity of the virus to propagate in a cell culture (Hamza *et al.*, 2011). Moreover, methods used to concentrate virus from environmental samples also concentrate contaminants that may inhibit cell culture infection, manifested by cell stress, cell death, or failure of matrix controls, and also causing false positive culture results (Julian & Schwab, 2012). In addition, some viruses do not form plaques, so they are not detected under agar (Hamza *et al.*, 2011).

Environment is a common source of HNoV contamination (Wang & Deng, 2012), but there is not an *in vitro* cell culture system for the detection of infectious virus. The feline calicivirus (FCV) and the murine norovirus (MNV) are common surrogate models used for HNoV (Bae & Schwab, 2008). Wobus *et al.*, (2004) developed a plaque assay for MNV, and Bae & Schwab (2008) improved the technique, concluding that MNV is the best choice as a HNoV surrogate due to its genetic similarity and environmental stability. MNV is now being used in stability and inactivation assays in environmental samples (Kahler *et al.*, 2011; Corrêa *et al.*, 2012 a).

Regarding HAdV, some serotypes can be difficult to grow in cell culture due lack the visible cytopathic effect. However, plaque assay for HAdV is one the most used when analyzing environmental samples. Cromeans *et al.*, (2008) developed a plaque assay for the fastidious HAdV 40 and 41, using the lung carcinoma cell line A549, methodologies that have been widely used in environmental samples determining the survival of HAdV 2 and 41 in ground and surface waters in different temperatures (Cromeans *et al.*, 2008; Cromeans, Kahler & Hill, 2010; Kahler el al., 2011; Garcia *et al.*, 2012; Fongaro *et al.*, 2013). The HAdV isolates used by the authors were first isolated in HeLa and primary CMK cells, followed by passages in G293 cells, but the plaque assay was better performed using A549 cells as described by Cromeans *et al.*, (2008). Rigotto *et al.*, (2011) determined the survival of HAdV 2 and 41 in ground and surface waters in different temperatures. Corrêa *et al.*, (2012 b) evaluated the kinetics of inactivation of murine norovirus and human adenovirus in natural and artificial seawater. After 30 min of contact with chlorine, human adenovirus showed a 2-log10 reduction and no MNV remained infectious.

2.2.2   Immunofluorescence Assay

Fluorescence antibody staining is widely employed for virus detection even for environmental samples. This cell culture method is based on the interaction of specific antibodies with an antigen. Thus, viable viruses that infected a permissive and susceptible cell can be detected by the use of specific antibodies labeled with fluorophores, with can be detected by a fluorescent microscopy using ultraviolet (UV) light with the proper wavelength needed to excite the fluorescent label. Immunofluorescence assay (IFA) is frequently the method of choice when sensitivity and specificity are required.

The most usual fluorophore used is the fluorescein isothiocyanate (FITC) (excitation/emission: 494 nm/519 nm), which emits a green fluorescence. Another fluorophores used are R-phycoerythrin (excitation/emission: 480 nm / 578 nm), and Rhodamine (excitation/emission: 547 nm /572 nm), which emits an orange fluorescence; Peridinin chlorophyll protein (PerCP) (excitation/emission: 490 nm / 675 nm) and Texas Red (excitation/emission: 589 nm / 615 nm), which emits a red fluorescence (Walker & Rapley, 2008). Considering that immunofluorescence methods are based on antibodies recognition, it is extremely important to ensure high quality and purity of the reagents in order to avoid cross reaction (non-specific binding) as well unwanted background. The IFA assay can be performed directly and indirectly. In the direct reaction, the viral antigen is detected by a specific antibody labeled with a fluorophore (primary antibody), while in the indirect reaction, the viral antigen is detected by a specific antibody which is detected by a second antibody labeled with a fluorophore and directed against the primary antibody. Although the direct reaction is faster, the main disadvantage is the need to conjugate each specific antibody with fluorophore. Especially for this reason, the indirect reaction is usually employed because only the secondary antibody has to be conjugated with the fluorescent label. In addition, the indirect IFA is slightly more sensitive and more versatile.

The detection of viruses in environmental matrices by IFA requires standardizing and optimization to know the best and exact conditions for each sort of sample (e.g.: river, lake, spring water, drinking water, seawater, sludge, sediment, bivalve mollusks).

The main questions need to be taken in standardizing includes:

- What is the non-cytotoxic sample dilution required?

- How many days of incubation does it need?

- What's the best way to block unspecific binding?

- How many steps of washing does it need?

- What are the best antibodies dilution?

- How long the antibody incubation steps need to be effective?

Also, the detection limit of each sample and virus needs to be known.

The adenovirus detection by immunofluorescence can be performed with a wide range of cell types, including primary human embryonic kidney cells (HEK), Graham 293 cells (HEK 293) and continuous epithelial lines (HEp-2, HeLa, KB, and A549). An important point to be aware is the susceptibility of each cell line for adenovirus detection. While HEK cells could support the entire range of human adenoviruses, HEK 293 is a good host for the two enteric adenoviruses (Ad40 and 41), HEp-2, HeLa, KB and A549 may be required to isolate some of the ocular adenovirus strains (Knipe & Howley, 2007). For an environmental detection, is important to work with a cell type appropriated for what is been searched, e.g., if the aim is detect general adenovirus, the HEK cell should be applied, whereas using A549 cells for this purpose can mask the real incidence of general adenovirus.

Likewise, the antibody specificity should be appropriated, directed against a common epitope for all adenovirus strains when is desired, or a specific epitope for a specific strain. The adenovirus proteins that provide useful antigens are the three coat proteins: hexon, penton base, and fiber. The most commonly antibody used is MAb8052, a mouse anti-adenovirus monoclonal antibody that is specific for a HAdV neutralizing epitope (Nihon Millipore™, Tokyo, Japan) (Calgua *et al.*, 2011; Corrêa *et al.*, 2012 a; Carratalà *et al.*, 2013).

Some studies have been performed for virus detection in environmental matrices by immunofluorescence. Recently, in Spain, authors employed IFA technique for HAdV 2 and HAdV 41 detection in river water (artificially contaminated) and raw sewage sample. The assay showed high sensitivity for HAdV in natural and spiked samples, and when compared with plaque assay and TCID50, IFA were 1 log10 greater. This difference may be due to the fact that IFA detects fluorescent foci in very early stages of virus replication because the virus can already be detected within the infected before cell lysis, whereas the plaque assay requires the infection of multiple neighboring cells, followed by lysis for subsequent display of the focus of infection (plaque forming). The optimal day of incubation for HAdV 2 was 4 days, and for HAdV 41 was 8 days. In raw sewage, all samples were positive for HAdV (Calgua *et al.*,

2011). The same group has applied IFA technique for HAdV 2 detection in mineral water, wastewater and seawater, also (Carratalà *et al.*, 2013). In Brazil, HAdV 5 was detected in oysters artificially contaminated after 3 days of incubation, showing the same sensitivity of ICC-PCR technique (Corrêa *et al.*, 2012 a).

2.2.3 Flow Cytometry

The application of the flow cytometry (FC) in virology studies remains the decade of 1990 were many studies are focused to evaluate the virus-cell interactions (McSharry, 1994). FC is a method that provide a simple, rapid and efficient quantitative assay by using labeled antibodies (MAbs), fluorescent dyes or fluorescent proteins (GFP) to detect virus-infected cells *in vitro* (Hamza, *et al.*, 2011). The FC is able to measure physical, morphological and/or chemical cells characteristics, counting and analyzing one cell at a time, while the cells pass through a single stream. The cells are intercepted by lasers that detect their morphological characteristics and/or fluorescent signals (McSharry, 1994; Li, He & Jiang, 2010).

In virology, this method has been used for titrating viruses or detect virus presence and infectivity in clinical samples (Chuan-Liang *et al.*, 2001; Barriga *et al.*, 2013). When compared with other methods to detect virus-cell infection such as plaque assay and indirect immunofluorescence, the FC is less time-consuming, allowing the detection of a single cell with fluorescent signal in the early stages of virus replication.

In environmental virology, the use of FC is still limited. Some studies were pioneers, employing the FC to evaluate the presence of infectious rotaviruses in clinical (fecal) samples, environmental waters and oysters meat samples by infection of permissive cells (MA104 or CaCo-2) to virus infection and labeled antibodies to detection (Abad, Pintó & Bosch, 1998; Barardi *et al.*, 1998, 1999). Li, He & Jiang (2010) using specific labeled antibodies for the hexon protein of the adenovirus (AdV), validate a FACS assay (Fluorescence-Activated Cell Sorting) showing AdV positive detection in primary sewage effluent and secondary sewage effluent samples with 3 days of incubation, using HEK293A cells (Li, He & Jiang, 2010).

These studies usually require many steps to evaluate virus infectivity (cell infection, fixation, permeabilization, primary and secondary antibody staining and quantification) (Philipson, 1961). To improve the accuracy and speed of flow cytometry detection in virology, some recent studies proposed the use of report genes, such as GFP (green fluorescent protein) incorporated in viral vectors. Many studies are using recombinant adenoviruses (rAdV), obtained by the excision of the E1A gene (early) of the adenovirus and replacing by the GFP gene, which can express GFP during viral replication. The GFP signals can be directly detect by FC, without fixation and staining steps by the infection of permissive cell line HEK293A, which express the E1A adenovirus gene, allowing the rAdV replication. The use of this method promote a rapid titration and quantification of adenoviral-GFP vectors by FC, being the results proportional to the titre obtained by plaque assay standard method (Hitt *et al.*, 2000, Gueret *et al.*, 2002, Li, He & Jiang, 2010). The rAdV can be also used as a surrogate on viral inactivation and stability studies in environmental waters.

Recently, an interesting assay, using an alternative approach to evaluate the infectivity of poliovirus was performed by Cantera, Chen & Yates (2010). This study used an engineered BGMK cells expressing fluorescent protein (CFP) and yellow fluorescent protein (YFP) linked by a peptide containing the poliovirus 2A protease cleavage site. The control of the fluorescence is maintained by the resonance energy transfer (FRET) that is disrupted during the cell infection by poliovirus, being the energy transferred of the excited donor fluorophore to the acceptor fluorophore. The change promoted by this energy transfer can be detected by flow cytometry due to the difference in the fluorescent signals during the infection cycle. Using this technology, this study showed that the titre obtained for poliovirus was similar by to the detected by plaque assay, and less time-consuming (8h). These results were reproducible using environmental waters spiked with poliovirus, were the values of the titer of poliovirus showed a linear correlation with the plaque assay (Cantera, Chen & Yates, 2010).

Despite the high sensibility, speed and accuracy of the FC to detect infectious virus, this method are still limited by the cost of the equipment and trained operators, as well the cost of specific antibodies and cell culture laboratory structure. The employment of this technology will be useful in future, regarding the importance of the inactivation and disinfection studies using environmental samples.

2.3   Cell Culture Integrated with Molecular Methods

2.3.1   Cell Culture Integrated with PCR or qPCR

The Integrate Cell Culture with PCR or qPCR (ICC-PCR) is a method that combine the high sensitivity of cell culture with the high specificity of PCR together and avoids the shortcomings of low specificity and long testing period of cell culture (Li *et al.*, 2002).

ICC-PCR method has still the possibility to detect nucleic acids of inactivated viruses from environmental samples simply adsorbed onto cell receptors without cell infection resulting in false positives infectious data (Sobsey *et al.*, 1988). Therefore, other strategies are required to confirm infectious viruses by assaying infection of the permissive cells; this can be based on the use of viral mRNA transcribed into infected cells as RT-PCR templates (ICC-RT-PCR). Thus, the detection of viral mRNA in cell culture indicates the presence of infectious viral particles; specificity and sensitivity are also important aspects to consider, as the ICC-RT-qPCR relies on mRNA and thus avoids false negatives or positives (Ko, Cromeans & Sobsey *et al.*, 2003; Rigotto *et al.*, 2010).

Studies emphasize the importance of using ICC-RT-PCR when is necessary to measure infectious pathogens, explaining that this technique is safe and accurate (Ko, Cromeans & Sobsey, 2003). However, the majority of studies using ICC-RT-qPCR attempt to estimate the viral infectivity of artificiality contaminated samples, but rarely employ such a technique to evaluate virus from environmental samples (Gallagher & Margolin, 2007; Lambertini *et al.*, 2010).

Compared with ICC-RT-PCR used for virus detection, PCR has several advantages: the time required for this test can be reduced from days or weeks to hours, costs for implementing this technique are substantially smaller, besides being a methodology easy to perform and has high specificity and sensitivity (Nuanualsuwan & Cliver, 2002; Carducci *et al.*, 2003). In addition, this method facilitates the identification of fastidious pathogen viruses that do not grow well in cell culture assays, such as rotavirus, calicivirus, adenoviruses and some HAV, and extends information previously available for enterovirus, which shows good growth in culture cells (Wyn-Jones & Sellwwod, 2001; Carducci *et al.*, 2003, Girones, *et al.*, 2010).

The use of the assay of ICC-RT-PCR or qPCR was reported as a rapid and accurate for detection of HAdV in environmental monitoring (Gallagher & Margolin 2007; Rigotto *et al.*, 2010; Fongaro *et al.*, 2013).

2.3.2   Molecular Beacons

[o]Molecular beacon (MB) is a nucleic acid probe developed by Tyagi & Kramer in 1996. Is composed by a labeled single-stranded oligonucleotide chain that present a strong affinity and specificity by a target acid nucleic sequence. It is usually constructed with approximately 25-35 nucleotides and a specific stem-loop conformation that allow the maintenance of the no fluorescence by resonance energy transfer (FRET) (Tyagi & Kramer, 1996; Li, Zhou & Ye, 2008). The loop portion contains the specific region that is complementary to the target; the stem portion is composed by 5-6 nucleotides that, in the absence of the target, hybridize together, allowing the hairpin conformation. In the 5′ end are attached a fluorophore group and a quencher in the 3′ end (Huang & Martí, 2012). When the probe is unbound, the close proximity between the fluorophore and the quencher, blocks the fluorescence. When the MB hybridizes with the target, there is a change in the loop conformation, resulting in an increase of the distance between the fluorophore and the quencher, breaking the FRET, allowing the fluorescence detection.

Due to their high specificity, MB have been used as a probe in quantitative PCR assays, as well as a tool to *in vitro* analysis, such as the accomplishment of a cell infection (McKillen *et al.*, 2007; Dunams *et al.*, 2012).

The use of this technology in the environmental virology are still recent and limited, a work conducted by McKillen *et al.*, (2007), evaluate the presence of four important swine viruses in clinical samples using MB technology in real time PCR assay. Using this method, the detection of this virus was highly improved showing to be a more specific diagnostic tool for the detection of viral DNA in clinical samples when compared with conventional PCR. Using this method, the detection of this virus was improved a high throughput detection, showing a specific diagnostic for the detection of viral DNA in clinical samples when compared with conventional PCR (Mckillen *et al.*, 2007).

In recent study, Dunams *et al.*, (2012) evaluate the simultaneous infection of echovirus and adenovirus in A549 cells using a multiplex MB designed to specific regions in the virus genome and carrying different fluorophores. The simultaneous infection was accomplishment by fluorescence microscopy within 3 hours post infection proving the specificity and rapidly of the assay. This methodology can be used in studies to evaluate the behavior of this important enteric virus during the cell infection, as well in assays to analyze the viral infectivity and stability in environmental matrices.

The MB method shows is an efficient tool to evaluate the infectivity of fastidious virus, or viruses that do not show cytopathic effects (CPE). Yeh *et al.*, (2008) designed a MB to the noncoding region of the hepatitis A virus (HAV). The probe was introduced in permeabilized FRhK-4 cells infected with HAV and after 6 hours post infection, it was possible the visualization of fluorescence signals, due to the probe hybridization with the newly mRNA synthetized during the virus replication. The use of this methodology, allow the detection limit a single one PFU, increasing significantly the time of detection (6h), when compared with one week, time usually required to the CPE visualization in normal conditions of cell culture infection (Yeh *et al.*, 2008).

The application of the MB technology, are still poor exploited in environmental virology, however, it is clear the importance of this method to improve the viral quantification and detection in environmental samples, which focuses particularly in samples with low concentration of viruses or samples contaminated by fastidious viruses, allowing the potential infectivity of these viruses, impairing epidemiological and quantitative microbial risk assessment (QMRA) studies.

3   Conclusion

Human adenoviruses (HAdV) are widely distributed in food and water samples and their presence can indicate fecal contamination and human health threat. Detection methods for HAdV in environmental samples are extensively described in literature and they are constantly improved aiming to improve sensitivity and to include detection methods for viable virus. Molecular methods are faster and less expensive, but, as they are based on genome detection, they are not able to differentiate inactivated from viable viruses. The enzymatic treatment with nuclease can ensure the undamaged HAdV presence, but also cannot ensure the viral infectivity since the damage can be partial, protecting the genome from enzymatic cleavage. Currently, cell culture based methods are the most used techniques for detection of viable adenovirus in environmental samples. However, it is more expensive and laborious, and not all serotypes of adenovirus are adapted to in vitro cell infection. Use of molecular methods coupled to cell culture can increase the probability to detect infectious virus in environmental samples and to assess the disinfections process efficiency.

Authors

Gislaine Fongaro, Vanessa Moresco, Lucas Ariel Totaro Garcia, Elmahdy Mohamed Elmahdy, Doris Sobral Marques Souza, Mariana de Almeida do Nascimento, Mariana Rangel Pilotto, Célia Regina Monte Barardi
Laboratorio de Virologia Aplicada, Departamento de Microbiologia, Imunologia e Parasitologia, Universidade Federal de Santa Catarina, Brazil, CEP 88040-900.

References

Abad, F. X., Pintó, R. M. & Bosch, A. (1998). *Flow cytometry detection of infectious rotaviruses in environmental and clinical samples. Applied and Environmental Microbiology, 64, 2392-2396.*

Abbaszadegan, M., Stewart, P. & LeChevallier, M. (1999). *A strategy for detection of viruses in groundwater by PCR. Applied and Environmental Microbiology, 65, 444-449.*

Baar, C., d'Abbadie, M., Vaisman, A., Arana, M. E., Hofreiter, M., Woodgate, R., Kunkel, T. A. & Holliger, P. (2011). *Molecular breeding of polymerases for resistance to environmental inhibitors. Nucleic Acids Research, 39, 51-63.*

Bae, J. & Schwab, K. J. (2008). *Evaluation of murine norovirus, feline calicivirus, poliovirus and MS2 as surrogates for human norovirus in a model of viral persistence in surface water and groundwater. Applied and Environmental Microbiology, 74, 477-484.*

Barardi C. R., Emsile, K. R., Vesey, G. & Williams K. L. (1998). *Development of a rapid and sensitive quantitative assay for rotavirus based on flow cytometry. Journal of Virological Methods, 74, 31-38.*

Barardi., C. R., Yip. H., Emsile. K. R., Vesey, G., Shanker, S. R. & Williams, K.L. (1999). *Flow cytometry and RT-PCR for rotavirus detection in artificially seeded oyster meat. International Journal of Food Microbiology, 49, 9-18.*

Barriga, G. P., Martínez-Valdebenito, C., Galeno, H., Ferrés, M., Lozach, P. Y. & Tischler, N. D. (2013). *A rapid method for infectivity titration of Andes hantavirus using flow cytometry. Journal of Clinical Virology, 193, 291-294.*

Berk, A.J. (2007). *Adenoviridae. The viruses and their replication. In: Knipe, D. M.; Howley, P. M. (Eds), Fields Virology. 5th. Philadelphia: Lippincott Williams & Wilkins (pp. 2356-2394).*

Bofill-Mas, S., Rusiñol, M., Fernandez-Cassi, X., Carratalà, A., Hundesa, A. & Girones, R. (2013). *Quantification of human and animal viruses to differentiate the origin of the fecal contamination present in environmental samples. Biomed Research International, 2013, pp.11.*

Bofill-Mas, S., Albinana-Gimenez, N., Clemente-Casares, P., Hundesa, A., Rodriguez-Manzano, J., Allard, A., Calvo, M. & Girones, R. (2006). *Quantification and stability of human adenoviruses and polyomavirus JCPyV in wastewater matrices. Applied and Environmental Microbiology, 72, 7894-7896.*

Bosch, A., Guix, S. Sano, D. & Pinto, R. M. (2008). *New tools for the study and direct surveillance of viral pathogens in water. Current Opinion in Biotechnology, 19, 295-301.*

Bosch, A., Sánchez, G., Abbaszadegan, M., Carducci, A., Guix, S., Le Guyader, F. S. L., Netshikweta, R., Pintó, R. M., Poel, W. H. M. v. d., Rutjes, S., Sano, D., Taylor, M. B., Zyl, W. B. v., Rodríguez-Lázaro, D., Kovač, K. & Sellwood, J. (2011). *Analytical Methods for Virus Detection in Water and Food. Food Analytical Methods 4, 4-12.*

Broman, M., Jokinen, S., Kuusi, M., Lappalainen, M., Roivainen, M., Liitsola, K. & Davidkin, I. (2010). *Epidemiology of Hepatitis A in Finland in 1990–2007. Journal of Medical Virology 82, 934-941.*

Bustin, S. A., Zaccara, S. & Nolan, T. (2012). *An introduction to the real-time polymerase chain reaction (qPCR). In: Quantitative real-time PCR in applied microbiology ed. Filion, M. Norwich: Caister Academic Press (pp. 3-26).*

Calgua, B., Barardi, C. R. M., Bofill-Mas, S., Rodriguez-Manzanoa, J. & Girones, R. (2011). *Detection and quantitation of infectious human adenoviruses and JC polyomaviruses in water by immunofluorescence assay. Journal of Virological Methods, 171, 1–7.*

Calgua, B., Mengewein, A., Grünert, A., Bofill-Mar, S., Clemente-Casares, P., Hundesa, A., Wyn-Jones, A. P., López-Pila, J. M. & Girones, R. (2008). *Development and application of a one-step low cost procedure to concentrate viruses from seawater samples. Journal of Virology Methods, 153, 79-83.*

Cantera, J. L., Chen, W. & Yates, M. V. (2010). *Detection of infective poliovirus by a single, rapid, and sensitive flow cytometry method based on fluorescence resonance energy transfer technology. Applied and Environmental Microbiology, 76, 584–588.*

Carducci, A., Casini, B., Bani, A., Rovini, E., Verani, M., Mazzoni, F. & Giuntini, A. (2003). *Virological control of groundwater quality using biomolecular tests. Water Science and Technology, 47, 261-266.*

Carter, M.J. (2005). *Enterically infecting viruses: pathogenicity, transmission and significance for food and waterborne infection. Journal of Applied Microbiology, 6, 1354–1380.*

Carratalà, A., Rusiñol, M., Rodriguez-Manzano, J., Guerrero-Latorre, L., Sommer, R. & Girones, R. (2013). *Environmental Effectors on the Inactivation of Human Adenoviruses in Water. Food and Environmental Virology. DOI: 10.1007/s12560-013-9123-3.*

CDC (2013). *Surveillance for Foodborne Disease Outbreaks – United States, 1998–2008. Atlanta, U.S. Department of Health and Human Services. 62, 40.*

Chuan-Liang, K., Meng-Chan, W., Yen-Hui, C., Jing-Lin, L., Yin-Chang, W., Yi-Yung, Y., Li-Kuang, C., Men-Fang, S. & Chwan-Chuen, K. (2001). *Flow cytometry with indirect immunofluorescence for rapid detection of dengue virus type 1 after amplification in tissue culture. Journal of Clinical Microbiology, 39, 3672-3677.*

Corrêa, A. A., Rigotto, C., Moresco, V., Kleemann, C. R., Teixeira, A. L., Poli, C. R., Simões, C. M. O & Barardi, C. R. M. (2012 a). *The depuration dynamics of oysters (Crassostrea gigas) artificially contaminated with hepatitis A virus and human adenovirus. Memórias do Instituto Oswaldo Cruz, 107, 11-17.*

Côrrea, A. A., Carratala, A., Barardi, C. R. M., Calvo, M., Girones, R. & Boffil-Mas, S. (2012 b). *Comparative inactivation of murine norovirus, human adenovirus and human JC polyomavirus by chlorine in seawater. Applied and Environmental Microbiology, 78, 6450-6457.*

Craun, G. F., Brunkard, J. M., Yoder, J. S., Roberts, V. A., Carpenter, J., Wade, T., Calderon, R. L., Roberts, J. M., Beach, M. J. & Roy, S. L. (2010). *Causes of Outbreaks Associated with Drinking Water in the United States from 1971 to 2006. Clinical Microbiology Reviews, 23, 507-528.*

Cromeans, T. L., Lu, X., Erdman, D. D., Humphrey, C. D. & Hill, V. R. (2008). *Development of plaque assays for adenoviruses 40 and 41. Journal of Virological Methods, 151, 140-145.*

Cromeans, T. L., Kahler, A. M. & Hill, V. R. (2010). *Inactivation of adenoviruses, enteroviruses, and murine norovirus in water by free chlorine and monochloramine. Applied and Environmental Microbiology, 76, 1028-1033.*

DiCaprio, E., Ma, Y., Purgianto, A., Hughes, J. & Lia, J. (2012). *Internalization and Dissemination of Human Norovirus and Animal Caliciviruses in Hydroponically Grown Romaine Lettuce. Applied and Environmental Microbiology 78, 6143–6152.*

Domingo, J. S., Schoen, M., Ashbolt, N. & Ryu, H. (2012). *Using qPCR for Water Microbial Risk Assessments. In: Quantitative real-time PCR in applied microbiology ed. Filion, M. Norwich: Caister Academic Press (pp. 121-148).*

Dong, Y., Kim, J. & Lewis, G.D. (2010). *Evaluation of methodology for detection of human adenoviruses in wastewater, drinking water, stream water and recreational waters. Journal of Applied Microbiology, 108, 800-809.*

Doré, B., Keaveney, S., Flannery, J. & Rajko-Nenow, P. (2010). *Management of health risks associated with oysters harvested from a norovirus contaminated area, Ireland, February–March 2010. Euro Surveillance, 15, 19567.*

Dulbecco, R. (1952). *Production of plaques in monolia yer tissue cultures by single particles of an animal virus. Pathology, 38, 747-752.*

Dunams, D., Sarkar, P., Chen, W. & Yates, M. V. (2012). *Simultaneous detection of infectious human echoviruses and adenoviruses by an in situ nuclease-resistant molecular beacon assay. Applied and Environmental Microbiology, 78,1584.*

Enriquez, C.E., Hurst, C.J. & Gerba, C.P. (1995). *Survival of the enteric adenoviruses 40 and 41 in tap, sea and wastewater. Water Research, 29, 2548-2553.*

Floyd, R. & Sharp, D. G. (1979). *Viral aggregation: buffer effects in the aggregation of poliovirus and reovirus at low and high pH. Applied and Environmental Microbiology, 38, 395-401.*

Fong, T. T., Griffin, D. W. & Lipp E. K. (2005). *Molecular assays for targeting human and bovine enteric viruses in coastal waters and application for library-independent source tracking. Applied and Environmental Microbiology, 71, 2070–2078.*

Fong, T.T. & Lipp, E.K. (2005). *Enteric viruses of human and animals in aquatic environments: health risks, detection, and potential water quality assessment tools. Microbiology Molecular Biology Review, 69, 357–371.*

Fong, T. T., Phanikumar, M. S., Xagoraraki, I. & Rose, J. B. (2010). *Quantitative detection of human adenoviruses in wastewater and combined sewer overflows influencing a Michigan River. Applied and Environmental Microbiology, 76, 715-723.*

Fongaro, G., Nascimento, M. A., Viancelli, A., Tonetta, D., Petrucio, M. M. & Barardi, C. R. M. (2012). *Surveillance of human viral contamination and physicochemical profiles in a surface water lagoon. Water Science and Technology, 66, 2682-2687.*

Fongaro, G., Nascimento, M. A, Rigotto, C., Ritterbusch, G., da Silva, A. D' A., Esteves P. A. & Barardi C. R. M. (2013). *Evaluation and molecular characterization of human adenovirus in drinking water supplies: viral integrity and viability assays. Virology Journal, 10, 166-175.*

Gallagher. E.M. & Margolin, A.B. (2007). *Development of an integrated cell culture--real-time RT-PCR assay for detection of reovirus in biosolids. Journal Virology Methods, 139, 195-202.*

Garcia, L. A. T, Viancelli, A., Rigotto, C., Pilotto, M. R., Esteves, P. A., Kunz, A. & Barardi, C. R. M. (2012). *Surveillance of human and swine adenovirus, human norovirus and swine circovirus in water samples in Santa Catarina, Brazil. Journal of Water and Health, 10, 445-452.*

Gassilloud, B. & Gantzer, C (2005). *Adhesion-Aggregation and Inactivation of Poliovirus 1 in Groundwater Stored in a Hydrophobic Container. Applied and Environmental Microbiology, 71, 912-920.*

Girones, R., Ferrús, M. A., Alonso, J. L., Rodriguez-Manzano, J., Calgua, B., Corrêa, A. A., Hundesa, A., Carratala, A. & Bofill-Mas, S. (2010). *Molecular detection of pathogens in water - the pros and cons of molecular techniques. Water Research, 44, 4325-4339.*

Glass, R. I., Parashar, U. D. & Estes, M. K. (2009). *Norovirus Gastroenteritis.The New England Journal of Medicine, 361, 1776-1785.*

Gofti-Laroche, L., Gratacap-Cavallier, B., Genoulaz, O., Joret, J. C., Harteman, P. h., Seigneurin, J. M., & Zmirou, D. (2001). *A new analytical tool to assess health risks associated with the virological quality of drinking water (EMIRA study). Water Science and Technology, 43, 39-48.*

Goyer, C. & Dandie, C. E. (2012). *Quantification of microorganisms targeting conserved genes in complex environmental samples using qPCR. In: Quantitative real-time PCR in applied microbiology ed. Filion, M. Norwich: Caister Academic Press (pp.87-106).*

Gueret, V., Negrete-Virgen, J. A., Lyddiatt, A. & Al-Rubeai, M. (2002). Rapid titration of adenoviral infectivity by flow cytometry in batch culture of infected HEK293 cells. Cytotechnology, 38, 87-97.

Guillois-Bécel, Y., Couturier, E., Saux, J. C. L., Roque-Afonso, A. M., Le Guyader, F. S. L., Goas, A. L., Pernès, J., Bechec, S. L., Briand, A., Robert, C., Dussaix, E., Pommepuy, M. & Vaillant, V. (2009). An oyster-associated hepatitis A outbreak in France in 2007. Euro Surveillance, 14, 19144.

Hamza, I. A., Jurzik, L., Überlab, K. & Wilhelm, M. (2011). Methods to detect infectious human enteric viruses in environmental water samples. International Journal of Hygiene and Environmental Health, 214, 424– 436.

Haramoto, E., Kitajimab, M., Katayamab, H., Asamic, M., Akibac, M. & Kunikaned, S. (2009). Application of real-time PCR assays to genotyping of F-specific phages in river water and sediments in Japan. Water Research, 43, 3759-3764.

Harley, D., Harrower, B., Lyon, M. & Dick, A. (2001). A primary school outbreak of pharyngoconjunctival fever caused by adenovirus type 3. Communicable Diseases Intelligence, 25 (1), 9 - 12.

He, X. Q., Cheng, L., Zhang, D. Y., Xie, X. M., Wang, D. H. & Wang, Z. (2011). One-year monthly survey of rotavirus, astrovirus and norovirus in three sewage treatment plants in Beijing, China and associated health risk assessment. Water Science and Technology, 63, 191-198.

Hijnen, W.A., Beerendonk, E.F. & Medema, G.J. (2006). Inactivation credit of UV radiation for viruses, bacteria and protozoan (oo)cysts in water: a review. Water Research, 40 (1), 3–22.

Hitt, D.C., Booth, J.L., Dandapani, V., Pennington, L. R., Gimble, J. M. & Metcalf, J. (2000). A flow cytometric protocol for titering recombinant adenoviral vectors containing the green fluorescent protein. Molecular Biotechnology, 14, 197-203.

Huang, K. & Martí, A. A. (2012). Recent trends in molecular beacon design and applications Analytical and Bioanalytical Chemistry, 40, 3091–3102.

Hundesa, A., Maluquer de Motes, C., Bofill-Mas, S., Albinana-Gimenez, N. & Girones, R. (2006). Identification of human and animal adenoviruses and polyomaviruses for determination of sources of fecal contamination in the environment. Applied and Environmental Microbiology, 72, 7886 - 7893.

Jiang, S. C. (2006). Human adenoviruses in water: occurrence and health implications: a critical review. Environmental Science and Technology, 40, 7132-7140.

Julian, T. R. & Schwab, K. J. (2012). Challenges in environmental detection of human viral pathogens. Current Opinion in Virology, 2, 78-83.

Kahler, A. M., Cromeans, T. L., Roberts, J. M. & Hill, V. R. (2011). Source water quality effects on monochloramine inactivation of adenovirus, coxsachievirus, echovirus, and murine norovirus. Water Research, 45, 1745-1751.

Kingsley, D. H. & Richards, G. P. (2003). Persistence of Hepatitis A Virus in Oysters. Journal of Food Protection 66, 331–334.

Knipe, D. M. & Howley, P. M. (2007). Fields Virology. Philadelphia: Lippincott Williams & Wilkins, 5th ed, V.1.

Ko, G., Cromeans, T. L., & Sobsey, M. D. (2003). Detection of infectious adenovirus in cell culture by mRNA reverse transcription-PCR. Applied and Environmental Microbiology, 69, 7377–7384.

Lambertini, E., Spencer, S.K., Bertz, P.D., Loge, F. & Borchardt, M.A. (2010). New mathematical approaches to quantify human infectious viruses from environmental media using integrated cell culture-qPCR. Journal Virology Methods, 163, 244–252.

Laverick, M.A., Wyn-Jones, A.P. & Carter, M.J. (2004). Quantitative RT-PCR for the enumeration of noroviruses (Norwalk-like viruses) in water and sewage. Letters in Applied Microbiology, 39, 127 - 136.

Le Guyader, F. S. ., Parnaudeau, S., Schaeffer, J., Bosch, A., Loisy, F., Pommepuy, M. & Atmar, R. L. (2009). Detection and quantification of noroviruses in shellfish. Applied and Environmental Microbiology, 75, 618-624.

Le Guyader, F. S., Loisy, F., Atmar, R. L., Hutson, A. M., Estes, M. K., Ruvoen-Clouet, N., Pommepuy, M., & Le Pendu, J. (2006). Norwalk virus specific binding to oyster digestive tissues. Emerging Infectious Diseases, 12, 931–936.

LeChevallier, M. W. & Au, K. (2004). Water Treatment and Pathogen Control Process - Efficiency in Achieving Safe Drinking Water. World Health Organization (WHO). Cornwall: TJ International, 1st ed. V.1.

Lee, C., Lee, S.H., Han, E. & Kim, S.J. (2004). Use of cell culture-PCR assay based on combination of A549 and BGMK cell lines and molecular identification as a tool to monitor infectious adenoviruses and enteroviruses in river water. Applied and Environmental Microbiology, 70, 6695 - 6705.

Li, D., He, M. & Jiang, S. C. (2010). Detection of infectious adenoviruses in environmental waters by Fluorescence activated-cell sorting assay. Applied and Environmental Microbiology, 76, 1442-1448.

Li, J.-W., Wang, X.-W., Yuan, C.-Q., Zheng, J.-L., Jin, M., Song, N., Shi, X.-Q., & Chao, F.-H. (2002). *Detection of enteroviruses and hepatitis a virus in water by consensus primer multiplex RT-PCR.* World Journal of Gastroenterology, 8, 699-702

Li, Y., Zhou, X. & Ye, D. (2008). *Molecular beacons: An optimal multifunctional biological probe.* Biochemical and Biophysical Research Communications, 373, 457–461.

Maalouf, H., Schaeffer, J, Parnaudeau, S., Le Pendu, J., Atmar, R. L., Crawford, S. E. & Le Guyader, F. S. (2011). *Strain-dependent norovirus bioaccumulation in oysters.* Applied and Environmental Microbioly, 77(10), 3189-3196.

Miagostovich, M.P., Ferreira, F.F.M., Guimarães, F.R., Fumian, T.M., Diniz-Mendes, L., Luz, S.L.B., Silva,L.A. & Leite, J.P.G. (2008). *Molecular Detection and Characterization of Gastroenteritis Viruses Occurring Naturally in the Stream Waters of Manaus, Central Amazônia, Brazil.* Applied and Environmental Microbiology, 74, 375-382.

Mcleod, C., Hay, B., Grant, C., Greening, G. & Day, D. (2009). *Localization of norovirus and poliovirus in Pacific oysters.* Journal of Applied Microbiology, 106, 1220-1230.

McKillen, J., Hjertner, B., Millar, A., Mcneilly, F., Belák, S., Adair, B. & Allan, G. (2007). *Molecular beacon real time PCR detection of swine viruses.* Journal of Virological Methods, 140, 155-164.

McSharry, J. J.(1994). *Uses of Flow Cytometry in Virology,* Clinical Microbiology Reviews, 7, 576-604.

Mena, K. D. & C. P. Gerba (2008). *Waterborne Adenovirus.* Reviews of Environmental Contamination and Toxicology, 198, 133-167.

Mesquita, J. R., Vaz, L., Cerqueira, S., Castilho, F., Santos, R., Monteiro, S., Manso, C. F., Romalde, J. L. & Nascimento, M. S. J. (2011). *Norovirus, hepatitis A virus and enterovirus presence in shellfish from high quality harvesting areas in Portugal.* Food Microbiology, 28, 936-941.

Moresco, V., Viancelli, A., Nascimento, M. A., Souza, D. S. M., Ramos, A. P. D., Garcia, L. A. T., Simões, C. M. O. & Barardi, C. R. M. (2012). *Microbiological and physicochemical analysis of the coastal waters of southern Brazil.* Marine Pollution Bulletin, 64, 40-48.

Noble, R. T., Lee, I. M. & Schiff, K. C. (2004). *Inactivation of indicator micro-organisms from various sources of faecal contamination in seawater and freshwater.* Journal of Applied Microbiology, 96, 464–472.

Nuanualsuwan, S. & Cliver, D. O. (2002). *Pretreatment to avoid positive RT-PCR results with inactivated viruses.* Journal Virology Methods, 104, 217–225.

Papapetropolou, M. & Vantarakis, A.C. (1995). *Detection of adenovirus outbreak at a municipal swimming pool by nested PCR amplification.* Journal of Infection, 36, 101 - 103.

Pina, S., Puig, N., Lucena, F., Jofre, J. & Girones, R. (1998). *Viral pollution in the environment and in shellfish: human adenovirus detection by PCR as an index of human viruses.* Applied and Environmental Microbiology, 64, 3376-3382.

Philipson, L. (1961). *Adenovirus assay by the fluorescent cell-counting procedure.* Virology, 15, 263-268.

Richards, G. P., McLeod, C. & Le Guyader, F. S. L. (2010). *Processing Strategies to Inactivate Enteric Viruses in Shellfish.* Food and Environmental Virology, 2, 183-193.

Rigotto. C., Victoria, M., Moresco. V., Kolesnikovas, C.K.M., Correa, A.A., Souza, D.S.M., Miagostovich, M., Simões, C.M. & Barardi, C.R. (2010). *Assessment of adenovirus, hepatitis A virus and rotavirus presence in environmental samples in Florianópolis South Brazil.* Jounal Applied Microbiology, 109, 1979–1987.

Rigotto, C, Hanley, K., Rochelle, P.A., De Leon, R., Barardi, C.R.M. & Yates, M.V. (2011). *Survival of Adenovirus types 2 and 41 in surface and ground waters measured by a plaque assay.* Environmental Science and Technology, 45, 4145-4150.

Rodríguez, R. A., Pepper, I.L. & Yerba, C.P. (2009): *Application of PCR-based methods to assess the infectivity of enteric viruses in environmental samples.* Applied Environmental Microbiology, 75, 297–307.

Rodríguez, R. A., Bounty, S. & Linden, K. G. (2013). *Long-range quantitative PCR for determining inactivation of adenovirus 2 by ultraviolet light.* Journal of Applied Microbiology, 114, 1854-1865.

Romalde, J. L., Estes, M. K., Szucs, G., Atmar, R. L., Woodley, C. M., & Metcalf, T. G. (1994). *In situ detection of hepatitis A virus in cell cultures and shellfish tissues.* Applied and Environmental Microbiology, 60, 1921–1926.

Scipioni, A., Mauroy, A., Ziant, D., Saegerman, C. & Thiry, E. (2008). *A SYBR Green RT-PCR assay in single tube to detect human and bovine noroviruses and control for inhibition.* Virology Journal, 5, 94-102.

Sinclair, R. G., Jones, E. L. & Gerba, C. P. (2009). *Viruses in recreational water-borne disease outbreaks: a review.* Journal of Applied Microbiology, 107, 1769-1780.

Sobsey, M.D., Battigelli, D.A., Shin, G.A. & Newland, S. (1988). RT-PCR amplification detects inactivated viruses in water and wastewater. Water Science and Technology, 38, 91–94.

Souza, D. S. M., Ramos, A. P. D., Nunes, F. F., Moresco, V., Taniguchi, S., Leal, D. A. G., Sasaki, S. T., Bícego, M. C., Montone, R. C., Durigan, M., Teixeira, A. L., Pilotto, M. R., Delfino, N., Franco, R. M. B., Melo, C. M. R. d., Bainy, A. C. D. & Barardi, C. R. M. (2012). Evaluation of tropical water sources and mollusks in southern Brazil using microbiological, biochemical, and chemical parameters. Ecotoxicology and Environmental Safety, 76, 153-161.

Sugden, D & Winter, P. (2008). Quantification of mRNA using real time RT-PCR: The SYBR solution. In: Molecular biomethods handbook ed. Walker, J. M & Rapley, R. Totowa: Humana Press.

Totsuka, A. Ohtaki, K. & Tagaya, I. (1978). Aggregation of enterovirus small plaque variants and polioviruses under low ionic strength conditions. Journal of General Virology, 38, 519-533.

Tyagi, S. & Kramer, F. R. (1996). Molecular beacons: probes that fluoresce upon hybridization. Nature Biotechnology, 14, 303-308.

Thurston-Enriquez, J.A., Haas, C.N., Jacangelo, J., Riley, K. & Gerba, C.P. (2003). Inactivation of feline calicivirus and adenovirus type 40 by UV radiation. Applied Environmental Microbiology, 69, 577–582.

USEPA – United States Environmental Protection Agency: Contaminant candidate list– CCL (2009). In http://water.epa.gov/scitech/drinkingwater/ dws/ccl/ccl3.cfm.

Voorthuizen, E. M., Ashbolt, N. J. & Schäfer, A. I.(2001). Role of hydrophobic and electrostatic interactions for initial enteric virus retention by MF membranes. Journal of Membrane Science, 194, 69-79.

Wang, J. & Deng, Z. (2012). Detection and forecasting of oyster norovirus outbreaks: recent advances and future perspectives. Marine Environmental Research, 80, 62-69.

Walker, J. M. & Rapley, R. (2008). Molecular Biomethods Handbook. Totowa: Humana Press, 2nd ed.

Wobus, C. E., Karst, S. M., Thackray, L. B., Chang, K. O., Sosnovtsev, S. V., Belliot, G., Krug, A., Mackenzie, J. M., Green, K. Y. & Virgin, H. W. (2004). Replication of norovirus in cell culture reveals a tropism for dendritc cells and macrophages. PLos Biology, 2, 2076-2084.

Wold, W.S.M. & Horwitz, M.S. (2007). Adenoviruses. In Fields virology. Edited by Knipe Howley, D.M., Philadelphia, P.M. Lippincott Williams & Wilkins (pp.2395–2436).

Wong, M., Kumar, L., Jenkins, T. M., Xagoraraki, I., Phanikumar, M. S. & Rose, J. B. (2009). Evaluation of public health risks at recreational beaches in Lake Michigan via detection of enteric viruses and a human-specific bacteriological marker. water research, 43, 1137 – 1149.

Wong, K. & Xagoraraki, I. (2011). Evaluating the prevalence and genetic diversity of adenovirus and polyomavirus in bovine waste for microbial source tracking. Applied Microbiology and Biotechnology, 90, 1521-1526.

Wyer, M. D., Wyn-Jones, A. P., Kay, D., Au-Yeung, H. K. C., Gironés, R., López-Pila, J., Husman, A. M. R., Rutjes, S. & Schneider, O. (2012). Relationships between human adenoviruses and faecal indicator organisms in European recreational waters. Water Research, 46, 4130 – 4141.

Wyn-Jones, A.P. & Sellwood J. (2001). Enteric viruses in the aquatic environment. Journal of Applied Microbiology, 91, 945–962.

Wyn-Jones, A. P., Carducci, A., Cook, N., D'Agostino, M., Divizia, M., Fleischer, J., Gantzer, C., Gawler, A., Girones, R., Höller, C., Husman, A. M. R., Kay, D., Kozyra, I., López-Pila, J., Muscillo, M., Nascimento, M. S. J., Papageorgiou, G., Rutjes S., Sellwood, J., Szewzyk, R. & Wyer, M. (2011). Surveillance of adenoviruses and noroviruses in European recreational waters. Water Research, 45, 1025-1038.

Ye, X. Y, Ming, X., Zhang, Y. L., Xiao, W. Q., Huang, X. N., Cao, Y. G. & Gu, K. D. (2012). Real-time PCR detection of enteric viruses in source water and treated drinking water in Wuhan, China. Current Microbiology, 65, 244-253.

Yeh, H. Y., Hwang, Y. C., Yates, M. V. Mulchandani, A. & Chen, W. (2008). Detection of Hepatitis A virus by using a combined cell culture-molecular beacon assay. Applied and Environmental Microbiology, 74, 2239-2243.

www.ingramcontent.com/pod-product-compliance
Lightning Source LLC
Chambersburg PA
CBHW050823220326
41598CB00006B/298

* 9 7 8 1 9 2 2 2 2 7 7 6 8 *